Eating Disorders and Addictive Behaviors: Implications for Human Health

Eating Disorders and Addictive Behaviors: Implications for Human Health

Editors

Roser Granero
Fernando Fernández-Aranda
Susana Jiménez-Murcia

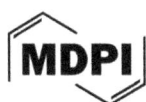

Basel • Beijing • Wuhan • Barcelona • Belgrade • Novi Sad • Cluj • Manchester

Editors

Roser Granero
Autonomous University
of Barcelona
Barcelona
Spain

Fernando Fernández-Aranda
University of Barcelona
Barcelona
Spain

Susana Jiménez-Murcia
University of Barcelona
Barcelona
Spain

Editorial Office
MDPI
St. Alban-Anlage 66
4052 Basel, Switzerland

This is a reprint of articles from the Special Issue published online in the open access journal *Nutrients* (ISSN 2072-6643) (available at: https://www.mdpi.com/journal/nutrients/special_issues/Eating_Disorders_and_Addictive_Behaviors_Implications_for_Human_Health).

For citation purposes, cite each article independently as indicated on the article page online and as indicated below:

Lastname, A.A.; Lastname, B.B. Article Title. *Journal Name* **Year**, *Volume Number*, Page Range.

ISBN 978-3-7258-0575-4 (Hbk)
ISBN 978-3-7258-0576-1 (PDF)
doi.org/10.3390/books978-3-7258-0576-1

© 2024 by the authors. Articles in this book are Open Access and distributed under the Creative Commons Attribution (CC BY) license. The book as a whole is distributed by MDPI under the terms and conditions of the Creative Commons Attribution-NonCommercial-NoDerivs (CC BY-NC-ND) license.

Contents

About the Editors vii

Fernando Fernández-Aranda, Roser Granero and Susana Jiménez-Murcia
Eating Disorders and Addictive Behaviors: Implications for Human Health
Reprinted from: *Nutrients* 2023, 15, 3718, doi:10.3390/nu15173718 1

Julia M. Rios, Martha K. Berg and Ashley N. Gearhardt
Evaluating Bidirectional Predictive Pathways between Dietary Restraint and Food Addiction in Adolescents
Reprinted from: *Nutrients* 2023, 15, 2977, doi:10.3390/nu15132977 9

Esther Via and Oren Contreras-Rodríguez
Binge-Eating Precursors in Children and Adolescents: Neurodevelopment, and the Potential Contribution of Ultra-Processed Foods
Reprinted from: *Nutrients* 2023, 15, 2994, doi:10.3390/nu15132994 19

Aneta Matusik, Mateusz Grajek, Patryk Szlacheta and Ilona Korzonek-Szlacheta
Comparison of the Prevalence of Eating Disorders among Dietetics Students and Students of Other Fields of Study at Selected Universities (Silesia, Poland)
Reprinted from: *Nutrients* 2022, 14, 3210, doi:10.3390/nu14153210 39

Mateusz Grajek, Karolina Krupa-Kotara, Agnieszka Białek-Dratwa, Wiktoria Staśkiewicz, Mateusz Rozmiarek, Ewa Misterska and Krzysztof Sas-Nowosielski
Prevalence of Emotional Eating in Groups of Students with Varied Diets and Physical Activity in Poland
Reprinted from: *Nutrients* 2022, 14, 3289, doi:10.3390/nu14163289 49

Juan Pedro López Siguero, Marta Ramon-Krauel, Gilberto Pérez López, Maria Victoria Buiza Fernández, Carla Assaf Balut and Fernando Fernández-Aranda
Attitudes, Behaviors, and Barriers among Adolescents Living with Obesity, Caregivers, and Healthcare Professionals in Spain: ACTION Teens Survey Study
Reprinted from: *Nutrients* 2023, 15, 3005, doi:10.3390/nu15133005 62

Ana Ibáñez-Caparrós, Isabel Sánchez, Roser Granero, Susana Jiménez-Murcia, Magda Rosinska, Ansgar Thiel, et al.
Athletes with Eating Disorders: Analysis of Their Clinical Characteristics, Psychopathology and Response to Treatment
Reprinted from: *Nutrients* 2023, 15, 3003, doi:10.3390/nu15133003 76

Janire Momeñe, Ana Estévez, Mark D. Griffiths, Patricia Macía, Marta Herrero, Leticia Olave and Itziar Iruarrizaga
Eating Disorders and Intimate Partner Violence: The Influence of Fear of Loneliness and Social Withdrawal
Reprinted from: *Nutrients* 2022, 14, 2611, doi:10.3390/nu14132611 92

Lindzey V. Hoover, Joshua M. Ackerman, Jenna R. Cummings and Ashley N. Gearhardt
The Association of Perceived Vulnerability to Disease with Cognitive Restraint and Compensatory Behaviors
Reprinted from: *Nutrients* 2023, 15, 8, doi:10.3390/nu15010008 104

Romina Miranda-Olivos, Zaida Agüera, Roser Granero, Susana Jiménez-Murcia, Montserrat Puig-Llobet, Maria Teresa Lluch-Canut, et al.
The Role of Food Addiction and Lifetime Substance Use on Eating Disorder Treatment Outcomes
Reprinted from: *Nutrients* 2023, 15, 2919, doi:10.3390/nu15132919 119

Neus Solé-Morata, Isabel Baenas, Mikel Etxandi, Roser Granero, Manel Gené, Carme Barrot, et al.
Underlying Mechanisms Involved in Gambling Disorder Severity: A Pathway Analysis Considering Genetic, Psychosocial, and Clinical Variables
Reprinted from: *Nutrients* **2023**, *15*, 418, doi:10.3390/nu15020418 . . . . **131**

Gemma Mestre-Bach and Marc N. Potenza
Potential Biological Markers and Treatment Implications for Binge Eating Disorder and Behavioral Addictions
Reprinted from: *Nutrients* **2023**, *15*, 827, doi:10.3390/nu15040827 . . . . **147**

Giulia Testa, Roser Granero, Alejandra Misiolek, Cristina Vintró-Alcaraz, Núria Mallorqui-Bagué, Maria Lozano-Madrid, et al.
Impact of Impulsivity and Therapy Response in Eating Disorders from a Neurophysiological, Personality and Cognitive Perspective
Reprinted from: *Nutrients* **2022**, *14*, 5011, doi:10.3390/nu14235011 . . . . **164**

Adoracion Nieto, Dan M. Livovsky and Fernando Azpiroz
Conditioning by a Previous Experience Impairs the Rewarding Value of a Comfort Meal
Reprinted from: *Nutrients* **2023**, *15*, 2247, doi:10.3390/nu15102247 . . . . **176**

Mikel Etxandi, Isabel Baenas, Bernat Mora-Maltas, Roser Granero, Fernando Fernández-Aranda, Sulay Tovar, et al.
Are Signals Regulating Energy Homeostasis Related to Neuropsychological and Clinical Features of Gambling Disorder? A Case–Control Study
Reprinted from: *Nutrients* **2022**, *14*, 5084, doi:10.3390/nu14235084 . . . . **189**

About the Editors

Roser Granero

Roser Granero has a PhD in Psychology (Autonomous University of Barcelona (AUB), 1999, with the distinction of "Extraordinary Doctorate Award"), a University Diploma in Statistics (AUB, 1996 year), a master's degree in Design and Statistics in Behavioral Sciences (AUB, 1997 year), and a master's degree in Child and Adolescent Psychopathology (AUB, 1997 year). Dr. Granero is a full professor of Methodology of Behavioral Sciences at the Psychobiology and Methodology Department. She is currently the principal investigator of the Neurosciences program *"Psychoneurobiology of Eating Disorders and Addictive Behaviors"* (at the Bellvitge Biomedical Research Institute, IDIBELL, Spain), and a researcher at the *CIBERobn* group (Center for Biomedical Research in Network, Physiopathology of Obesity and Nutrition, Instituto Carlos III, Spain). She has more than 360 published studies in the Web of Science (WoS), 150 of which are empirical papers indexed in the first quartile (Q1) of the *Journal Citation Reports* (JCR). Two awards for excellence in research stand out: the ICREA-Acadèmia award (2021) and the "Doctora-Alcalà" national award (2023).

Fernando Fernández-Aranda

Fernando Fernandez-Aranda, Full Professor (School of Medicine and Health Sciences, University of Barcelona, Spain), Specialist in Clinical Psychology, has been the Director of the Eating Disorders (ED) unit at the Clinical Psychology Department (University Hospital Bellvitge, Barcelona, Spain), a Scientific Director of the research institute IDIBELL, Vicedirector of CIBERobn (Excellence Spanish Research Network for Obesity and Nutrition), co-Head of the research group CIBERobn and co-Head of the group Psychoneurobiology of Eating and Addictive Behaviours (IDIBELL). He is a past president of the Eating Disorders Research Society (EDRS) and a current co-Chair of the Eating Disorders Section of the World Psychiatric Association. He obtained his PhD in Psychology in 1996 at the University of Hamburg (Germany). His previous appointments were as a Clinical Psychologist at the Psychiatric University Hospital of Hamburg (1994–1995), a long-term predoctoral Research Fellowship in Hannover, Germany (1992–1993), and as a Consultant Psychologist at the Department of Psychiatry, University Hospital Bellvitge, Barcelona (1996–03). He has given more than 450 invited lectures at international or national professional psychology, psychiatry, and nutrition/endocrinology conferences. He is a fellow of the Academy for Eating Disorders and was the Editor-in-Chief of *European Eating Disorders Review* (2011–2022). He was awarded with the Meehan Hartley Award for Public Service and/or Advocacy in 2004, a Leadership Research Award in 2015, and the Hilde Bruch Lecture Award in 2017 (University of Tübingen, Germany). He has received several additional development and innovation awards (Best European Video Game for Health, 2011; Best Spanish Research Ideas, *Diario Médico*, 2011). He has been PI in 12 international/EU grants and 22 national grants. He has published more than 500 English peer-reviewed manuscripts in international journals.

Susana Jiménez-Murcia

Susana Jiménez-Murcia is a specialist in Clinical Psychology and an Associate Professor at the School of Medicine and Health Sciences (University of Barcelona, Spain). She has served as the Director of the Pathological Gambling and Behavioral Addictions Unit at the University Hospital Bellvitge (Barcelona, Spain) and is currently the Head of the Department of Clinical Psychology at the same hospital and Director of the Territorial Mental Health Plan MetroSud. She has been the Faculty Director of the Psychology Clinic of the University of Barcelona and the Co-Chair of the group CIBERobn (Excellent Spanish Research Network for Obesity and Nutrition) and of the IDIBELL Group on Psychoneurobiology of Eating and Addictive Behaviours. She obtained her PhD in Psychology in 2004 at the Autonomous University of Barcelona, a master's degree in Clinical Psychology and Behavioral Medicine in 1992, and her BP in 1988 (Clinical Psychology) at the same university. She has published more than 400 articles in peer-reviewed journals with impact factors. She has given more than 300 invited lectures at international/national conferences. She has completed over 35 competitive research projects at both national and European agencies. Awards: Sanitarias, 2024; Best European Video Game for Health, 2011; Best Spanish Research Ideas, *Diario Médico*, 2011 and 2019.

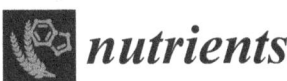

Editorial

Eating Disorders and Addictive Behaviors: Implications for Human Health

Fernando Fernández-Aranda [1,2,3,4,*], Roser Granero [1,2,5] and Susana Jiménez-Murcia [1,2,3,4]

1. CIBER Physiology of Obesity and Nutrition (CIBEROBN), Carlos III Health Institute, 28029 Madrid, Spain; roser.granero@uab.cat (R.G.); sjimenez@bellvitgehospital.cat (S.J.-M.)
2. Psychoneurobiology of Eating and Addictive Behaviors Group, Neurosciences Programme, Bellvitge Biomedical Research Institute (IDIBELL), 08908 Barcelona, Spain
3. Clinical Psychology Unit, University Hospital of Bellvitge, 08907 Barcelona, Spain
4. Department of Clinical Sciences, School of Medicine and Health Sciences, University of Barcelona, 08907 L'Hospitalet de Llobregat, Spain
5. Department of Psychobiology and Methodology, Autonomous University of Barcelona, 08193 Barcelona, Spain
* Correspondence: ffernandez@bellvitgehospital.cat; Tel.: +34-932-607-227

1. Introduction

Eating disorders (EDs) are mental health diseases characterized by dysfunctional eating patterns, including restrictive eating, avoidance of foods, binge eating, and compensative behaviors to avoid weight increases and promote thinness (purging, vomiting, laxative/diuretics misuse, and compulsive exercise). These eating-related behaviors occur with concurrent severe negative consequences which affect physical, psychological, and social function [1]. As a consequence, the onset and progression of EDs often lead to comorbidity with other multiple psychiatric disorders, disabilities, and mortality rates [2].

There are a diverse range of ED types, with the most common being anorexia nervosa, bulimia nervosa, binge-eating disorder, and other specified feeding and eating disorders [3]. Overall, lifetime EDs have been identified in around 5% of the general population among developed societies [4]. EDs are now on the rise worldwide, and the large increases in estimated prevalence during recent decades (rates more than doubled between 2000 and 2020 among all people) have pointed to the need for new studies assessing the etiology and underlying mechanisms of these complex eating-related problems among clinical and population-based samples [5].

Behavioral addictions (BAs) are non-substance-related addictions characterized by an incapacity to resist impulses toward rewarding stimuli despite the adverse consequences. Aside from gambling and gaming disorder (the two most frequent conditions within the spectrum of behavioral addictions), other maladaptive and uncontrolled behaviors include compulsive sexual behaviors and compulsive buying, among other clinical conditions. The estimated prevalence differs depending on the BA subtype, geographical area, and measurement tools, with values ranging between 0.1% and 6.0% for gambling-related problems [6], 3% and 6% for gaming disorder [7,8], and 5% for compulsive buying [9]. The high prevalence of BAs over the last two decades has attracted increased scientific interest, mostly towards those related to the use of technology [10].

This Special Issue aims to identify the underlying triggers of EDs and BAs, two complex conditions with different diagnostic criteria but that exhibit common clinical features and functional processes. In the following sections, we present the studies and contents covered in this topic, which provide a new empirical basis for developing reliable assessment tools and evidence-based intervention plans (tailored to the individual needs of patients) from a multidisciplinary perspective.

2. Young People: A High-Vulnerability Group for EDs

Etiological research has identified multiple risk factors as predictors of ED onset and progression, with age being one of the variables receiving special attention. The stage between adolescence and early adulthood has been described as a typical age of onset for EDs since this is a crucial period for significant changes [11]. At the biological level, significant changes are observed in morphological, physiological, hormonal, and cognitive functions. At the psychological level, this is a key period of emotional adjustment aimed at facilitating the formation of an identity. At the social level, young people typically challenge parental authority. They make great efforts to be accepted in certain social groups. During this complex process, increased self-awareness contributes to dysfunctional self-doubts and unfavorable social comparisons, which are also highly impacted by sociocultural pressures related to self-image and lifestyle habits (resulting in body dissatisfaction, dieting, and other compensatory behaviors). Individuals with high emotional hyperreactivity and low executive control of their own behaviors can exhibit dysfunctional behavioral patterns that can be conceptualized as precursors of behavioral problems and psychopathology. Finally, young people represent a vulnerable group for developing and progressing mental illness.

Five manuscripts in this Special Issue analyzed data collected among children and adolescents. First, Rios et al. explored the relationships between food addiction and dietary restraint within a sample of adolescents between 13 and 16 years of age in a longitudinal study over a 2-year period of follow-up [12]. A cross-lagged panel revealed that early food addiction more strongly predicted future dietary restraint than the inverse relationship. The authors concluded that their results validated models of addiction among adolescents, particularly those sustaining that restraining behavior constitutes a way to control addictive behaviors. Consequently, strategic plans specifically aiming to ameliorate food addiction (such as nutritional-health-promoting school and home settings) may be crucial during adolescence to prevent later dietary restraint behaviors and the onset of EDs.

Second, the study by Via and Contreras-Rodríguez was a narrative review of the brain basis of binge-eating disorder among children and adolescents, a critical period for neurodevelopment [13]. The review's scope points special attention to the deficits in the emotional regulatory mechanisms identified in this disorder, mostly involving reward-based processing and inhibitory mechanisms related to self-regulation. Similar findings in adult studies, neurocognitive tests, and MRI tasks among youths suggest that hypoactivation in inhibitory control circuits and the hyperactivation of hug regions of reward systems are signals of binge-eating patterns. The study also suggests that ultraprocessed food and drink exposure during childhood may promote changes in the frontolimbic brain circuits, which then contribute to dysfunctional emotional regulation processes during adolescence.

Continuing with the study of youth, another work in this Special Issue, conducted by Matusik and colleagues, also suggests that within this period, specific groups that a priori could be considered as low-vulnerability can, in turn, trigger a nascent obsession with food, eating styles, and body image. The authors estimated a high prevalence of subjects with a positive score in screening tests for EDs among university dietetics students (close to 46%) [14]. Although it may seem inconsistent, these (young) students, who receive extensive education on proper nutrition and healthy, fashionable eating styles, could also develop abnormal relationships with food, and the authors suggest that this is probably due to their exacerbated desire to become perfect role models in eating and body appearance. These individuals are also often prone to stressful events including moving to college, making decisions about their future, or simply taking exams. The authors also observed that around 14% of nutrition students were in the range of overweight to obese at the start of university, and this evidence suggests that ED problems could be underlying in these concrete individuals prior to the beginning of their studies (individuals may view their studies as a way to deal with their inappropriate eating styles, but in the end, they increase their preoccupation with healthy eating).

Similar results were observed in the fourth study of this issue analyzing data among a young population. Grajek et al. compared university students distinguished by their fields of study: health-related areas versus non-health-related areas [15]. They observed a high prevalence of young individuals reporting behaviors characterized by a lack of control over intake (20.7%) and emotional eating (37.9%), independent of their course. This study concluded that among university students, those with lifestyles characterized by inappropriate diets, low rates of physical activity, and high levels of perceived stress are likely to develop unhealthy eating patterns independent of their chosen subject. Ultimately, arrival at university is one of the most important changes that take place in the lives of young people. This period of liberation is usually accompanied by an increase in stress levels, and students' initially high expectations of study motivation can be hampered because they find themselves experiencing concurrent changes that overall affect their lifestyle.

This Special Issue also includes a multicenter, cross-sectional study aimed at exploring behaviors, attitudes, perceptions, and barriers to engagement among children and adolescents (12 to 17 years old) with obesity, caregivers, and healthcare professionals [16]. The results showed that around one-quarter of children with obesity and around half of caregivers perceived that the child's weight was in the normal range; additionally, almost 95% of caregivers perceived the child in their care to be in good health. These results evidence the tendency for parents/caregivers to misperceive their child's weight (they underestimate overweight status), and therefore, their severe inability to recognize obesity as a disease during this stage. Given that many caregivers in the study (around 40%) also felt that possibly being overweight was not a relevant problem because the children would get thinner as they grew up, this will lead to a denial of the problem and delay early intervention. The authors recommend improved communication systems between all the individuals involved in the process (children and adolescents living with obesity, caregivers, and healthcare professionals), an adequate identification of the multiple barriers to addressing weight-related problems, and improved health education on nutrition and its correlates.

3. Other Risks for EDs (Affecting Any Age Group)

The prevalence of EDs has increased across all social sectors in developed countries. In addition to the risks that are typically present at different points in the life course, epidemiological research has identified additional threats to EDs that can have an impact at any age/stage of life, depending on the broader sociocultural and psychological context. For example, participating in competitive sports may increase the chances of developing ED outcomes [17]. Professional athletes focus most of their lives on sports and they can relate their athletic performance to restricted dietary and dysfunctional nutritional intake. These individuals can also emphasize appearance and overvalue the belief that lower body weight will improve performance [18]. The study by Ibañez-Caparrós and colleagues included in this issue observed that, when comparing ED patients who were professional athletes with those who were not, the athletes showed less body dissatisfaction and better psychological performance [19]. However, within the athlete group, individual sport activity and aesthetic sports (such as gymnastics, diving, and figure skating) were associated with worse clinical profiles (higher eating-disorder symptom levels and more comorbid psychological problems) and poorer therapy outcomes. The authors outlined the need for adequate prevention plans for sports organizations and professionals to support athletes. Special attention must be paid to aesthetic sports, which involve judging individual/team performance based on a complex set of rules including appearance. Weight-dependent sports (which divide athletes into weight classes) also deserve special attention, since athletes could normalize the use of compensatory behaviors like vomiting, laxatives, diuretics, and even dehydration as weight control mechanisms.

Stress can impact eating patterns and trigger EDs. Concretely, stressful events occurring in the social and family domains have been identified as powerful risk factors for the onset and evolution of eating-related problems. And, simultaneously, studies have observed that EDs also greatly impact family and social functioning. In this Special Issue, the study carried out by Momeñe and colleagues used path analysis to analyze the underlying relationships between dysfunctional features strongly related to ED profiles (the perception and fear of loneliness, inadequate coping mechanisms to regain control over stressful events, and social isolation) and the likelihood of suffering intimate partner violence (IPV) throughout life [20]. Among a population-based sample composed of young participants, it was observed that specific ED symptoms were directly related to IPV (high drive for thinness, ineffectiveness, perfectionism, interoceptive awareness, impulsiveness, and social insecurity). The study also showed that fear of loneliness was a mediating link between ED symptoms and received violence, but specifically among the high social withdrawal stratum. The authors concluded that the results were consistent with a bidirectional model between EDs and IPV, with central features such as fear of loneliness and social withdrawal acting as mediating links. In this sense, EDs may be interpreted as the consequence of employing dysfunctional mechanisms for coping with the highly adverse consequences of received violence. In addition, with the progression of the disorder, the severity of eating symptoms and other individual characteristics (such as fear of loneliness and social withdrawal) contribute to reinforcing the likelihood of establishing violent partner relationships.

The study by Hoover and colleagues was also focused on how individuals cope with stress levels as a potential risk for ED-related problems [21]. Using a mediational model, these authors tested the relationships between elevated perceived vulnerability to disease and increased fear of fat and cognitive restraint (defined as the control over food intake with the aim of regulating body weight) and compensatory behaviors. Among a sample of $n = 247$ adults (men and women aged from 21 to 70 years), it was found that perceived infectability and germ aversion directly predicted compensatory behaviors, while fear of obesity partially mediated the association. In addition, the participants' sex was not identified as a moderator variable, indicating invariance in the structural coefficients for men and women. This suggested that reducing fear of fat among individuals who experience high perceived vulnerability to infection and disease may be a way to reduce disordered eating (e.g., delivering interventions and cognitive–behavioral techniques to cope with internalized weight stigma).

Finally, persons exposed to comorbid mental conditions represent a further group at significantly elevated risk of EDs. The presence of psychological problems is associated with a set of risks and vulnerabilities, and therefore, the onset and progression of a mental condition raise the odds of concurrent psychiatric diseases. A range of factors have been identified for the comorbid presence of mental disorders, including elevated rates of substance consumption to cope with distress and negative mood states, an unhealthy diet, and unhealthy lifestyles (diminished physical activity and disturbed sleep patterns). Current systematic reviews confirm that, for some individuals, EDs may be chronic disorders that persist from childhood to adulthood, and that patients with EDs are at a higher risk of developing multiple comorbid mental clinical states [22]. The study carried out by Miranda-Olivos and coworkers, included in this Special Issue, assessed how the presence of EDs with comorbid addictions (food addiction and/or substance use) impacts clinical profiles and treatment outcomes [23]. The results showed that the presence of addictive behaviors at baseline was associated with a higher risk of dropout during therapy, and that within the patients with poor treatment outcomes, a comorbid ED plus at least one addiction-related behavior was linked to a clinical profile characterized by greater ED symptom severity, a worse psychopathological state, and more dysfunctional personality traits. The authors concluded that while the presence of addictive behaviors could show a low direct impact on treatment efficacy among ED patients, these comorbid conditions could exert an indirect effect on interventions acting as mediating variables, contributing to worsening clinical profiles at baseline (global distress and ED severity).

4. The Biology of EDs and BAs: Genetic and Neuropsychological Markers

Evidence suggests the existence of multiple biological markers related to the onset and progression of EDs and BAs, including genetic and neuropsychological processes. The study by Solé-Morata et al. [24], included in this issue, tested the underlying mechanisms contributing to BA severity through path analysis, specifically among patients seeking treatment for gambling disorder. Overall, 183 nucleotide polymorphisms (SNPs) of several neurotrophic factors (NFTs) were genotyped, and 4 were selected and analyzed based on the results obtained in previous research: (1) rs796189, the presence of genotypes "AG/GG" (dominant model) and "AG" (overdominant model); (2) rs3763614, the presence of genotypes "CC" (codominant and dominant models) and "CC/TT" (overdominant model); (3) rs11140783, the presence of genotype "CC" (codominant model); and (4) rs3739570, the presence of genotypes "CC" (dominant model) and "CC/TT" (overdominant model). The results showed a complex vulnerability model including the direct and indirect impacts of both the genotype (single SNPs but also haplotype blocks) and phenotype (sociodemographic, psychosocial, and clinical factors) on the severity of gambling symptoms, which is consistent with etiological models of this disorder that include genetic and environmental factors [25].

The etiology of gambling disorder also identified neurocognition as a key domain in characterizing and maintaining the disease. Overall, BAs are associated with a distinct pattern of neurocognitive functioning differentiated by impaired top–down executive control and bias risk–reward processing. Theoretical models of addiction propose a hyperactive drive/reward salience network (a particular affectation was observed in the orbitofrontal cortex, striatum, and dorsal anterior cingulate cortex), in parallel with reduced executive functioning and cognitive control over behavior (related to decreased activity in the inferior frontal cortex and ventral anterior cingulate cortex) [26]. As a consequence, behavioral disinhibition and reward-driven decision making are observed in treatment-seeking patients at baseline (the dysfunctional level is interpreted as a measure of the addictive severity), and are also predictive of treatment relapse [27]. The manuscript by Mestre-Bach and Potenza [28] included in this issue is a state-of-the-art review about specific changes in the brain as a consequence of interventions in both BA- and ED-related conditions (specifically food addiction and binge eating). Specific attention was paid to ventral striatal activation and the related circuitry as a biomarker for these clinical conditions and their recovery, due to their role in reward processing systems. One main implication of the research is that neuropsychological performance should be considered in early detection plans, as well as potentially viable targets for designing novel, more effective interventions (pharmacological, psychobehavioral, and neuromodulatory), aimed towards the activation of specific brain areas involved in reward processing and its connectivity with others.

Turning to the field of EDs, one key domain in their etiology and development is impulsivity [29,30]. This is a complex transdiagnostic construct implied in multiple separate neuropsychological and behavioral dimensions [31] and strongly related to inhibitory control responses and cognitive decision-making processes [32,33]. Impulsivity has also proved to impact therapy response in both short- and long-term outcomes. The study by Testa and colleagues carried out in a sample of $n = 37$ female ED patients using cognitive behavioral therapy (a treatment recommended by most evidence-based guidelines) [34] found that poor inhibitory control at baseline (measured in a Stroop task) was a predictor of poor remission of ED symptom levels at the end of the therapy, while higher novelty seeking (a personality trait defined as the preference for new experiences with intense emotional sensations and risk taking) and poorer inhibition in event-related potentials registered in an emotional go/no-go task negatively impacted symptomatology remission at 2-year follow-up after the treatment [35]. This empirical evidence is consistent with other studies that showed associations between lower cognitive and behavioral control and poor remission (a high risk of dropout and suboptimal remission) in the short term and at follow-up in patients with EDs [36]. The empirical evidence obtained in the study by Testa et al. urges the need of the early detection of ED signals, including lack of inhibition, with the aim to plan precise intervention plans to improve treatment effectiveness. Therapeutic approaches with inhibitory control training with general or food-specific stimuli could be good candidates for ED patients with difficulties in inhibition [37–39].

5. Signals Regulating Energy Homeostasis among EDs and BAs

The homeostatic system is implied in control of feeding based on the regulation of the energy balance (motivation to eat is increased following a reduction in energy stores). Contrarily, the hedonic system implied in feeding is based on the reward-based regulation system and can override homeostatic signals during periods of energy abundance through a rise in the desire for highly palatable foods. Studies have analyzed the control of energy homeostasis and the pathogenesis of EDs, but new empirical evidence is required to further understand energy balance.

In this vein, the study by Nieto et al. [40] included in this issue analyzed the association between the digestive process that follows meal ingestion and a postprandial experience that involves homeostatic sensations (satiety and fullness) with a hedonic dimension (digestive well-being and mood). Based on the Pavlovian conditioning model and the hypothesis that the postprandial experience depends on the characteristics of the individual (intestinal sensitivity, digestive function, and other cognitive/emotive factors) and the meal (organoleptic and the amount and composition), the authors observed that pairing a pleasant meal with an experimentally induced aversive sensation conditions the postprandial response to the subsequent consumption of the same meal. The study also observed that aversive conditioning did not contribute to a homeostatic sensation and physiological digestive response, but significantly impaired the hedonic practice. As a consequence, it was suggested that aversive postprandial conditioning may be considered for the treatment of diverse health conditions, such as obesity, hypercholesterolemia, diabetes, and functional gut disorders. Also, the reinforcement of postprandial rewards and food balance could help counteract natural neophobias of new/unknown foods (for example, in children or patients with autism spectrum disorders) and promote ingestion in individuals with nutritional deficits (for example, patients with anorexia as a consequence of oncological treatments).

Another study included in this Special Issue was also focused on the study of signals involved in energy homeostasis, specifically in patients who met diagnostic criteria for gambling disorder [41]. An analysis of diverse gut hormones (ghrelin (an appetite-stimulator) and liver-expressed antimicrobial peptide2 (LEAP2, an endogenous antagonist of growth hormone secretagogue receptor)) and adipocytokines (leptin and adiponectin) revealed that, compared with a healthy control group, patients with gambling problems presented increased plasma ghrelin and lower LEAP2 and adiponectin concentrations, while no differences in leptin levels were found. The authors concluded that endocrine functions are related to reward processing involved in substance- and non-substance-related addictive processes, and therefore, they may have therapeutic implications because of the relationship with intensifying craving and relapsing.

Author Contributions: Conceptualization, writing—original draft preparation, writing—review and editing: F.F.-A., R.G. and S.J.-M. All authors have read and agreed to the published version of the manuscript.

Funding: This research was funded by Instituto de Salud Carlos III (ISCIII) (FIS PI20/00132) and co-funded by FEDER funds/European Regional Development Fund (ERDF), a way to build Europe. CIBERobn is an initiative of ISCIII. This work was additionally supported by a grant from the Ministerio de Ciencia, Innovación y Universidades (grant RTI2018-101837-B-100), the Delegación del Gobierno para el Plan Nacional sobre Drogas (2019I47 and 2021I031). This study was also funded by the European Union's Horizon 2020 research and innovation program under grant agreement no. 847879 (PRIME/H2020, Prevention and Remediation of Insulin Multimorbidity in Europe). Additional funding was received from AGAUR-Generalitat de Catalunya (2021-SGR-00824). R.G. was supported by the Catalan Institution for Research and Advanced Studies (ICREA-Academia, 2021-Programme).

Acknowledgments: We thank CERCA Programme/Generalitat de Catalunya for institutional support. We also thank Instituto de Salud Carlos III (ISCIII), CIBERobn (an initiative of ISCIII), FEDER funds/European Regional Development Fund (ERDF), and a way to build Europe and European Social Fund (ESF, investing in your future).

Conflicts of Interest: F.F.-A. and S.J.-M. received consultancy honoraria from Novo Nordisk, and F.F.-A. received editorial honoraria from Wiley as the EIC. R.G. declares no conflicts of interest. The funders had no role in the design of the study; in the interpretation of data; in the writing of the manuscript; or in the decision to publish the results.

References

1. Treasure, J.; Duarte, T.A.; Schmidt, U. Eating disorders. *Lancet* **2020**, *395*, 899–911. [CrossRef]
2. Tan, E.J.; Raut, T.; Le, L.K.; Hay, P.; Ananthapavan, J.; Lee, Y.Y.; Mihalopoulos, C. The association between eating disorders and mental health: An umbrella review. *J. Eat. Disord.* **2023**, *11*, 51. [CrossRef]
3. American Psychiatric Association. *Diagnostic and Statistical Manual of Mental Disorders*; American Psychiatric Publishing: Washington, DC, USA, 2013.
4. Galmiche, M.; Déchelotte, P.; Lambert, G.; Tavolacci, M.P. Prevalence of eating disorders over the 2000–2018 period: A systematic literature review. *Am. J. Clin. Nutr.* **2019**, *109*, 1402–1413. [CrossRef]
5. Le, L.K.-D.; Barendregt, J.J.; Hay, P.; Mihalopoulos, C. Prevention of eating disorders: A systematic review and meta-analysis. *Clin. Psychol. Rev.* **2017**, *53*, 46–58. [CrossRef]
6. World Health Organization. The Epidemiology and Impact of Gambling Disorder and Other Gambling-Related Harm. 2017. Available online: https://www.who.int/docs/default-source/substance-use/the-epidemiology-and-impact-of-gambling-disorder-and-other-gambling-relate-harm.pdf (accessed on 27 July 2023).
7. Meng, S.Q.; Cheng, J.L.; Li, Y.Y.; Yang, X.Q.; Zheng, J.W.; Chang, X.W.; Shi, Y.; Chen, Y.; Lu, L.; Sun, Y.; et al. Global prevalence of digital addiction in general population: A systematic review and meta-analysis. *Clin. Psychol. Rev.* **2022**, *92*, 102128. [CrossRef]
8. Stevens, M.W.; Dorstyn, D.; Delfabbro, P.H.; King, D.L. Global prevalence of gaming disorder: A systematic review and meta-analysis. *Aust. N. Z. J. Psychiatry* **2021**, *55*, 553–568. [CrossRef]
9. Black, D.W. Compulsive shopping: A review and update. *Curr. Opin. Psychol.* **2022**, *46*, 101321. [CrossRef]
10. Sixto-Costoya, A.; Castelló-Cogollos, L.; Aleixandre-Benavent, R.; Valderrama-Zurián, J.C. Global scientific production regarding behavioral addictions: An analysis of the literature from 1995 to 2019. *Addict. Behav. Rep.* **2021**, *14*, 100371. [CrossRef]
11. Hochberg, Z.E.; Konner, M. Emerging Adulthood, a Pre-adult Life-History Stage. *Front. Endocrinol.* **2020**, *10*, 918. [CrossRef]
12. Rios, J.; Berg, M.; Gearhardt, A. Evaluating Bidirectional Predictive Pathways between Dietary Restraint and Food Addiction in Adolescents. *Nutrients* **2023**, *15*, 2977. [CrossRef]
13. Via, E.; Contreras-Rodríguez, O. Binge-Eating Precursors in Children and Adolescents: Neurodevelopment, and the Potential Contribution of Ultra-Processed Foods. *Nutrients* **2023**, *15*, 2994. [CrossRef]
14. Matusik, A.; Grajek, M.; Szlacheta, P.; Korzonek-Szlacheta, I. Comparison of the Prevalence of Eating Disorders among Dietetics Students and Students of Other Fields of Study at Selected Universities (Silesia, Poland). *Nutrients* **2022**, *14*, 3210. [CrossRef]
15. Grajek, M.; Krupa-Kotara, K.; Białek-Dratwa, A.; Staśkiewicz, W.; Rozmiarek, M.; Misterska, E.; Sas-Nowosielski, K. Prevalence of Emotional Eating in Groups of Students with Varied Diets and Physical Activity in Poland. *Nutrients* **2022**, *14*, 3289. [CrossRef]
16. López Siguero, J.; Ramon-Krauel, M.; Pérez López, G.; Buiza Fernández, M.; Assaf Balut, C.; Fernández-Aranda, F. Attitudes, Behaviors, and Barriers among Adolescents Living with Obesity, Caregivers, and Healthcare Professionals in Spain: ACTION Teens Survey Study. *Nutrients* **2023**, *15*, 3005. [CrossRef]
17. Torstveit, M.K.; Rosenvinge, J.H.; Sundgot-Borgen, J. Prevalence of eating disorders and the predictive power of risk models in female elite athletes: A controlled study. *Scand. J. Med. Sci. Sports* **2008**, *18*, 108–118. [CrossRef]
18. Marí-Sanchis, A.; Burgos-Balmaseda, J.; Hidalgo-Borrajo, R. Eating disorders in sport. Update and proposal for an integrated approach. *Endocrinol. Diabetes Nutr.* **2022**, *69*, 131–143. [CrossRef]
19. Ibáñez-Caparrós, A.; Sánchez, I.; Granero, R.; Jiménez-Murcia, S.; Rosinska, M.; Thiel, A.; Zipfel, S.; de Pablo, J.; Camacho-Barcia, L.; Fernandez-Aranda, F. Athletes with Eating Disorders: Analysis of Their Clinical Characteristics, Psychopathology and Response to Treatment. *Nutrients* **2023**, *15*, 3003. [CrossRef]
20. Momeñe, J.; Estévez, A.; Griffiths, M.; Macía, P.; Herrero, M.; Olave, L.; Iruarrizaga, I. Eating Disorders and Intimate Partner Violence: The Influence of Fear of Loneliness and Social Withdrawal. *Nutrients* **2022**, *14*, 2611. [CrossRef]
21. Hoover, L.; Ackerman, J.; Cummings, J.; Gearhardt, A. The Association of Perceived Vulnerability to Disease with Cognitive Restraint and Compensatory Behaviors. *Nutrients* **2023**, *15*, 8. [CrossRef]
22. Filipponi, C.; Visentini, C.; Filippini, T.; Cutino, A.; Ferri, P.; Rovesti, S.; Lattela, E.; Di Lorenzo, R. The Follow-Up of Eating Disorders from Adolescence to Early Adulthood: A Systematic Review. *Int. J. Environ. Res. Public. Health* **2022**, *19*, 16237. [CrossRef]
23. Miranda-Olivos, R.; Agüera, Z.; Granero, R.; Jiménez-Murcia, S.; Puig-Llobet, M.; Lluch-Canut, M.; Gearhardt, A.; Fernández-Aranda, F. The Role of Food Addiction and Lifetime Substance Use on Eating Disorder Treatment Outcomes. *Nutrients* **2023**, *15*, 2919. [CrossRef]

24. Solé-Morata, N.; Baenas, I.; Etxandi, M.; Granero, R.; Gené, M.; Barrot, C.; Gómez-Peña, M.; Moragas, L.; Ramoz, N.; Gorwood, P.; et al. Underlying Mechanisms Involved in Gambling Disorder Severity: A Pathway Analysis Considering Genetic, Psychosocial, and Clinical Variables. *Nutrients* **2023**, *15*, 418. [CrossRef]
25. Stefanovics, E.A.; Potenza, M.N. Update on Gambling Disorder. *Psychiatr. Clin. N. Am.* **2022**, *45*, 483–502. [CrossRef]
26. Hüpen, P.; Habel, U.; Votinov, M.; Kable, J.W.; Wagels, L. A Systematic Review on Common and Distinct Neural Correlates of Risk-taking in Substance-related and Non-substance Related Addictions. *Neuropsychol. Rev.* **2023**, *33*, 492–513. [CrossRef]
27. Christensen, E.; Brydevall, M.; Albertella, L.; Samarawickrama, S.K.; Yücel, M.; Lee, R.S.C. Neurocognitive predictors of addiction-related outcomes: A systematic review of longitudinal studies. *Neurosci. Biobehav. Rev.* **2023**, *152*, 105295. [CrossRef]
28. Mestre-Bach, G.; Potenza, M. Potential Biological Markers and Treatment Implications for Binge Eating Disorder and Behavioral Addictions. *Nutrients* **2023**, *15*, 827. [CrossRef]
29. Miranda-Olivos, R.; Testa, G.; Lucas, I.; Sánchez, I.; Sánchez-González, J.; Granero, R.; Jiménez-Murcia, S.; Fernández-Aranda, F. Clinical factors predicting impaired executive functions in eating disorders: The role of illness duration. *J. Psychiatr. Res.* **2021**, *144*, 87–95. [CrossRef]
30. Stoyanova, S.; Ivantchev, N.; Giannuoli, V. Functional, Dysfunctional Impulsivity and Sensation Seeking in Medical Staff-PubMed. *Psychiatr. Danub.* **2021**, *33*, 25–29.
31. Lavender, J.M.; Mitchell, J.E. Eating Disorders and Their Relationship to Impulsivity. *Curr. Treat. Options Psychiatry* **2015**, *2*, 394–401. [CrossRef]
32. Bartholdy, S.; Dalton, B.; O'Daly, O.G.; Campbell, I.C.; Schmidt, U. A systematic review of the relationship between eating, Weight and inhibitory control using the stop signal task. *Neurosci. Biobehav. Rev.* **2016**, *64*, 35–62. [CrossRef]
33. Lavagnino, L.; Arnone, D.; Cao, B.; Soares, J.C.; Selvaraj, S. Inhibitory control in obesity and binge eating disorder: A systematic review and meta-analysis of neurocognitive and neuroimaging studies. *Neurosci. Biobehav. Rev.* **2016**, *68*, 714–726. [CrossRef]
34. Linardon, J.; Wade, T.D.; de la Piedad Garcia, X.; Brennan, L. The efficacy of cognitive-behavioral therapy for eating disorders: A systematic review and meta-analysis. *J. Consult. Clin. Psychol.* **2017**, *85*, 1080–1094. [CrossRef]
35. Testa, G.; Granero, R.; Misiolek, A.; Vintró-Alcaraz, C.; Mallorqui-Bagué, N.; Lozano-Madrid, M.; Heras, M.; Sánchez, I.; Jiménez-Murcia, S.; Fernández-Aranda, F. Impact of Impulsivity and Therapy Response in Eating Disorders from a Neurophysiological, Personality and Cognitive Perspective. *Nutrients* **2022**, *14*, 5011. [CrossRef]
36. Kaidesoja, M.; Cooper, Z.; Fordham, B. Cognitive behavioral therapy for eating disorders: A map of the systematic review evidence base. *Int. J. Eat. Disord.* **2023**, *56*, 295–313. [CrossRef]
37. Chami, R.; Treasure, J.; Cardi, V.; Lozano-Madrid, M.; Eichin, K.N.; McLoughlin, G.; Blechert, J. Exploring Changes in Event-Related Potentials After a Feasibility Trial of Inhibitory Training for Bulimia Nervosa and Binge Eating Disorder. *Front. Psychol.* **2020**, *11*, 1056. [CrossRef]
38. Keeler, J.L.; Chami, R.; Cardi, V.; Hodsoll, J.; Bonin, E.; MacDonald, P.; Treasure, J.; Lawrence, N. App-based food-specific inhibitory control training as an adjunct to treatment as usual in binge-type eating disorders: A feasibility trial. *Appetite* **2022**, *168*, 105788. [CrossRef]
39. Turton, R.; Nazar, B.P.; Burgess, E.E.; Lawrence, N.S.; Cardi, V.; Treasure, J.; Hirsch, C.R. To Go or Not to Go: A Proof of Concept Study Testing Food-Specific Inhibition Training for Women with Eating and Weight Disorders. *Eur. Eat. Disord. Rev.* **2018**, *26*, 11–21. [CrossRef]
40. Nieto, A.; Livovsky, D.; Azpiroz, F. Conditioning by a Previous Experience Impairs the Rewarding Value of a Comfort Meal. *Nutrients* **2023**, *15*, 2247. [CrossRef]
41. Etxandi, M.; Baenas, I.; Mora-Maltas, B.; Granero, R.; Fernández-Aranda, F.; Tovar, S.; Solé-Morata, N.; Lucas, I.; Casado, S.; Gómez-Peña, M.; et al. Are Signals Regulating Energy Homeostasis Related to Neuropsychological and Clinical Features of Gambling Disorder? A Case and Control Study. *Nutrients* **2022**, *14*, 5084. [CrossRef]

Disclaimer/Publisher's Note: The statements, opinions and data contained in all publications are solely those of the individual author(s) and contributor(s) and not of MDPI and/or the editor(s). MDPI and/or the editor(s) disclaim responsibility for any injury to people or property resulting from any ideas, methods, instructions or products referred to in the content.

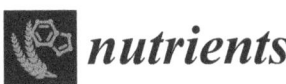

Article

Evaluating Bidirectional Predictive Pathways between Dietary Restraint and Food Addiction in Adolescents

Julia M. Rios *, Martha K. Berg and Ashley N. Gearhardt

Department of Psychology, University of Michigan, 530 Church St., Ann Arbor, MI 48109, USA; bergmk@umich.edu (M.K.B.); agearhar@umich.edu (A.N.G.)
* Correspondence: jsmr@umich.edu

Abstract: The relationship between food addiction, an important emerging construct of excessive eating pathology, and dietary restraint has yet to be fully understood. Eating disorder models commonly posit that dietary restraint exacerbates loss of control eating (e.g., binge episodes) and may also play a causal role in the development of food addiction. However, dietary restraint as a reaction to consequences of food addiction (e.g., uncontrollable eating or weight gain) represents another plausible pathway. Existing studies indicate that the association between food addiction and dietary restraint may be more significant during adolescence than adulthood, but are limited by cross-sectional study designs. A longitudinal study using an adolescent sample is ideal for investigating potential pathways underlying links between food addiction and dietary restraint. This study examined temporal pathways between food addiction and dietary restraint in a sample of one hundred twenty-seven adolescents (M = 14.8, SD = 1.1) at three timepoints spanning two years. This is the first study to examine longitudinal cross-lagged panel associations between food addiction and dietary restraint. In this adolescent sample, food addiction significantly predicted future dietary restraint (b = 0.25, SE = 0.06, $p < 0.001$), but dietary restraint did not significantly predict future food addiction (b = 0.06, SE = 0.05, $p > 0.05$). These findings support the theory that dietary restraint may be a reaction to deleterious effects of food addiction during adolescence.

Keywords: food addiction; dietary restraint; adolescence; longitudinal analysis

1. Introduction

Food addiction is an emerging classification of compulsive overeating, characterized by "excessive overeating of high-calorie food accompanied by loss of control and intense food cravings" [1,2]. Alongside empirical support for the concept of food addiction, remaining questions regarding its mechanisms and clinical utility have stimulated scholarly debate. A leading critique of the food addiction construct is that existing models do not adequately account for contributions of dietary restraint [3]. Dietary restraint has often been defined as a self-imposed restriction of food intake in order to lose weight or avoid weight gain [4]. However, empirical evidence suggests that individuals who report high levels of dietary restraint do not always appear to be actually reducing or restricting caloric intake [5,6]. More recently, dietary restraint has been better understood to also encompass cognitive efforts to reduce overall intake or avoid certain types of food regardless of success [7,8].

Eating disorder models have traditionally held that maladaptive (e.g., rigid or excessive) dietary restraint is a critical antecedent to binge eating [9,10]. According to many eating disorder models, dietary restraint creates a state of physiological and psychological deprivation which is difficult to maintain and ultimately induces pathological overeating [11]. In contrast with traditional eating disorder models, food addiction models do not currently centralize dietary restraint as a causal etiological factor [9,12,13]. Because food addiction and binge eating share key features (e.g., loss of control eating and food cravings [14]), it stands to reason that findings on dietary restraint and related eating

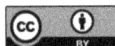

disorders (e.g., BED and BN) provide valuable theoretical insight regarding how dietary restraint may influence similar eating pathology in food addiction. Based on the dietary restraint literature in eating disorders, it is plausible that dietary restraint may also contribute to food addiction pathology or occur as a reaction to negative consequences of food addiction. However, addictive eating and binge eating are nonidentical pathologies and restraint is not a central causal feature in known addiction pathways (e.g., substance use disorders [12]). Numerous prior cross-sectional studies have failed to find evidence for an association between food addiction and dietary restraint in adults [15–17], though findings have been mixed in a small number of international studies [18,19]. Thus, it is also possible that dietary restraint may not be strongly associated with food addiction, highlighting the need to examine their distinct relationship. However, the existing literature on associations between food addiction and dietary restraint is overall sparse, and potential relations or directional pathways have received limited empirical investigation. Therefore, this study aims to shed light on potential temporal pathways and directionality in the relationship between these constructs.

Adolescence is a potentially key period during which to investigate the relationship between food addiction and dietary restraint. Adolescence is a high-risk period for both the emergence of dieting behaviors and heightened vulnerability to addictive behaviors [20,21]. However, few existing studies, to our knowledge, have explored food addiction and dietary restraint in adolescents. In one study, food addiction symptoms assessed by the dimensional Yale Food Addiction Scale for Children 2.0 (dYFAS-C 2.0), a version of the YFAS adapted to reflect age-appropriate symptoms (e.g., problems at school instead of work) and reading level [22], were positively correlated with dietary restraint scores on the DEBQ-R ($r = 0.32$ [23]). A second study showed that YFAS scores were significantly correlated with the Three Factors Eating Questionnaire dietary restraint subscale in Turkish adolescents (OR = 1.01 [24]). Of note, the effect size of these associations were small. Nonetheless, these studies suggest that food addiction and dietary restraint may be related in adolescents but are limited by cross-sectional research design.

According to restraint-based theories for eating pathology, these prior findings could be interpreted as evidence that dietary restraint increases the risk for addictive eating behaviors. However, these results could also signify that adolescents with higher propensity for addictive eating may be more likely to engage in dietary restraint as a reaction to patterns of overconsumption and possible weight gain. If dietary restraint is a stronger predictor of future food addiction, this may support restraint-based theories for a causal role of dietary restraint. Alternatively, if food addiction is a stronger predictor of future dietary restraint, this may support a model of food addiction in which risk is primarily underlied by exposure to HP foods, and dietary restraint occurs as a consequence, rather than a cause, of addictive eating. If neither dietary restraint nor food addiction predicts longitudinal change in either construct, this may indicate that dietary restraint is a less relevant construct in food addiction than binge-type eating disorders.

The limitations of cross-sectional prior studies make it difficult to speculate on the nature of the relationship between food addiction and dietary restraint over time. This study aims to determine whether food and dietary restraint are correlated in a sample of adolescents (N = one hundred twenty-seven) in a longitudinal design over a two-year period of repeated assessment. This will increase understanding of the temporal associations and possible directionality between food addiction and dietary restraint that appears during adolescence.

2. Materials and Methods

2.1. Participants

Recruitment. As part of a larger longitudinal study examining adolescent eating behavior and responsivity to food advertisements (Project Media), adolescent participants (i.e., 13–16 years of age) were recruited from southeast Michigan using print and online advertisements. A parent or guardian provided written informed consent and adolescents provided written informed assent prior to enrollment. Adolescents (N = 127), ranging from 13 to 16 years of age (M = 14.8, SD = 1.1), were recruited for the full study. The dimensional YFAS-C 2.0 (dYFAS-C 2.0) was added to the questionnaire battery later in data collection, and 127 participants completed the measure at the initial wave of data collection (Time 1). Participants completed self-report measures at baseline (Time 1) and follow-ups after one year (Time 2) and two years (Time 3). Participants provided demographics at baseline (Time 1; participant descriptives are summarized in Table 1). Due to the sensitive nature of some of the self-reported content, additional protocols were implemented to reduce potential bias and increase validity of responses. Participants were provided a private space to complete all measures and were informed that all researchers were blind to their de-identified responses. This study was approved by the University of Michigan Institutional Review Board (IRB) and complied with the ethical standards of the APA (APA, 2013).

Table 1. Adolescent Participant Demographics, Descriptives, and Sample Size at Each Wave (N = 127).

	Total (n)	Percent (%)
Gender		
Male	61	48.0
Female	66	52.0
Race		
American Indian/Alaska Native	3	2.4
Black/African American	19	15.0
White	91	71.7
Other	1	0.8
Mixed	8	6.3
Unknown	5	3.9
Parental Education		
Less than High School	15	11.8
High School Degree	5	3.9
Some College	19	15
Associates Degree	11	8.7
Bachelor's Degree	35	27.6
Advanced Degree	42	33.1
Sample Size at Each Wave		
Time 1	127	100.0
Time 2	92	72.4
Time 3	88	69.3
	Mean (SD)	Range (min, max)
Age (months) at Time 1	177.3 (12.4)	(156.0, 202.5)
BMI z-score	0.95 (0.9)	(−1.2, 2.7)

Note. SD = standard deviation; BMI = body mass index. Data missingness was determined by availability of data for primary variables included in the cross-lagged panel analysis (i.e., food addiction (YFAS) and dietary restraint (DEBQ-R) at each time point).

Inclusion and Exclusion Criteria. Due to the aims of the larger study investigating eating behavior and reward response to food marketing in adolescents, participant exclusion criteria included the following factors known to influence reward functioning: (1) a history of or a current eating disorder diagnosis, (2) current mood, anxiety, trauma, or psychotic disorders, (3) current prescription for a psychotropic medication, and (4) underweight BMI status.

2.2. Measures

Demographics and Anthropometry. Participants were asked to complete a demographics questionnaire at the first study visit (Time 1). Participants were asked to self-report their date of birth (which was used to calculate age in months), race, gender (as male, female, other gender identity, or prefer not to identify), and parental education level. Participant height and weight measurements were taken at the first study visit (Time 1). Participants were asked to remove any shoes, hats, and outerwear. Participant heights and weights were taken twice to confirm accuracy. Participants were weighed to the nearest 0.1 kg using a Detecto Portable Scale. If weights differed by more than 0.1 kg, the measurements were repeated. Participant height was measured using an O'Leary Acrylic Stadiometer to the nearest 1 cm. If height measurements differed by more than 1 cm, the measurements were repeated. Participant BMI z-scores were calculated using percentiles determined by the Center for Disease for Control's assessment for children and teens [25]. Participant demographics and anthropometry measures are summarized in Table 1.

dYFAS-C 2.0. The dYFAS-C 2.0 is a 16-item self-report measure that operationalizes food addiction characteristics in children and adolescents based on the same DSM-5 criteria for substance use disorders as the YFAS ([16,23]. When completing the dYFAS-C 2.0, participants are instructed to think about foods high in refined carbohydrates and/or fats, as these foods have been most evidenced in food addiction [26]. All items are reported on a 5-point Likert scale (from 0 = never to 4 = always). Prior research suggests that problematic substance use in adolescence is more accurately conceptualized as a continuous rather than a categorical syndrome [27]. Thus, the dYFAS-C 2.0 utilizes a dimensional scoring approach. Item scores are summed with higher scores indicating more severe food addiction. The dYFAS-C 2.0 demonstrates good convergent and incremental validity, as well as internal consistency [23]. In the current sample, dYFAS-C 2.0 scores demonstrated good internal consistency ($\alpha = 0.90$).

Dutch Eating Behaviors Questionnaire Restraint Subscale. The Dutch Eating Behaviors Questionnaire Restraint Subscale (DEBQ) is a 33-item self-report survey designed to capture various aspects of eating style including external eating, emotional eating, and restrained eating. The 10-item restrained eating subscale (DEBQ-R) measures intentions and attempts to reduce food intake or to avoid certain food types. All items were reported on a 5-point Likert scale (from 1 = never to 5 = very often). Scores on the DEBQ-R reflect the average of all items, with higher scores indicating a greater degree of dietary restraint. The DEBQ demonstrates good predictive validity and internal consistency in adults [28,29], as well as adolescents [30,31]. In the current sample, DEBQ-R scores demonstrated excellent internal consistency ($\alpha = 0.93$).

2.3. Data Analytic Plan

Statistical tests were completed using R version 4.1.2 and the *lavaan* package [32]. Preliminary analyses were completed to verify that these data did not violate assumptions for cross-lagged panel analysis including normality, stationarity, and synchronicity [31]. Individuals who completed all measures at all time points (n = 91) did not significantly differ from individuals who did not complete measures at Time 2 and/or Time 3 of the study (n = 36) on any of our variables of interest (i.e., food addiction or dietary restraint, all $p > 0.05$), covariates (i.e., age, gender, or BMI z-score, all $p > 0.05$), or demographics (i.e., race or parental education; all $p > 0.05$). Full information maximum likelihood estimation was also used to maximize sample size, given an assumption that all missing data was missing at random [33]. Prior to analysis, outlier values from both primary variables (food addiction and dietary restraint) were winsorized [34], and both variables were standardized.

Temporal associations between food addiction and dietary restraint were examined using a cross-lagged panel design across three waves (Time 1, Time 2, and Time 3). To control for possible confounding effects of differences in baseline age, gender, or BMI z-score [35,36], these were considered as covariates in the model. Age and BMI z-score variables were mean-centered, and gender variable was contrast-coded. Zero-order correlations among variables of interest and covariates were tested at Time 1, Time 2, and Time 3. Inclusion of covariates did not change the patterns of significance for any findings in the cross-lagged panel analysis but did result in poorer model fit (unadjusted CFI = 0.95, SRMR = 0.054, adjusted CFI = 0.86, SRMR = 0.14). Thus, for ease of interpretation and improved model fit, results and figures reported here reflect the unadjusted structural equation models (SEM; see Figure 1). The model simultaneously estimated the cross-lagged relationships between the two variables, as well as auto-regressive paths for each variable across time. All effects were assumed to be constant across the three time points; therefore, a single estimate was computed for each cross-lagged and auto-regressive relationship, independent of time (see Figure 1 for labeled path diagram). Pathways and results from the adjusted SEM are provided as Supplemental Materials (see Supplemental Materials Figure S1 and Table S2). We also conducted exploratory imputation analyses to account for missingness in the data at Time 2 and Time 3. However, no substantial differences were observed in the correlations or cross-lagged panel analyses between the non-imputed and imputed data sets. Thus, the results from the non-imputed data are reported here.

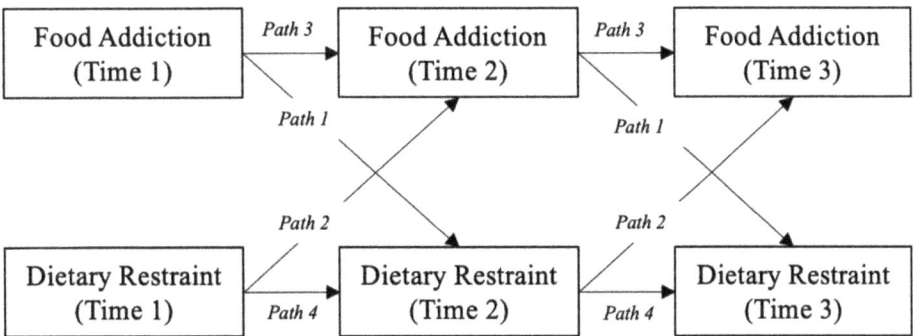

Figure 1. Path Diagram for Unadjusted Cross-lagged Panel Analysis between Food Addiction and Dietary Restraint.

3. Results

Food addiction and dietary restraint were significantly associated with each other at all time points ($r = 0.34$, $p = <.001$; $r = 0.36$, $p = < 0.001$; $r = 0.47$, $p = < 0.001$), and were each associated with age, gender, and BMI z-score at most time points (see Supplemental Table S1).

Cross-lagged panel analysis revealed that food addiction significantly predicted future dietary restraint ($b = 0.25$, SE = 0.06, $p < 0.001$). Dietary restraint did not significantly predict future food addiction ($b = 0.06$, SE = 0.05, $p > 0.05$; see Table 2 for all model estimates). In comparing the difference between coefficients for each of the cross-lagged paths, Path 1 (food addiction predicting dietary restraint) was significantly stronger than Path 2 (dietary restraint predicting food addiction; $b = 0.18$, SE = 0.08, $p < 0.05$). Auto-regressive paths were significant for both food addiction ($b = 0.61$, SE = 0.05, $p < 0.001$) and dietary restraint ($b = 0.59$, SE = 0.056, $p < 0.001$) over time, suggesting both constructs showed test-retest reliability over time.

Table 2. Standardized Regression Coefficients for Food Addiction and Dietary Restraint from Unadjusted Structural Equation Models.

							CI (95%)	
Path	Predictor	Outcome	b	SE	z	p	Lower	Upper
1	Food addiction	Dietary restraint	0.25	0.06	4.51	<0.001	0.14	0.37
2	Dietary restraint	Food addiction	0.06	0.05	1.24	0.21	−0.04	0.16
3	Food addiction	Food addiction	0.74	0.05	15.32	<0.001	0.64	0.83
4	Dietary restraint	Dietary restraint	0.58	0.06	10.48	<0.001	0.47	0.68

Model Fit: $X^2(8) = 21.14$ ($p < 0.01$); SRMR = 0.04; CFI = 0.95. CI = confidence interval. A post-hoc sensitivity analysis using pwrSEM ([37] with ten thousand simulations and a seed of twenty-three indicated that our model had 100% power to detect an effect of this size for Path 1, and 41% power to detect an effect of this size for Path 2. Predictor variables were measured at T1, outcome variables were measured at times T2 and T3.

4. Discussion

In a longitudinal study of one hundred twenty-seven adolescents, we assessed and compared the strength of predictive pathways between food addiction symptoms and dietary restraint across two years. Cross-lagged panel analyses showed that food addiction significantly predicted future dietary restraint over time. In contrast, dietary restraint did not predict future food addiction. To address our primary research question, we computed the difference between the coefficients for each of the cross-lagged paths. The path for food addiction predicting dietary restraint (Path 1) was stronger than the path for dietary restraint predicting food addiction (Path 2). Auto-regressive paths for food addiction (Path 3) and dietary restraint (Path 4) were both significant, indicating the stability of these predictors over time.

The present findings provide additional support to the existing literature that food addiction and dietary restraint demonstrate some association in adolescents [22–24]. While some researchers have thereby speculated that dietary restraint plays a causal role in the development or progression of food addiction [38], these longitudinal findings show that food addiction is a stronger predictor of future dietary restraint than dietary restraint is of future food addiction. This suggests that food addiction may be more likely to emerge prior to dietary restraint, and that dietary restraint occurs as a consequence rather than a cause of food addiction. This finding is consistent with other models of addiction (e.g., substance use disorders) in which individuals exhibit restraint in an effort to control addictive behaviors or substance use [12,13].

This is in contrast to some predominant models for binge eating, which have historically suggested that dietary restraint is a causal preceding factor [9,10]. However, findings from more recent empirical studies on binge eating and dietary restraint have been mixed. While dietary restraint appears to be a relevant factor in binge-type eating pathology for some individuals (e.g., about half of individuals who develop BED [39–41]), binge-type eating behaviors are reported to precede dietary restraint for many others [39,42,43]. The present findings suggest that the relationship between food addiction and dietary restraint in adolescence may be more consistent with the subgroup of individuals for whom dietary restraint appears to occur as a reaction to binge-type eating pathology (e.g., in an effort to avoid weight gain [44,45]). It may be that an addictive response to HP foods results in a greater tendency to engage in reactionary dietary restriction (e.g., due to social pressures and beauty ideals about thinness) to offset excessive food intake. A recent study demonstrated that repeated exposure to HP foods in healthy, normal-weight participants led to increased sensitization to the rewarding properties of HP foods and related neurobehavioral dysfunction, such as decreased preference for minimally processed foods and increased consumption of HP foods [46]). Thus, individuals who exhibit addictive eating of HP foods may be more likely to engage in dietary restriction in order to combat increased consumption of HP foods or related weight gain. Future research utilizing latent class growth analyses may provide more specific insights into latent pathways or subgroup differences for associations or temporal relationships among these constructs.

In sum, while these constructs do appear to be related during this stage of development, longitudinal analyses do not support a causal role of dietary restraint in mechanistic models of food addiction. Rather, the present findings provide stronger empirical support for a model of food addiction in which risk may be underlied by alternative factors, such as exposure to HP foods [44,45], clinical co-morbidities and psychological risk factors (e.g., addiction proneness [47]), stronger reward sensitivity [46,48], vulnerability for weight gain [44,45], or addiction risk factors (e.g., family history of addiction [49]). Therefore, evidenced associations between food addiction and dietary restraint in adolescents may reflect attempts to manage an addictive response to HP foods. The present study provides empirical evidence for a direct temporal pathway between food addiction and dietary restraint. It will be important for future research to investigate theoretical risk factors (e.g., proneness to addiction or exposure to HP foods) or mediators (e.g., weight or shape concerns) in the model.

If food addiction is a stronger predictor of future dietary restraint, strategies aimed specifically at ameliorating food addiction symptoms may be most effective for reducing future dietary restraint and any amplifying effects on future food addiction. The implementation of prevention (e.g., health-promoting school and home settings [50]), treatment (e.g., adapted addiction treatment programs, treatment of comorbid psychopathology [51]), and policy (e.g., restrictions on HP food marketing that targets teens [52]) interventions during the crucial stage of adolescence may have substantial benefits for reducing both food addiction and dietary restraint behaviors in adolescents. Currently, the majority of prior research has been dedicated to evaluating the food addiction construct, and much less research has explored or tested intervention approaches. This will be an important future direction for food addiction research.

There is a critical need for research-guided public health recommendations for dietary restraint that address the impairment and distress related to symptoms of food addiction [1] and living in a social environment that stigmatizes weight gain and fatness [53]. Importantly, existing research suggests that not all forms of dietary restraint are associated with equally poor eating outcomes. For example, rigid dietary restraint (e.g., all-or-nothing dieting approach) compared with flexible dietary restraint (e.g., graduated dieting approach) appears to be more strongly associated with binge-type eating when dieting rules are violated [54]. Prior research also shows improvements in eating outcomes (e.g., reduced external eating and emotional eating) when dietary restraint is implemented regularly and proactively (e.g., routine restraint) compared to irregularly and retroactively (e.g., compensatory restraint following diet noncompliance [55]). It is therefore possible that the type of dietary restraint which occurs in reaction to food addiction may have differential impacts on health and well-being. Intervention strategies that promote more flexible and proactive dietary restraining behaviors may have some pro-health utility. However, additional research is needed to better understand which forms of dietary restraint may be most harmful, neutral, or beneficial for promotion of healthy eating behaviors and how this may interact with a propensity for food addiction. It will be critical for future research to explore and develop dietary recommendations for individuals who endorse food addiction symptoms and struggle to control their eating.

This study offers a number of important strengths and contributions to the empirical literature. This is the first longitudinal study design exploring temporal pathways between food addiction and dietary restraint allowing for inferences regarding the nature and directionality of the relationship between these constructs. Furthermore, this study involved adolescent participants and utilized developmentally appropriate psychometrics, which provided an assessment of food addiction and dietary restraint during a key developmental period in which eating pathology and dieting behaviors often emerge [21,56]. However, because this study was limited to a two-year span during adolescence, much remains unknown about early life risk factors and long-term progression of both food addiction and dietary restraint. Existing research indicates that by adulthood, food addiction and dietary restraint have a weaker association [19] or may no longer be associated [16,18,57]. Without longitudinal data spanning adolescence and adulthood, it is difficult to pinpoint why this association seems to diminish over time. Ongoing research is needed to better understand additional factors which may contribute to risk for both food addiction and dietary restraint, as well as how associations between these constructs change throughout various stages of development.

The present study was also limited to a relatively small and well-resourced sample. Additional research is needed to test how these findings may generalize to larger and more diverse populations. The use of a larger sample size would also provide more power to examine possible moderating effects of key covariates (i.e., age, gender, and BMI z-score) or explore latent class analyses to assess for individual differences or subgroups of pathway directionality. This study utilized data collected from a larger study with aims to examine eating behavior and reward response to food marketing in adolescents that excluded participants with psychiatric conditions including eating disorders or underweight BMI status. This allowed us to consider bidirectional effects of food addiction and dietary restraint more precisely, minimizing possible confounding effects of other eating pathology (e.g., binge eating). However, it should be noted this removes participants with the most extreme presentations of dietary restraint and limits the generalizability of the findings.

5. Conclusions

The current results utilizing longitudinal data indicate that dietary restraint may be more likely to occur as a reaction or consequence to food addiction symptoms. These findings highlight the potential utility of food addiction as a research target for intervention or prevention efforts towards improving eating behavior. Future research is needed to better understand the bidirectional mechanisms that drive the association between food addiction and dietary restraint in adolescents.

Supplementary Materials: The following supporting information can be downloaded at: https://www.mdpi.com/article/10.3390/nu15132977/s1, Figure S1: Path Diagram for Adjusted Cross-lagged Panel Analysis among Food Addiction, Dietary Restraint, and Covariates (Age, Gender, and BMI z-score); Table S1: Summary of Bivariate Correlations Among Adolescent Food Addiction, Dietary Restraint, and Associated Covariates; Table S2: Standardized Regression Coefficients from Adjusted Structural Equation Models with Covariates.

Author Contributions: Conceptualization, J.M.R. and A.N.G.; Methodology, J.M.R.; A.N.G. and M.K.B.; Formal analysis, J.M.R. and M.K.B.; Writing—original draft, J.M.R. and A.N.G.; Writing—review & editing, J.M.R. and A.N.G.; Supervision, A.N.G.; Funding acquisition, A.N.G. All authors have read and agreed to the published version of the manuscript.

Funding: This research was funded by National Institute of Health, Grant/Award Number: R01 DK102532.

Institutional Review Board Statement: This study was approved by the University of Michigan Institutional Review Board, and research complied with the ethical standards of the American Psychological Association (American Psychiatric Association, 2013).

Informed Consent Statement: Informed consent was obtained from all subjects involved in the study.

Data Availability Statement: The data presented in his study are available on request from Dr. Ashley Gearhardt (agearhar@umich.edu).

Conflicts of Interest: The authors declare no conflict of interest.

References

1. Gearhardt, A.N.; Corbin, W.R.; Brownell, K.D. Preliminary validation of the Yale Food Addiction Scale. *Appetite* **2009**, *52*, 430–436. [CrossRef]
2. Maxwell, A.L.; Gardiner, E.; Loxton, N.J. Investigating the relationship between reward sensitivity, impulsivity, and food addiction: A systematic review. *Eur. Eat. Disord. Rev.* **2020**, *28*, 368–384. [CrossRef] [PubMed]
3. Wiss, D.; Brewerton, T. Separating the Signal from the Noise: How Psychiatric Diagnoses Can Help Discern Food Addiction from Dietary Restraint. *Nutrients* **2020**, *12*, 2937. [CrossRef]
4. Herman, C.P.; Polivy, J. Anxiety, restraint, and eating behavior. *J. Abnorm. Psychol.* **1975**, *84*, 666–672. [CrossRef]
5. Lowe, M.R. The effects of dieting on eating behavior: A three-factor model. *Psychol. Bull.* **1993**, *114*, 100–121. [CrossRef]
6. Stice, E.; Fisher, M.; Lowe, M.R. Are Dietary Restraint Scales Valid Measures of Acute Dietary Restriction? Unobtrusive Observational Data Suggest Not. *Psychol. Assess.* **2004**, *16*, 51–59. [CrossRef]
7. Lowe, M.R.; Annunziato, R.A.; Markowitz, J.T.; Didie, E.; Bellace, D.L.; Riddell, L.; Maille, C.; McKinney, S.; Stice, E. Multiple types of dieting prospectively predict weight gain during the freshman year of college. *Appetite* **2006**, *47*, 83–90. [CrossRef]
8. Polivy, J.; Herman, C.P.; Mills, J.S. What is restrained eating and how do we identify it? *Appetite* **2020**, *155*, 104820. [CrossRef]
9. Herman, C.; Polivy, J. From dietary restraint to binge eating: Attaching causes to effects. *Appetite* **1990**, *14*, 123–125. [CrossRef]
10. Telch, C.F.; Agras, W.S. The effects of a very low calorie diet on binge eating. *Behav. Ther.* **1993**, *24*, 177–193. [CrossRef]
11. Kirkley, B.G.; Burge, J.C.; Ammerman, A. Dietary restraint, binge eating, and dietary behavior patterns. *Int. J. Eat. Disord.* **1988**, *7*, 771–778. [CrossRef]
12. Schulte, E.M.; Grilo, C.M.; Gearhardt, A.N. Shared and unique mechanisms underlying binge eating disorder and addictive disorders. *Clin. Psychol. Rev.* **2016**, *44*, 125–139. [CrossRef] [PubMed]
13. Ziauddeen, H.; Fletcher, P.C. Is food addiction a valid and useful concept? *Obes. Rev.* **2012**, *14*, 19–28. [CrossRef] [PubMed]

14. Gearhardt, A.N.; Grilo, C.M.; Dileone, R.J.; Brownell, K.D.; Potenza, M.N. Can food be addictive? Public health and policy implications. *Addiction* **2011**, *106*, 1208–1212. [CrossRef]
15. Carter, J.C.; Van Wijk, M.; Rowsell, M. Symptoms of 'food addiction' in binge eating disorder using the Yale Food Addiction Scale version 2.0. *Appetite* **2019**, *133*, 362–369. [CrossRef]
16. Gearhardt, A.N.; Corbin, W.R.; Brownell, K.D. Development of the Yale Food Addiction Scale Version 2.0. *Psychol. Addict. Behav.* **2016**, *30*, 113–121. [CrossRef]
17. Rios, J.M.; Miller, A.L.; Lumeng, J.C.; Rosenblum, K.; Appugliese, D.P.; Gearhardt, A.N. Associations of maternal food addiction, dietary restraint, and pre-pregnancy BMI with infant eating behaviors and risk for overweight. *Appetite* **2023**, *184*, 106516. [CrossRef]
18. Imperatori, C.; Fabbricatore, M.; Lester, D.; Manzoni, G.M.; Gianluca, C.; Raimondi, G.; Innamorati, M. Psychometric properties of the modified Yale Food Addiction Scale Version 2.0 in an Italian non-clinical sample. *Eat. Weight. Disord. Stud. Anorex. Bulim. Obes.* **2018**, *24*, 37–45. [CrossRef]
19. Legendre, M.; Bégin, C. French validation of the addiction-like eating behavior scale and its clinical implication. *Eat. Weight. Disord. Stud. Anorex. Bulim. Obes.* **2020**, *26*, 1893–1902. [CrossRef]
20. Crews, F.; He, J.; Hodge, C. Adolescent cortical development: A critical period of vulnerability for addiction. *Pharmacol. Biochem. Behav.* **2007**, *86*, 189–199. [CrossRef]
21. Stice, E.; Mazotti, L.; Krebs, M.; Martin, S. Predictors of adolescent dieting behaviors: A longitudinal study. *Psychol. Addict. Behav.* **1998**, *12*, 195–205. [CrossRef]
22. Gearhardt, A.N.; White, M.; Masheb, R.M.; Grilo, C.M. An examination of food addiction in a racially diverse sample of obese patients with binge eating disorder in primary care settings. *Compr. Psychiatry* **2013**, *54*, 500–505. [CrossRef] [PubMed]
23. Schiestl, E.T.; Gearhardt, A.N. Preliminary validation of the Yale Food Addiction Scale for Children 2.0: A dimensional approach to scoring. *Eur. Eat. Disord. Rev.* **2018**, *26*, 605–617. [CrossRef]
24. Alim, N.; Gokustun, K.; Caliskan, G.; Besler, Z. Do Disordered Eating Behaviors Have an Effect on Food Addiction? *Health Behav. Policy Rev.* **2021**, *8*, 319–330. [CrossRef]
25. Kuczmarski, R.J.; Ogden, C.L.; Guo, S.S.; Grummer-Strawn, L.M.; Flegal, K.M.; Mei, Z.; Wei, R.; Curtin, L.R.; Roche, A.F.; Johnson, C.L. 2000 CDC Growth Charts for the United States: Methods and Development. *Vital Health Stat.* **2002**, *11*, 1–190.
26. Schulte, E.M.; Avena, N.M.; Gearhardt, A.N. Which Foods May Be Addictive? The Roles of Processing, Fat Content, and Glycemic Load. *PLoS ONE* **2015**, *10*, e0117959. [CrossRef] [PubMed]
27. Lui, C.K.; Sterling, S.A.; Chi, F.W.; Lu, Y.; Campbell, C.I. Socioeconomic Differences in Adolescent Substance Abuse Treatment Participation and Long-Term Outcomes. *Addict. Behav.* **2017**, *68*, 45–51. [CrossRef]
28. van Strien, T.; Frijters, J.E.; Bergers, G.P.; Defares, P.B. The Dutch Eating Behavior Questionnaire (DEBQ) for Assessment of Restrained, Emotional, and External Eating Behavior. *Eat. Disord.* **1986**, *5*, 295–315. Available online: https://onlinelibrary.wiley.com/doi/epdf/10.1002/1098-108X%28198602%295%3A2%3C295%3A%3AAID-EAT2260050209%3E3.0.CO%3B2-T (accessed on 6 June 2023). [CrossRef]
29. van Strien, T.; Herman, C.P.; Anschutz, D. The predictive validity of the DEBQ-external eating scale for eating in response to food commercials while watching television. *Int. J. Eat. Disord.* **2011**, *45*, 257–262. [CrossRef]
30. Banasiak, S.J.; Wertheim, E.H.; Koerner, J.; Voudouris, N.J. Test-retest reliability and internal consistency of a variety of measures of dietary restraint and body concerns in a sample of adolescent girls. *Int. J. Eat. Disord.* **2001**, *29*, 85–89. [CrossRef]
31. Kenny, D.A.; Harackiewizc, J.M. Cross-lagged panel correlation: Practice and promise. *J. Appl. Psychol.* **1979**, *64*, 372–379. [CrossRef]
32. Rosseel, Y. lavaan: AnRPackage for Structural Equation Modeling. *J. Stat. Softw.* **2012**, *48*, 1–36. [CrossRef]
33. Tabachnick, B.G.; Fidell, L.S. Using Multivariate Statistics Title: Using Multivariate Statistics. 2019. Available online: https://lccn.loc.gov/2017040173 (accessed on 6 June 2023).
34. Wilcox, R. Trimming and Winsorization. In *Encyclopedia of Biostatistics*; John Wiley & Sons, Ltd.: Hoboken, NJ, USA, 2005. [CrossRef]
35. Snoek, H.M.; van Strien, T.; Janssens, J.M.A.M.; Engels, R.C.M.E. Restrained Eating and BMI: A Longitudinal Study Among Adolescents. *Health Psychol.* **2008**, *27*, 753–759. [CrossRef] [PubMed]
36. Wiedemann, A.A.; Carr, M.M.; Ivezaj, V.; Barnes, R.D. Examining the construct validity of food addiction severity specifiers. *Eat. Weight. Disord. Stud. Anorex. Bulim. Obes.* **2020**, *26*, 1503–1509. [CrossRef] [PubMed]
37. Wang, Y.A.; Rhemtulla, M. Power Analysis for Parameter Estimation in Structural Equation Modeling: A Discussion and Tutorial. *Adv. Methods Pract. Psychol. Sci.* **2021**, *4*, 1–17. [CrossRef]
38. Wiss, D.; Avena, N.M. Food Addiction, Binge Eating, and the Role of Dietary Restraint: Converging Evidence from Animal and Human Studies. In *Binge Eating: A Transdiagnostic Psychopathology*; Springer: Cham, Switzerland, 2020; pp. 193–209. [CrossRef]
39. Grilo, C.; Masheb, R. Onset of dieting vs. binge eating in outpatients with binge eating disorder. *Int. J. Obes.* **2000**, *24*, 404–409. [CrossRef] [PubMed]
40. Hilbert, A.; Pike, K.M.; Goldschmidt, A.B.; Wilfley, D.E.; Fairburn, C.G.; Dohm, F.-A.; Walsh, B.T.; Weissman, R.S. Risk factors across the eating disorders. *Psychiatry Res.* **2014**, *220*, 500–506. [CrossRef]
41. Reas, D.L.; Grilo, C.M. Timing and sequence of the onset of overweight, dieting, and binge eating in overweight patients with binge eating disorder. *Int. J. Eat. Disord.* **2006**, *40*, 165–170. [CrossRef]

42. Brewerton, T.; Brewerton, T.D.; Dansky, B.S.; Kilpatrick, D.G.; O'neil, P.M. Which Comes First in the Pathogenesis of Bulimia Nervosa: Dieting or Bingeing? *Int. J. Eat. Disord.* **2000**, *28*, 259–2640. [CrossRef]
43. Tanofsky-Kraff, M.; Faden, D.; Yanovski, S.Z.; Wilfley, D.E.; Yanovski, J.A. The Perceived Onset of Dieting and Loss of Control Eating Behaviors in Overweight Children. *Int. J. Eat. Disord.* **2005**, *38*, 112. [CrossRef]
44. Lowe, M.R. Dieting: Proxy or Cause of Future Weight Gain? *Obes. Rev.* **2015**, *16*, 19–24. [CrossRef] [PubMed]
45. Lowe, M.R.; Doshi, S.D.; Katterman, S.N.; Feig, E.H. Dieting and Restrained Eating as Prospective Predictors of Weight Gain. *Front. Psychol.* **2013**, *4*, 577. [CrossRef] [PubMed]
46. Thanarajah, S.E.; DiFeliceantonio, A.G.; Albus, K.; Br€, J.C.; Tittgemeyer, M.; Small, D.M. Habitual daily intake of a sweet and fatty snack modulates reward processing in humans. *Cell Metab.* **2023**, *35*, 571–584.e6. [CrossRef] [PubMed]
47. Davis, C.; Curtis, C.; Levitan, R.D.; Carter, J.C.; Kaplan, A.S.; Kennedy, J.L. Evidence That 'Food Addiction' Is a Valid Phenotype of Obesity. *Appetite* **2011**, *57*, 711–717. [CrossRef]
48. Loxton, N.J.; Tipman, R.J. Reward sensitivity and food addiction in women. *Appetite* **2017**, *115*, 28–35. [CrossRef]
49. Hoover, L.V.; Yu, H.P.; Cummings, J.R.; Ferguson, S.G.; Gearhardt, A.N. Co-occurrence of food addiction, obesity, problematic substance use, and parental history of problematic alcohol use. *Psychol. Addict. Behav. J. Soc. Psychol. Addict. Behav.* **2022**. [CrossRef]
50. Lee, A.; Ho, M.; Keung, V. Healthy School as an Ecological Model for Prevention of Childhood Obesity. *Res. Sports Med.* **2010**, *18*, 49–61. [CrossRef]
51. Cassin, S.; Sockalingam, S. *The Clinical Utility of Food Addiction and Eating Addiction*; MDPI: Basel, Switzerland, 2021. [CrossRef]
52. Harris, J.L.; Yokum, S.; Fleming-Milici, F. Hooked on Junk: Emerging Evidence on How Food Marketing Affects Adolescents' Diets and Long-Term Health. *Curr. Addict. Rep.* **2021**, *8*, 19–27. [CrossRef]
53. Brown, A.; Flint, S.W.; Batterham, R.L. Pervasiveness, impact and implications of weight stigma. *Eclinicalmedicine* **2022**, *47*, 101408. [CrossRef]
54. Westenhoefer, J.; Stunkard, A.J.; Pudel, V. Validation of the Flexible and Rigid Control Dimensions of Dietary Restraint. *Int. J. Eat. Disord.* **1999**, *26*, 53–64. [CrossRef]
55. Schembre, S.; Greene, G.; Melanson, K. Development and validation of a weight-related eating questionnaire. *Eat. Behav.* **2009**, *10*, 119–124. [CrossRef] [PubMed]
56. Mussell, M.P.; Mitchell, J.E.; Weller, C.L.; Raymond, N.C.; Crow, S.J.; Crosby, R.D. Onset of binge eating, dieting, obesity, and mood disorders among subjects seeking treatment for binge eating disorder. *Int. J. Eat. Disord.* **1995**, *17*, 395–401. [CrossRef] [PubMed]
57. Gearhardt, A.N.; Miller, A.L.; Sturza, J.; Epstein, L.H.; Kaciroti, N.; Lumeng, J.C. Behavioral Associations with Overweight in Low-Income Children. *Obesity* **2017**, *25*, 2123–2127. [CrossRef] [PubMed]

Disclaimer/Publisher's Note: The statements, opinions and data contained in all publications are solely those of the individual author(s) and contributor(s) and not of MDPI and/or the editor(s). MDPI and/or the editor(s) disclaim responsibility for any injury to people or property resulting from any ideas, methods, instructions or products referred to in the content.

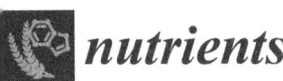

Review

Binge-Eating Precursors in Children and Adolescents: Neurodevelopment, and the Potential Contribution of Ultra-Processed Foods

Esther Via [1,2,*] and Oren Contreras-Rodríguez [3,4,5,*]

1. Child and Adolescent Mental Health Research Group, Institut de Recerca Sant Joan de Déu, Santa Rosa 39-57, 08950 Esplugues de Llobregat, Spain
2. Department of Child and Adolescent Mental Health, Hospital Sant Joan de Déu, Passeig Sant Joan de Déu, 2, 08950 Esplugues de Llobregat, Spain
3. Medical Imaging, Girona Biomedical Research Institute (IdIBGi), Parc Hospitalari Martí i Julià-Edifici M2, Salt, 17190 Girona, Spain
4. Health Institute Carlos III (ISCIII) and CIBERSAM, 28029 Madrid, Spain
5. Department of Psychiatry and Legal Medicine, Faculty of Medicine, Universitat Autònoma de Barcelona, 08193 Bellaterra, Spain
* Correspondence: esther.via@sjd.es (E.V.); ocontreras@idibgi.org (O.C.-R.)

Abstract: Binge-eating disorder (BED) is a highly prevalent disorder. Subthreshold BED conditions (sBED) are even more frequent in youth, but their significance regarding BED etiology and long-term prognosis is unclear. A better understanding of brain findings associated with BED and sBED, in the context of critical periods for neurodevelopment, is relevant to answer such questions. The present narrative review starts from the knowledge of the development of emotional self-regulation in youth, and the brain circuits supporting emotion-regulation and eating behaviour. Next, neuroimaging studies with sBED and BED samples will be reviewed, and their brain-circuitry overlap will be examined. Deficits in inhibition control systems are observed to precede, and hyperactivity of reward regions to characterize, sBED, with overlapping findings in BED. The imbalance between reward/inhibition systems, and the implication of interoception/homeostatic processing brain systems should be further examined. Recent knowledge of the potential impact that the high consumption of ultra-processed foods in paediatric samples may have on these sBED/BED-associated brain systems is then discussed. There is a need to identify, early on, those sBED individuals at risk of developing BED at neurodevelopmental stages when there is a great possibility of prevention. However, more neuroimaging studies with sBED/BED pediatric samples are needed.

Keywords: binge eating; emotional eating; ultra-processed food; reward; inhibition; MRI; children; adolescents

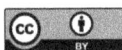

1. Introduction

Binge-eating disorder (BED) has been a diagnosis on its own only since the last edition of the Diagnostic and Statistical Manual of Mental Disorders (DSM-5) [1] in 2013. However, data on prevalence already suggest it is the most-prevalent eating disorder worldwide [2]. The first peak of prevalence occurs in adolescence [3], at 1–3% in children and adolescents [3], and 3% for subclinical presentations [4]. BED prevalence rises to 37% in populations of adolescents with obesity [5,6]. Despite the high prevalence, full comprehension of the diagnosis and its pathophysiological mechanisms is still in its infancy, particularly regarding youths, who frequently have a different clinical presentation compared to adults [7].

BED involves at-least-weekly episodes of binge eating, which imply eating a large amount of food in a discrete time period and with a sense of lack of control over it [1]. It is associated with physical and psychiatric comorbidities and a high impact on quality of life and disability-adjusted life-years (DALYs) [2,8]. Regarding physical comorbidity, BED is most frequently associated with obesity, which confers a risk of other medical conditions such as metabolic and cardiovascular diseases, leading causes of death worldwide [9]. Psychiatric comorbidities are the norm more than the exception, representing more than 60% lifetime prevalence in subjects with BED, mostly anxiety and mood disorders [10,11]. While BED is a recognized disorder, other related presentations have attracted interest in the literature. These presentations are either subclinical or precursor forms of BED (from now on, sBED), which are defined by different but clinically overlapping terminology throughout the scientific literature. Such constructs are not validated, are mostly descriptive, and most do not use operationalized criteria. In some cases, but not all, individuals with these conditions might be diagnosed with specified or unspecified DSM-5 eating disorder categories ("other specified feeding or eating disorder", OSFED, or "eating disorder not otherwise specified", EDNOS) [1]. Some examples are *disordered eating* [12], *dysregulated eating behaviour* [13], *uncontrolled eating* [14,15], *emotional eating* [16], *overeating disorder* [15], *disinhibited eating* [17], *LOC eating* (loss of control overeating), the latter being the sole condition with operationalized criteria [5,18,19]. Another closely related concept is *food addiction*, a construct under considerable debate for the last 10 years that entails compulsive and dysregulated intake of high-calorie foods [20–23]. Food addiction is a transdiagnostic construct; it is present in non-clinical and clinical samples. For example, it is found in high percentages in clinical samples of eating disorders (between 41.5% and 72.2% in BED) [24].

In comparison with adults, incomplete sBED forms are more frequent in youths, which is partially explained by the developmental differences between the two groups [7]. For example, binges in children generally entail lower energy intake, and unadjusted behaviour is likely limited by the environment (i.e., limited access to food) [7]. Considering this, adapted criteria have been proposed to detect BED in youths, although this is not a DSM-5 validated diagnosis and it is not widely used in the literature (see refs. [25–28]). BED diagnoses are frequently preceded by sBED in paediatric populations, with symptoms such as *LOC eating*, eating in response to emotions, eating without hunger, and overeating being associated with a higher risk for later BED development in different studies [18,19,29,30]. Of note, the prevalence of sBED in children is stable across childhood [31] and the presence of sBED in childhood is associated with a higher risk, compared to adulthood, for more severe binge eating and other eating disorders such as bulimia nervosa [19,32]. The rate of diagnostic conversion from sBED to BED is not clear, and to our knowledge, only one study has evaluated this matter, reporting 28% transition from sBED to BED in a group of adolescents during a 8-year of follow-up [33]. Given that it was a community study, the sample of sBED was very small ($n = 18$).

The most important known underlying factor in BED and sBED is deficiency in emotional regulation strategies [34,35], which refers to the ability to regulate emotional responses and to inhibit impulses for immediate gratification in the service of waiting for larger, delayed rewards [36]. In this scenario, binge-eating episodes are considered maladaptive strategies to cope with negative affections (e.g., sadness, boredom, restlessness) and/or to obtain rewarding experiences [7,37]. Indeed, difficulties in emotional identification and awareness, impulsivity, reward sensitivity, depressive symptoms, low self-esteem, anxiety, ruminative tendencies, and the presence of an attention deficit and hyperactivity disorder (ADHD) have been found to predict sBED or to be associated with binge-eating scores [19,22,35,38–42]. For ADHD, the overlapping of implicated brain circuits in the two pathologies suggests common neurological substrates or pathophysiological processes [15]. Notably, brain circuits underlying emotional regulation processes develop during childhood and adolescence, coinciding with the emergence of sBED. While some research has been conducted on these circuits in the context of sBED/BED, for example, to evaluate prefrontal responses to inhibition-processing demands, or reward processes at the level of the nucleus accumbens—among other regions—our understanding of the relationship between the development of underlying emotion-regulation brain systems in youth and sBED/BED remains limited. In this regard, some studies have suggested that sBED and

BED are mediated by premorbid deficits in neural systems regulating emotions which confer a vulnerability for sBED/BED development [19,35,43].

In contrast, other studies have suggested that dietary restraint is involved in the development of BED (restraint model) [44–47], while others have implied that sBED, and possibly BED, originate in long-term hypercaloric food consumption [35]. The literature supporting the former is rather mixed, and results might depend on the evaluated outcome (i.e., bulimia nervosa, BED or sBED), the sample characteristics (i.e., subjects with obesity vs. community samples), the variables studied (i.e., fasting, low-calorie diets, regularity of meals), and the evaluation of other concomitant factors (i.e., dieting due to internal motivations related to body dissatisfaction vs. other reasons for dieting) [44–50]. Once BED is established, however, regular eating and no skipping of meals are two of the most important factors to overcome the disorder [49]. Regarding the long-term hypercaloric food consumption hypothesis, recent evidence points towards an association between high consumption and exposure to ultra-processed foods and drinks (UPF in advance) and the development of sBED and BED [51,52]. In addition, current evidence links UPF consumption with sBED/BED-associated brain systems (see further). Children and adolescents show high rates of UPF consumption, with estimates indicating that they obtain between 29% and 68% of their total energy intake from UPF consumption, a figure which increased by 5.6% between 1999 and 2018 [53,54]. In Spain, the percentage of UPF among all food purchases almost tripled between 1990 and 2010 (from 11.0% to 31.7%) [55]. Notably, this previous data are concurrent with the alarming rise in obesity prevalence in youth [9,53,56,57].

Given that eating disorders are better understood from a biopsychosocial framework [58], it is important to note that other factors are also important contributors to the development of sBED and BED. The etiology of eating disorders is indeed multifactorial and complex, characterized by a dynamic interplay among biological factors (e.g., inheritable traits, neurodevelopmental influences, neuroendocrinological factors), as well as psychological (e.g., personality traits such as low self-esteem) and environmental factors (e.g., sociocultural expectations) [58,59]. Moreover, all of these factors can both trigger and perpetuate eating disorders [59]. In the context of children and adolescents and sBED/BED, one important factor includes food-learning habits, for example through parental style (extensively studied, as in [60–62]); parents might use practices such as restricting food access to the child, pressuring the child to eat, or using food as a reward or in an attempt to regulate negative emotions [62]. Such a relationship, however, is seen to be complex and bilaterally associated with child behaviour [60]. Nevertheless, the contribution of all these variables to sBED/BED are beyond the scope of this review and will not be covered here.

A better comprehension of the link between sBED conditions and BED pathophysiology, both clinically and at the level of the brain, as well as the long-term trajectory of these two forms during vulnerable neurodevelopmental periods, might help to detect and treat those individuals at greater risk for BED [63]. In addition, it is also necessary to review the evidence of the association between the consumption of UPF, BED, and sBED forms, in order to identify and examine new factors that may contribute to increasing the clinical and subclinical presentation of this eating disorder.

Review Scope

In the present narrative review, we aim to provide a clear picture of the convergence between brain alterations in sBED in children and adolescence, and those under full BED forms. To that end, we will first provide a brief review of the brain circuit's underlying eating behaviour (Section 2), as well as of the neurodevelopment of emotional self-regulation processes (Section 3). In Section 4, we will synthetize the neuroimaging studies conducted on sBED and BED, and draw conclusions regarding the convergence and divergence of the findings, if possible. The preliminary evidence linking the high consumption of UPF, sBED, and BED is reviewed in Section 5. In Section 6, we conclude by suggesting lines of research for future studies. Despite not conducting a systematic review (while others exist, such as [13]), a selection of reviewed articles has been conducted using a systematic search on three different databases (Pubmed, Scopus, WoS), specifically looking for magnetic resonance studies in children and adolescents and on binge eating or subthreshold conditions such as emotional eating or food addiction. We apologize in advance to our colleagues whose work has been omitted unintentionally or due to space constraints.

2. Eating Brain Circuitry

Eating behaviour is driven by several psychobiological factors that include homeostatic factors, the coding of rewarding properties of food, and other individual psychosocial factors associated with eating [64]. Food is processed through ascending sensory pathways that bring information about the properties of food (smell, taste, texture) to the brain. For example, gustatory information is processed by the cranial nerves, the nucleus of the solitary tract, and the gustatory thalamus [65]. Information from different sensory channels is then largely integrated to the frontal opercula and insular cortex [65–69]. Next, the orbitofrontal region (its caudolateral parts considered the secondary cortical taste) assigns reinforcement values to food [70,71]. Other limbic and cognitive neural systems involved in eating behaviour modulate this primary response, for example, in the anticipation of the food stimulus, in the hedonic or emotional response, and in approaching behaviour related to food stimuli [72]. These regions might be conceptualized as a ventral system (emotional, excitatory) and a dorsal system (cognitive, inhibitory). This model has been used to explain other eating disorders, such as anorexia nervosa [73].

The ventral system is composed of the striato-limbic and ventral parts of the prefrontal cortex, and it sends information to more dorsal prefrontal pathways (bottom-up). It is involved in the monitorization of internal and external responses, such as the identification of emotional significance, encoding the value for a choice, and in hedonically motivated eating behaviours, including craving [72,74–77]. For example, the orbitofrontal cortex and the striatum (dorsal- and ventral-encompassing the nucleus accumbens, the hub area of the reward system) are involved in both the anticipation and the consummatory food reward [78–81]. Within this circuit, the insular cortex is a multimodal region that integrates primary sensory and interoceptive information with emotional, cognitive, and motivational signals in a posterior-to-anterior anatomical progression [69,82,83]. Together with the thalamus, it encodes the organoleptic properties of food and food energy, and regulates energy balance, feeding, and satiety [67,84]. As an example, the response of the insular cortex is associated with gut hormone responses and peripheral blood glucose levels [84,85]. Thus, the insular cortex plays an important role in homeostasis and interoceptive processes involved in eating behaviour [86,87]. In addition, anterior parts of the insula have been consistently involved in craving, including food craving [88–90].

The dorsal system (top-down), in turn, includes prefrontal regions, and it exerts control over subcortical striato-limbic structures [73,91]. This neural system is in charge of executive functions, such as planning and organization for problem solving, which are crucial to direct behaviours toward objectives, and to inhibit behaviours [73]. For instance, it is critically involved in the decision to eat or to inhibit the desire (or craving) to eat [92]. Under physiological conditions, the balance functioning between these ventral and dorsal neural systems, and their interaction with homeostatic regulatory circuits in the hypothalamus, will finally determine food intake (for a review, see [93,94]). Alterations within the ventral and dorsal systems are thought to characterize sBED/BED [95]. The next section will provide a review of our knowledge regarding the standard neurodevelopment of brain systems involved in emotional self-regulation and the potential implication for the risk of developing BED.

3. Neurodevelopment of Emotional Self-Regulation

As mentioned, deficits in emotional regulation processes crucially underlie sBED and BED [34,35]. Adaptive self-emotional regulation is achieved over life by learning processes, with cognitive reappraisal being the most studied. Cognitive reappraisal entails deliberately altering the self-relevant meaning (an appraisal) of an emotion-inducing stimulus to change its emotional impact [96]. Its frequent use is linked to an improved control of emotions, cognitive performance, and interpersonal functioning [97]. Children can engage in cognitive reappraisal with adult guidance between the ages of three and five but it is not until middle childhood, around 6–7 years of age, that they are able to independently reappraise emotional stimuli if instructed to do so (for a review see [98]).

The effective employment of cognitive reappraisal is dependent on underlying executive functions, such as working memory and attentional shifting [99]. In congruence with the normal development of prefrontal-supporting executive systems, neuropsychological and neuroimaging studies suggest that this strategy is not effective until adolescence [98]. Such studies indicate that from middle childhood into late adolescence, the use of reappraisal effectively downregulates the activity within core limbic brain structures involved in emotion generation (e.g., amygdala) [98] (for a review of the network implicated in cognitive reappraisal, see [100]). Among the diverse prefrontal areas implicated in cognitive reappraisal, the ventrolateral and medial prefrontal cortices have been repeatedly associated with the effectiveness of reappraisal in studies, with samples ranging from middle to young adulthood [101]. These regions are associated with the appropriate inhibition of automatic appraisals and the selection of alternate ones, and with the representation of the reward value of goal-directed behaviours [100]. Children, with a yet immature prefrontal system, are more dependent on external regulation, mostly from parents [102]. Other factors, such as the temperament of the child and biological factors such as functional non-pathological differences in neurotransmitter receptors (serotonin, dopamine) contribute to these processes [103–105].

Thus, childhood and adolescence are key periods for learning emotional regulatory strategies, which are supported differentially across ages. While young children depend greatly on the presence of consistent environment control over the predominance of more limbic and reward-based own drivers, middle children and adolescents rely more on their own self-regulatory strategies, supported by their prefrontal cortex systems and built on temperament characteristics and learning experiences [106]. Although the emergence of sBED and BED may be more evident in adolescents, when autonomy is gained [13], altered relationship with food- and brain-based dysfunction might have started earlier, for example, with learning processes fostered by the immediate environment.

4. sBED-Related Brain Vulnerability Markers and BED

This section will first review the studies conducted with samples presenting sBED conditions, and then summarize those conducted with subjects with a BED diagnosis across the main clinical domains of dysfunction.

4.1. Response and Behavioral Inhibition Deficits

Several studies suggest that primary deficits in inhibitory functions, supported by prefrontal regions, may underlie the deficits in emotional regulation that confer a vulnerability for sBED and BED [19]. In particular, children or adolescents with such deficits might feel overwhelmed and might fail to cope using adaptative responses [19] when exposed to stressful and negativity-inducing situations (e.g., threats and social losses). In such situations, vulnerable subjects may show a rush for eating (usually palatable) food, which avoids facing emotions and initially reduces the negative affect by the obtainment of pleasure [19,107–109]. While this model has been more extensively studied in binges occurring in bulimia nervosa [99], there is some limited evidence for sBED and BED.

At the neural level, some studies give support to deficits in behavioural inhibitory functions in sBED. For example, in adolescents with sBED, one study showed evidence of decreased activation of the frontoparietal and temporal regions during inhibitory processing in a functional magnetic resonance (fMRI) study using the go/no-go task [110]. Similarly, in another study, adolescent girls with sBED and obesity failed to engage prefrontal regions (ventromedial and dorsolateral prefrontal cortices) in an emotion regulation task in the context of negative mood induction through a peer-interaction paradigm [111]. In another pilot study, preadolescents with overweight or obesity and sBED were exposed to an intermittent food restriction paradigm during a magnetic resonance session, in which they received different milkshake flavours in a restricted vs. unrestricted manner [112]; sBED subjects, compared to weight- and sex-matched controls, presented increased activity in self-regulatory and attention regions (right prefrontal regions, left cingulate, and left cuneus) during restricted conditions. Hyperactivations were suggested as representing an increased cognitive effort to regulate emotions under such restrictive conditions [112].

Longitudinal studies using community samples might be more informative in disentangling whether these alterations are or are not primary deficits. Most of these studies come from large longitudinal cohorts in healthy children and adolescents, such as the ABCD study (United States population [113]) or the IMAGEN study (European population [114]). For example, a study from the IMAGEN cohort ($n = 1607$) showed that greater responses of the anterior cingulate cortex and medial prefrontal cortex during failed inhibition trials in a stop signal task at 14 years of age were associated with the development of disordered eating behaviours at 16 (self-reported binge eating and purging episodes), compared to healthy controls [107]. The authors suggested that the increased activation may work as an early compensatory mechanism for inhibitory deficits, which could point towards a potential early biomarker of sBED. Importantly, the brain alterations reported by all these studies were not accompanied by deficits in task-behavioural responses, suggesting inhibitory control performance is not necessarily impaired in sBED, and it also indicates that compensatory mechanisms may be effective. Further studies should elucidate whether such prefrontal hyperactivation is or is not a useful biomarker of sBED and/or its transition to BED.

In BED, evidence of poor impulse control or decreased inhibitory control comes mostly from limited examinations of adult samples (see reviews in [43,91,115]). In the systematic review and meta-analysis in obesity of Lavagnino et al. [43], the authors concluded that, while subjects with obesity (adults and youths) showed decreased inhibitory control performance, such performance did not differ between subjects (only adults) with BED and those without BED. In contrast, a decreased neural activation in prefrontal areas during inhibitory tasks characterized adult subjects with BED and obesity compared to subjects with obesity and without BED in two other studies [116,117].

In conclusion, the very limited literature found in children and adolescents gives some support for alterations in brain regions involved in inhibition control as a potential early dysfunction that facilitates sBED. Based on the reviewed studies, the different directions of the findings (i.e., hypo- vs. hyperactivations) might depend on age (i.e., younger ages presenting hyperactivations), the premorbid stage vs. consolidated sBED (i.e., hyperactivations prior to sBED development) or even the nature and potential triggering effects of the tasks used (i.e., hyperactivations during a simulation of intermittent restriction vs. hypoactivation during tasks purely evaluating cold-cognition, such as the go/no-go task). There is a lack of information in BED on youths, and the literature is mixed on adult samples.

4.2. Reward-Based Deficits

Other studies have suggested that some youth, considered vulnerable to sBED/BED and to obesity, might present either a hypo- or hyperresponsive reward system, which can drive them towards developing sBED or BED [118,119]. However, according to Stice and Burger [118], there is little support for the reward deficit theory [14], while the hyperresponsiveness hypothesis is nowadays the theory with the largest support. In this respect, some authors have suggested that the impulsivity that characterizes children with sBED may be explained by an increased sensitivity to reward and decreased ability to delay gratification [120]. Subjects with full BED forms clinically present increased preference for immediate (food or other stimuli) reward as opposed to delayed [109], greater food-reward sensitivity, and greater rash-spontaneous behaviour in the context of food [121].

Some studies have reported neural differences in response to reward in samples with sBED conditions. For example, in one study of healthy children, the symptom "eating in the absence of hunger" was positively associated with the activation of the nucleus accumbens [74]. In community-based cohorts, one study of the ABCD project observed that certain structural differences of key reward brain regions (i.e., cellular density in the nucleus accumbens) during childhood (9–10 years old) were associated with body mass index at the one-year follow-up (n = 2212) [122]. The authors discussed the results in the context of obesity and possibly unhealthy eating, although the percentage of obesity or presence of unhealthy eating could not be reported [122]. Another study of the same cohort of children evidenced that higher functional resting state connectivity between the nucleus accumbens and the frontoparietal network was predictive of BMI increase over time, although only for the female group [123]. In adolescents, one study in a community sample (n = 122) observed that those with BED symptoms (possibly a mixed sample sBED/BED), compared to those without, showed an increased reward-receipt response in the caudate in a reward-guessing task when money was won [95]. In this same study, the activation of both the ventromedial prefrontal cortex and of the caudate during reward receipt correlated positively with binge symptoms severity; in addition, there were no between-group activity differences during the anticipation of reward in any of the selected regions (striatum, medial prefrontal cortex, orbitofrontal cortex, and amygdala) [95].

BED has received more attention in the study of reward-based neural responses, but mostly in adults. A recent systematic review concluded that BED and sBED were characterized by lower resting frontostriatal connectivity, but higher activation of this neural system when anticipating or receiving food (see [75], adult BED studies [124–132], with only one including adolescents with BED, a resting-state study [133]). In this review, studies in adults with BED also showed the hyperactivation of the insula during the anticipation of reward, but a lower activation when receiving the reward [75]. Another study in a mixed sample of adults with bulimia nervosa and binge-eating disorder suggested differential reward-receipt responses depending on the stimulus: increased activity in reward-processing regions when receiving food, but no differences in response to monetary reward [134]. Other studies also reported that reward-based responses might vary according to homeostatic state [87]; for example, in preclinical models of BED, the normal decreases in food reward value at the orbitofrontal cortex when satiated [135] are attenuated [87], akin to what is observed in humans in bulimia nervosa [136]. However, to our knowledge, the interaction between homeostatic and reward processes has not been explored in BED or sBED samples.

In summary, and in accordance with the existing literature, the observed behavioural increased sensitivity to reward in sBED and BED is complemented by some evidence of the hyperactivation of hub regions of the reward system, or hyperconnectivity between these and prefrontal regions in sBED and BED. Research is again very scarce in youth BED samples, and studies evaluating brain responses to reward in its different processes (e.g., anticipation, receipt, learning, delay), homeostatic states (i.e., fasting, satiety), and in response to different stimuli (i.e., money, food, others) are lacking.

4.3. Beyond Inhibition and Reward

Although we described the different processes that may be implicated in sBED conditions and full BED forms (e.g., inhibition and reward-based processes) independently, they are, however, interrelated, with reciprocal influences of one brain system with another, and partially reliant on overlapping brain systems [77,137]. Indeed, based on the restricted literature on youth and the larger body of literature on adults, one possibility is that BED is better explained by an imbalance between the two systems, rather than independent alterations in either of them. Interestingly, one preclinical study provides support for this idea; the researchers found evidence that changes in the connectivity between prefrontal (i.e., medial prefrontal cortex) and nucleus accumbens might lead either to vulnerability or resilience to an addiction-like behaviour with food intake [138]. In particular, the enhancement of synaptic excitatory transmission in this circuit (both at the dorsolateral prefrontal cortex and nucleus accumbens) prevented such behaviour, while the inhibition of neuronal activity in this pathway (dorsolateral prefrontal cortex, in its projections to the nucleus accumbens) led to compulsive food seeking [138]. This provides specific brain targets of vulnerability to be evaluated in humans.

In turn, the presence of sBED conditions is also believed to challenge the homeostatic regulation of eating behaviour (and thus the balance between hunger and satiety), thereby increasing the risk of food overconsumption and health problems (e.g., obesity, diabetes) [139]. Connections from the basolateral amygdala to the lateral hypothalamus during satiety have been implicated in susceptibility to weight gain both in rodents and humans [140], and in one study in adolescents with excess weight, increased resting-state connectivity between the lateral hypothalamus and midbrain was associated with sBED [141]. In a systematic review in children and adolescents, sBED conditions were associated with alterations in frontostriatal and frontoparietal regions involved in self-regulatory processes, but also in regions involved in satiety signalling and interception [13].

Other studies support the idea that alterations in limbic regions would significantly contribute to the expression of full BED forms. This is congruent with clinical observations that binges take place in response to stress and negative affects [19,91] and with, for example, evidence for greater secretion of stress hormones and enzymes (i.e., salivary cortisol, alpha-amylase) in women with BED compared to healthy controls in response to a social stress-inducing task [142]. The few studies that have assessed the limbic system in full BED forms point toward alterations in the amygdala, the anterior insula, the hippocampus, ventral regions of the anterior cingulate cortex, and ventromedial prefrontal and orbitofrontal cortices [91,143]. For example, a neuroimaging study with a small sample of BED women showed a decreased activation of the hippocampus when exposed to unpleasant (physical, social) stressors [144]. Finally, a recent study evaluated connectivity between different brain systems during the resting state in pre-adolescent children with BED compared to healthy children, finding aberrant connectivity in prefrontal to amygdala and in anterior cingulate cortex to orbitofrontal cortex regions [133]. However, to our knowledge, there is no other information on youth with BED in this respect.

4.4. Relevant Considerations

A final point needs to be made regarding obesity. Obesity is estimated to be comorbid in 87% of individuals with BED, over the course of their lives [145]. This condition is a potential confounder in studies in BED; it is associated with gliosis and neuroinflammation in reward brain regions [146], and obesity in adulthood has been associated with similar brain inhibitory processing alterations (e.g., lower prefrontal activity) to obesity with BED [43,118]. Some authors found greater reward response to food cues in obesity (reviewed here [147]), but others, for example in children, failed to observe differences in reward regions' activity [148]. In addition, body interoceptive awareness is attenuated in overweight and obese individuals [149], and some authors suggest that excess weight in youth could be associated with a decreased insula response to interoceptive signals (i.e., satiation) but increased response toward external food cues [150].

Obesity has frequently been associated with similar neuropsychological and neuroimaging alterations to those in BED, and it is difficult to disentangle common and differing vulnerability and maintaining factors. Control groups in studies need to consider obesity as an important confounder factor. As previously mentioned, the literature is mixed on the independent contribution of obesity and sBED/BED to alterations in brain circuitry (Lavagnino et al. [43], as opposed to other studies [116,117]). Of note, a larger number of studies in obesity exist, when compared to sBED and BED. Due to the high comorbidity between conditions, it is likely that most studies in obesity include a significant number of subjects with sBED/BED; however, such clinical characterization is frequently lacking.

5. Ultra-Processed Food and Drinks and BED?

According to the NOVA classification, one of the most commonly used definitions of ultra-processed foods (UPFs) [151] is ingredient formulations that result from series of industrial processes [152] and that are characterized by no or relatively small amounts of minimally processed foods that conserve their nutritional properties. In general, they have low nutrient densities, and they are poor in protein, dietary fibre, and micronutrients. At the same time, they have a high energy density, high contents of saturated and trans fatty acids, added sugars, and salt [151]. Moreover, UPFs have a high content of additives (i.e., sweeteners, colorants, emulsifiers) intended to intensify their sensory qualities, palatability, and attractiveness [153]. They may also contain chemicals acquired through contact materials, such as sophisticated packaging (e.g., bisphenol), and neo-formed contaminants generated during food processing (e.g., acrylamide, acrolein) [154]. UPFs are engineered to be highly rewarding and they are easily accessible, inexpensive, heavily marketed, and habit forming [155]. These characteristics make UPFs different from processed foods, which are identified by the NOVA classification as being made by adding culinary ingredients (e.g., sugar, oil, salt) to simple unprocessed or minimally processed natural foods. In addition, while these foods may contain additives to preserve the original food properties or resist microbial contamination, they do not aim to imitate the sensory qualities of natural foods. Finally, several industrial processes with no domestic equivalents are used in the manufacture of UPF products (e.g., extrusion and moulding, and pre-processing for frying).

UPF consumption is associated with negative health outcomes among children and adolescents, including cardiometabolic risk, asthma [156], and obesity [157,158]. Also, growing evidence in both animals and humans suggests that highly processed foods may trigger addictive processes that drive compulsive patterns of intake. A study by Ayton and colleagues [51] was the first to objectively show that patients with a BED diagnosis, as well as bulimia nervosa, consumed approximately 70% UPF, and that foods consumed in a binge pattern were 100% UPF. This was then substantiated by a second study with a large sample of participants [52]. In adolescents from the general population, UPF consumption has also been associated with sBED conditions, including food addiction [159–161], but in addition to internalizing problems [162], depressive symptoms [163], and anxiety-induced disturbances [164]. However, despite these associations, the potential effect of the consumption of UPFs on the brain systems implicated in BED and sBED remains to be understood. This is worrying considering that, in some countries, children are highly exposed to unhealthy foods from two years of age [53], a sensitive period because of the unbalanced neurodevelopment between subcortical and prefrontal brain systems [165].

The first evidence that the consumption of UPFs may be associated with changes in the brain systems underlying sBED and BED came from studies showing that the viewing or anticipation of unhealthy foods in children changes the activation in brain regions implicated in reward and cognitive processes (e.g., the orbitofrontal cortex, and inferior frontal gyrus) [166,167]. These results are congruent with alterations in these brain systems in BED and sBED sample groups [26,91,95,107,133]. In addition, it is also of interest to consider that dietary exposure to high levels of foods rich in saturated fats, added sugar, and salt shifts preference to foods with a higher concentration of these substances [168,169]. The reshaping of the gustatory systems induced by these substances, a mechanism known as chemosensory plasticity, may also affect the processing of taste, and reward processes through interactions with the brain [168]. However, these studies provide generic evidence of the effect of UPF. More compelling evidence comes from the few studies that have explored the direct effect of UPF consumption. The first clinical trial showed that a UPF diet increases fasting glucose, insulin levels, and the hunger hormone ghrelin [170]. Also, a recent study reported prenatal UPF consumption to be negatively associated with verbal functioning, including verbal expression and concept reasoning, in early childhood (4–5 years of age) [171], skills that can predict emotional regulation abilities in early adolescence [172]. Of note, albeit in an adult sample, a recently published study showed the consumption of UPF to be positively associated with depressive symptoms but negatively associated with the grey matter volume within the frontolimbic brain circuits, which in those with obesity also encompassed reward-related brain networks (i.e., the ventral striatum) [173]. These preliminary studies indicate that the consumption of UPFs may interact with emotional processes, as previously suggested in the context of the consumption of unhealthy foods in BED [7,19]. However, to our knowledge, no previous studies have investigated this in pediatric samples.

Regarding the effects of specific components and features of UPF, the content of low-/no-calorie sweeteners (LNCSs) [174–176], their organoleptic properties (i.e., taste, texture) [177], and design (e.g., ready to consume) [153] have been associated with reduced satiety and overeating [51]. Regarding LNCSs, neuroimaging studies have provided evidence that the sweet taste in the absence of nutritive carbohydrates may not lead to changes in the functioning of the hypothalamus [178,179] and brain regions of the ventral system (i.e., the nucleus accumbens, and the insula) [180]. Another study found that those subjects that lacked activation of the insula following a non-nutritive sweetened drink also showed higher total energy intake in a subsequent libitum buffet [181], and a recent review showed that subcortical limbic brain regions are among the most commonly reported in neuroimaging studies evaluating the processing of sugars and LNCSs. In addition, the soft texture that characterizes some UPFs makes them easier to chew and swallow, with lower satiation, increased eating rate, and higher overall food intake [177,182]. UPFs are designed to be eaten fast, and it is well known that foods that can be ingested rapidly increase subjective appetite and food intake [183], as well as the risk of overconsumption [184].

Finally, some preliminary studies have reported that the adverse effects of UPF additives on gut health (see a review in [92]) may affect eating behaviours through induced alterations in brain neurotransmission. In this line, a study showed that 6 months of consumption of the artificial sweetener sucralose in drinking water in mice altered host microbiota and related metabolites, including those belonging to the serotonin(5-HT)-precursor tryptophan [185]. Inflammation and oxidative stress associated with a high content of additives [186–188], trans fats [189–191], and advanced glycation end-products can also alter neurotransmission in the ventral and dorsal systems [192]. This is of concern if we consider that a proinflammatory immune profile has been reported by some studies in people with BED and sBED forms [193]. In addition, higher doses or exposure to certain nanoparticles (like those contained in food additives) in mice are associated with induced impairment in DA and 5-HT neurotransmitters [194,195], cytotoxicity in glial cells and hippocampal neurons [196], and hippocampal neuroinflammation [197]. Their accumulation has been demonstrated in the hippocampus, hypothalamus, and cerebral cortex [186,198]. However, further studies should explore whether food-grade nanoparticles have similar effects.

6. Conclusions: Future

Despite the scarce existing literature on sBED and BED in youths, the present review established a parallelism in the impaired brain systems between these conditions (see Figure 1). In particular, some evidence points towards a lack of emotional regulatory mechanisms in BED and sBED, mostly involving reward-based processing and inhibitory mechanisms involved in self-regulation, although studies may be biased by the neurocognitive test or MRI task selected. Specifically, evidence of deficits in inhibitory control regions has been found in youth with sBED and prior to sBED development, suggesting them as potential early markers of sBED and possibly of BED. Additionally, studies have indicated that hyperactivation in these regions among youth with sBED may represent potential early brain compensatory mechanisms. In the case of BED, findings come from adult studies, which indicate hypoactivation in inhibitory control circuits. In contrast, hyperactivation of hub regions of the reward system seems to characterize both sBED and BED, as indicated by data from adult studies and some studies involving youth. Of note, obesity is an important confounding factor in most of these findings, but it is rarely taken into account. However, because the diagnosis of BED is mostly based on behaviour (except for the loss of control item), it is possible that different mechanisms involving an imbalance of inhibition and reward-based systems could lead to a similar phenotypic presentation [199]. This is, however, speculative at this point. It is likely that a more complex interplay between brain systems is present, and other systems, such as those involved in interoceptive processes and emotional identification, as well as emotional response, are gaining evidence. More complex analysis regarding brain dynamics will probably help improve our understanding of such altered patterns in BED, particularly during changing neurodevelopmental periods.

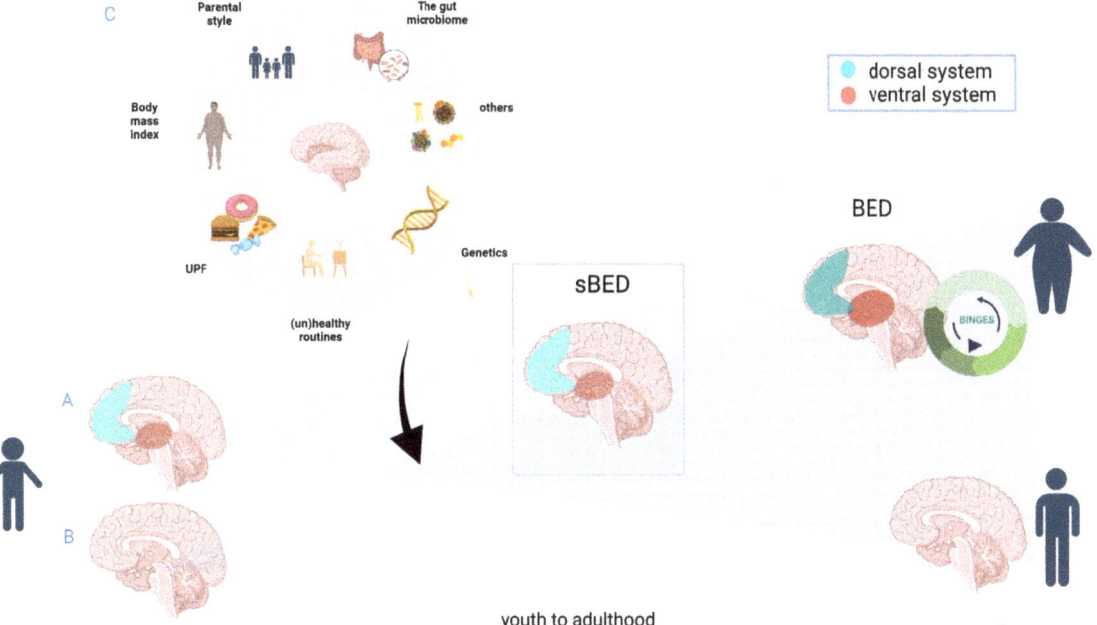

Figure 1. Summary of theoretical approaches to BED emergence in the context of neurodevelopment. From either a vulnerable (**A**) or healthy (**B**) starting point, and subject to external factors (**C**), a sBED condition may or may not develop. From sBED, one group of subjects will develop BED, while others will not.

A critical evaluation must be conducted regarding the potential association between UPF consumption and the development of primary emotional regulation strategies, and eating behaviours [98]. Excessive UPF exposure prior to adolescence may induce changes in the frontolimbic brain circuits, as well as difficulties in emotional regulation processes at adolescent stages. The risks should not be minimized regarding sBED/BED, and given that UPF consumption is a modifiable factor, preventive and more strictly holistic strategies should be enforced. This is even more important, considering that behavioural interventions remain modest for BED [200]. Information about the potential interaction between UPF consumption and age-related development vulnerability windows, as well as the 'toxic quantity' of UPF that each subject might tolerate, should be examined in future studies.

With all the information reviewed in the present manuscript, it becomes apparent that more clarity must be achieved in respect to groups of subjects with sBED conditions that might be more vulnerable to the development of BED. More information about longitudinal trajectories, and the risks and protective factors of BED development is needed. In this regard, neuroimaging biomarkers might prove more valuable in clinical practice for prognostic, rather than diagnostic purposes [201], and they might open up opportunities to develop target-directed treatments (e.g., cognitive rehabilitation, neuromodulation strategies). Finally, one other important question will need to be addressed in future studies:

whether sBED is part of a dimensional continuum with BED or, rather, sBEDs are non-pathological traits present in the general population that confer a risk for BED only in vulnerable subjects.

Author Contributions: Conceptualization, investigation, writing—original draft preparation, writing—review and editing, E.V. and O.C.-R. All authors have read and agreed to the published version of the manuscript.

Funding: This research was funded by the Project Grants PREC-BED (PI22/00655, E Via) and UP-PREdev (PI22/00645, O Contreras-Rodríguez), both from Health Institute Carlos III (ISCIII). Partial support was also obtained from the CIBERSAM—Consorcio Centro de Investigación Biomédica en Red Salud Mental—Proyectos Intramurales, Health Institute Carlos III (ISCIII) (O Contreras-Rodríguez). O Contreras-Rodriguez is funded by a "Miguel Servet" contract (CP20/00165) from the Health Institute Carlos III (ISCIII). E. Via thanks the CERCA Progamme, Generalitat de Catalunya.

Institutional Review Board Statement: Not applicable.

Informed Consent Statement: Not applicable.

Data Availability Statement: Not applicable.

Acknowledgments: We thank Tom Yohannan for language editing and proofreading of the final version of the manuscript.

Conflicts of Interest: The authors declare no conflict of interest.

References

1. American Psychiatric Association. *Diagnostic and Statistical Manual of Mental Disorders*, 5th ed.; American Psychiatric Association: Washington, DC, USA; Arlington, VA, USA, 2013; ISBN 9780890425541.
2. Santomauro, D.F.; Melen, S.; Mitchison, D.; Vos, T.; Whiteford, H.; Ferrari, A.J. The hidden burden of eating disorders: An extension of estimates from the Global Burden of Disease Study 2019. *Lancet Psychiatry* **2021**, *8*, 320–328. [CrossRef] [PubMed]
3. Smink, F.R.E.; Van Hoeken, D.; Oldehinkel, A.J.; Hoek, H.W. Prevalence and severity of DSM-5 eating disorders in a community cohort of adolescents. *Int. J. Eat. Disord.* **2014**, *47*, 610–619. [CrossRef]
4. Kjeldbjerg, M.L.; Clausen, L. Prevalence of binge-eating disorder among children and adolescents: A systematic review and meta-analysis. *Eur. Child Adolesc. Psychiatry* **2021**, *32*, 549–574. [CrossRef] [PubMed]
5. Tanofsky-Kraff, M.; Marcus, M.D.; Yanovski, S.Z.; Yanovski, J.A. Loss of control eating disorder in children age 12 years and younger: Proposed research criteria. *Eat. Behav.* **2008**, *9*, 360–365. [CrossRef]
6. Decaluwé, V.; Braet, C. Prevalence of binge-eating disorder in obese children and adolescents seeking weight-loss treatment. *Int. J. Obes.* **2003**, *27*, 404–409. [CrossRef] [PubMed]
7. Marzilli, E.; Cerniglia, L.; Cimino, S. A narrative review of binge eating disorder in adolescence: Prevalence, impact, and psychological treatment strategies. *Adolesc. Health Med. Ther.* **2018**, *9*, 17–30. [CrossRef]
8. Ágh, T.; Kovács, G.; Supina, D.; Pawaskar, M.; Herman, B.K.; Vokó, Z.; Sheehan, D.V. A systematic review of the health-related quality of life and economic burdens of anorexia nervosa, bulimia nervosa, and binge eating disorder. *Eat. Weight Disord.* **2016**, *21*, 353–364. [CrossRef]
9. World Health Organization (WHO). Obesity and Overweight. Available online: https://www.who.int/news-room/fact-sheets/detail/obesity-and-overweight (accessed on 11 June 2023).
10. Guerdjikova, A.I.; Mori, N.; Casuto, L.S.; McElroy, S.L. Update on Binge Eating Disorder. *Med. Clin. N. Am.* **2019**, *103*, 669–680. [CrossRef]
11. Kessler, R.C.; Berglund, P.A.; Chiu, W.T.; Deitz, A.C.; Hudson, J.I.; Shahly, V.; Aguilar-Gaxiola, S.; Alonso, J.; Angermeyer, M.C.; Benjet, C.; et al. The prevalence and correlates of binge eating disorder in the World Health Organization World Mental Health Surveys. *Biol. Psychiatry* **2013**, *73*, 904–914. [CrossRef]
12. Neumark-Sztainer, D.; Wall, M.; Guo, J.; Story, M.; Haines, J.; Eisenberg, M. Obesity, disordered eating, and eating disorders in a longitudinal study of adolescents: How do dieters fare 5 years later? *J. Am. Diet. Assoc.* **2006**, *106*, 559–568. [CrossRef]
13. Smith, K.E.; Luo, S.; Mason, T.B. A systematic review of neural correlates of dysregulated eating associated with obesity risk in youth. *Neurosci. Biobehav. Rev.* **2021**, *124*, 245–266. [CrossRef]
14. Vainik, U.; Neseliler, S.; Konstabel, K.; Fellows, L.K.; Dagher, A. Eating traits questionnaires as a continuum of a single concept. Uncontrolled eating. *Appetite* **2015**, *90*, 229–239. [CrossRef]
15. Hebebrand, J.; Gearhardt, A.N. The concept of "food addiction" helps inform the understanding of overeating and obesity: NO. *Am. J. Clin. Nutr.* **2021**, *113*, 268–273. [CrossRef]
16. Eldredge, K.L.; Agras, W.S. Weight and shape overconcern and emotional eating in binge eating disorder. *Int. J. Eat. Disord.* **1996**, *19*, 73–82. [CrossRef]

17. Nakamura, Y.; Koike, S. Association of Disinhibited Eating and Trait of Impulsivity with Insula and Amygdala Responses to Palatable Liquid Consumption. *Front. Syst. Neurosci.* **2021**, *15*, 647143. [CrossRef]
18. Tanofsky-Kraff, M.; Shomaker, L.B.; Olsen, C.; Roza, C.A.; Wolkoff, L.E.; Columbo, K.M.; Raciti, G.; Zocca, J.M.; Wilfley, D.E.; Yanovski, S.Z.; et al. A Prospective study of pediatric loss of control eating and psychological outcomes. *J. Abnorm. Psychol.* **2011**, *120*, 108–118. [CrossRef] [PubMed]
19. Vannucci, A.; Nelson, E.E.; Bongiorno, D.M.; Pine, D.S.; Yanovski, J.A.; Tanofsky-Kraff, M. Behavioral and neurodevelopmental precursors to binge-type eating disorders: Support for the role of negative valence systems. *Psychol. Med.* **2015**, *45*, 2921–2936. [CrossRef]
20. Davis, C.; Carter, J.C. Compulsive overeating as an addiction disorder. A review of theory and evidence. *Appetite* **2009**, *53*, 1–8. [CrossRef] [PubMed]
21. Von Deneen, K.M.; Liu, Y. Obesity as an addiction: Why do the obese eat more? *Maturitas* **2011**, *68*, 342–345. [CrossRef] [PubMed]
22. Hauck, C.; Cook, B.; Ellrott, T. Food addiction, eating addiction and eating disorders. *Proc. Nutr. Soc.* **2020**, *79*, 103–112. [CrossRef]
23. Gearhardt, A.N.; Corbin, W.R.; Brownell, K.D. Preliminary validation of the Yale Food Addiction Scale. *Appetite* **2009**, *52*, 430–436. [CrossRef] [PubMed]
24. Imperatori, C.; Fabbricatore, M.; Vumbaca, V.; Innamorati, M.; Contardi, A.; Farina, B. Food Addiction: Definition, measurement and prevalence in healthy subjects and in patients with eating disorders. *Riv. Psichiatr.* **2016**, *51*, 60–65. [CrossRef] [PubMed]
25. Cebolla, A.; Perpiñá, C.; Lurbe, E.; Alvarez-Pitti, J.; Botella, C. Prevalencia del trastorno por atracón en una muestra clínica de obesos. *An. Pediatría* **2012**, *77*, 98–102. [CrossRef] [PubMed]
26. Shapiro, J.R.; Woolson, S.L.; Hamer, R.M.; Kalarchian, M.A.; Marcus, M.D.; Bulik, C.M. Evaluating binge eating disorder in children: Development of the children's binge eating disorder scale (C-BEDS). *Int. J. Eat. Disord.* **2007**, *40*, 82–89. [CrossRef]
27. Marcus, M.D.; Kalarchian, M.A. Binge eating in children and adolescents. *Int. J. Eat. Disord.* **2003**, *34*, S47–S57. [CrossRef]
28. Chamay-Weber, C.; Combescure, C.; Lanza, L.; Carrard, I.; Haller, D.M. Screening Obese Adolescents for Binge Eating Disorder in Primary Care: The Adolescent Binge Eating Scale. *J. Pediatr.* **2017**, *185*, 68–72.e1. [CrossRef]
29. Balantekin, K.N.; Birch, L.L.; Savage, J.S. Eating in the absence of hunger during childhood predicts self-reported binge eating in adolescence. *Eat. Behav.* **2017**, *24*, 7–10. [CrossRef]
30. Herle, M.; Stavola, B.; De Hübel, C.; Abdulkadir, M.; Ferreira, D.S.; Loos, R.J.F.; Bryant-Waugh, R.; Bulik, C.M.; Micali, N. A longitudinal study of eating behaviours in childhood and later eating disorder behaviours and diagnoses. *Br. J. Psychiatry* **2020**, *216*, 113–119. [CrossRef]
31. Ashcroft, J.; Semmler, C.; Carnell, S.; Van Jaarsveld, C.; Wardle, J. Continuity and stability of eating behaviour traits in children. *Eur. J. Clin. Nutr.* **2008**, *62*, 985–990. [CrossRef]
32. Brewerton, T.D.; Rance, S.J.; Dansky, B.S.; O'Neil, P.M.; Kilpatrick, D.G. A comparison of women with child-adolescent versus adult onset binge eating: Results from the National Women's Study. *Int. J. Eat. Disord.* **2014**, *47*, 836–843. [CrossRef]
33. Stice, E.; Nathan Marti, C.; Rohde, P. Prevalence, incidence, impairment, and course of the proposed DSM-5 eating disorder diagnoses in an 8-year prospective community study of young women. *J. Abnorm. Psychol.* **2013**, *122*, 445–457. [CrossRef] [PubMed]
34. Brockmeyer, T.; Skunde, M.; Wu, M.; Bresslein, E.; Rudofsky, G.; Herzog, W.; Friederich, H.C. Difficulties in emotion regulation across the spectrum of eating disorders. *Compr. Psychiatry* **2014**, *55*, 565–571. [CrossRef] [PubMed]
35. Favieri, F.; Marini, A.; Casagrande, M. Emotional regulation and overeating behaviors in children and adolescents: A systematic review. *Behav. Sci.* **2021**, *11*, 11. [CrossRef]
36. Mischel, W.; Shoda, Y.; Rodriguez, M.L. Delay of Gratification in Children. *Science.* **1989**, *244*, 933–938. [CrossRef]
37. Stein, R.I.; Kenardy, J.; Wiseman, C.V.; Dounchis, J.Z.; Arnow, B.A.; Wilfley, D.E. What's driving the binge in binge eating disorder?: A prospective examination of precursors and consequences. *Int. J. Eat. Disord.* **2007**, *40*, 195–203. [CrossRef] [PubMed]
38. Penzenstadler, L.; Soares, C.; Karila, L.; Khazaal, Y. Systematic Review of Food Addiction as Measured with the Yale Food Addiction Scale: Implications for the Food Addiction Construct. *Curr. Neuropharmacol.* **2019**, *17*, 526–538. [CrossRef]
39. Bleck, J.R.; DeBate, R.D.; Olivardia, R. The Comorbidity of ADHD and Eating Disorders in a Nationally Representative Sample. *J. Behav. Health Serv. Res.* **2015**, *42*, 437–451. [CrossRef]
40. Goldschmidt, A.B.; Lavender, J.M.; Hipwell, A.E.; Stepp, S.D.; Keenan, K. Emotion Regulation and Loss of Control Eating in Community-Based Adolescents. *J. Abnorm. Child Psychol.* **2017**, *45*, 183–191. [CrossRef]
41. Levin, R.L.; Rawana, J.S. Attention-deficit/hyperactivity disorder and eating disorders across the lifespan: A systematic review of the literature. *Clin. Psychol. Rev.* **2016**, *50*, 22–36. [CrossRef]
42. Kalarchian, M.A.; Marcus, M.D. Psychiatric comorbidity of childhood obesity. *Int. Rev. Psychiatry* **2012**, *24*, 241–246. [CrossRef]
43. Lavagnino, L.; Arnone, D.; Cao, B.; Soares, J.C.; Selvaraj, S. Inhibitory control in obesity and binge eating disorder: A systematic review and meta-analysis of neurocognitive and neuroimaging studies. *Neurosci. Biobehav. Rev.* **2016**, *68*, 714–726. [CrossRef] [PubMed]
44. Stice, E.; Davis, K.; Miller, N.P.; Marti, C.N. Fasting Increases Risk for Onset of Binge Eating and Bulimic Pathology: A 5-Year Prospective Study. *J. Abnorm. Psychol.* **2008**, *117*, 941. [CrossRef] [PubMed]
45. Da Luz, F.Q.; Hay, P.; Gibson, A.A.; Touyz, S.W.; Swinbourne, J.M.; Roekenes, J.A.; Sainsbury, A. Does severe dietary energy restriction increase binge eating in overweight or obese individuals? A systematic review. *Obes. Rev.* **2015**, *16*, 652–665. [CrossRef]

46. Elran-Barak, R.; Sztainer, M.; Goldschmidt, A.B.; Crow, S.J.; Peterson, C.B.; Hill, L.L.; Crosby, R.D.; Powers, P.; Mitchell, J.E.; Le Grange, D. Dietary Restriction Behaviors and Binge Eating in Anorexia Nervosa, Bulimia Nervosa and Binge Eating Disorder: Trans-diagnostic Examination of the Restraint Model. *Eat. Behav.* **2015**, *18*, 192–196. [CrossRef]
47. Racine, S.E.; Burt, S.A.; Iacono, W.G.; McGue, M.; Klump, K.L. Dietary Restraint Moderates Genetic Risk for Binge Eating. *J. Abnorm. Psychol.* **2011**, *120*, 119. [CrossRef]
48. Conceição, E.M.; Moreira, C.S.; de Lourdes, M.; Ramalho, S.; Vaz, A.R. Exploring Correlates of Loss of Control Eating in a Nonclinical Sample. *Front. Psychol.* **2022**, *12*, 787558. [CrossRef] [PubMed]
49. Fairburn, C.G. *Overcoming Binge Eating: The Proven Program to Learn Why You Binge and How You Can Stop*; Barnes & Noble, Ed.; Guilford Publications Inc.: New York, NY, USA, 2013; ISBN 1572305614.
50. Ricciardelli, L.A.; McCabe, M.P. Dietary restraint and negative affect as mediators of body dissatisfaction and bulimic behavior in adolescent girls and boys. *Behav. Res. Ther.* **2001**, *39*, 1317–1328. [CrossRef]
51. Ayton, A.; Ibrahim, A.; Dugan, J.; Galvin, E.; Wright, O.W. Ultra-processed foods and binge eating: A retrospective observational study. *Nutrition* **2021**, *84*, 111023. [CrossRef] [PubMed]
52. Figueiredo, N.; Kose, J.; Srour, B.; Julia, C.; Kesse-Guyot, E.; Péneau, S.; Allès, B.; Paz Graniel, I.; Chazelas, E.; Deschasaux-Tanguy, M.; et al. Ultra-processed food intake and eating disorders: Cross-sectional associations among French adults. *J. Behav. Addict.* **2022**, *11*, 588–599. [CrossRef]
53. Wang, L.; Martínez Steele, E.; Du, M.; Pomeranz, J.L.; O'Connor, L.E.; Herrick, K.A.; Luo, H.; Zhang, X.; Mozaffarian, D.; Zhang, F.F. Trends in Consumption of Ultraprocessed Foods Among US Youths Aged 2–19 Years, 1999–2018. *JAMA* **2021**, *326*, 519–530. [CrossRef]
54. Marino, M.; Puppo, F.; Del Bo', C.; Vinelli, V.; Riso, P.; Porrini, M.; Martini, D. A systematic review of worldwide consumption of ultra-processed foods: Findings and criticisms. *Nutrients* **2021**, *13*, 2778. [CrossRef] [PubMed]
55. Latasa, P.; Louzada, M.L.D.C.; Martinez Steele, E.; Monteiro, C.A. Added sugars and ultra-processed foods in Spanish households (1990–2010). *Eur. J. Clin. Nutr.* **2018**, *72*, 1404–1412. [CrossRef] [PubMed]
56. Pagliai, G.; Dinu, M.; Madarena, M.P.; Bonaccio, M.; Iacoviello, L.; Sofi, F. Consumption of ultra-processed foods and health status: A systematic review and meta-analysis. *Br. J. Nutr.* **2021**, *125*, 308–318. [CrossRef] [PubMed]
57. Mitchison, D.; Touyz, S.; González-Chica, D.A.; Stocks, N.; Hay, P. How abnormal is binge eating? 18-Year time trends in population prevalence and burden. *Acta Psychiatr. Scand.* **2017**, *136*, 147–155. [CrossRef]
58. Bulik, C.M.; Sullivan, P.F.; Kendler, K.S. Genetic and environmental contributions to obesity and binge eating. *Int. J. Eat. Disord.* **2003**, *33*, 293–298. [CrossRef]
59. Frank, G.K.W. The Perfect Storm—A Bio-Psycho-Social Risk Model for Developing and Maintaining Eating Disorders. *Front. Behav. Neurosci.* **2016**, *10*, 44. [CrossRef]
60. Costa, A.; Oliveira, A. Parental Feeding Practices and Children's Eating Behaviours: An Overview of Their Complex Relationship. *Healthcare* **2023**, *11*, 400. [CrossRef]
61. Paroche, M.M.; Caton, S.J.; Vereijken, C.M.J.L.; Weenen, H.; Houston-Price, C. How Infants and Young Children Learn about Food: A Systematic Review. *Front. Psychol.* **2017**, *8*, 1046. [CrossRef]
62. Vaughn, A.E.; Ward, D.S.; Fisher, J.O.; Faith, M.S.; Hughes, S.O.; Kremers, S.P.J.; Musher-Eizenman, D.R.; O'Connor, T.M.; Patrick, H.; Power, T.G. Fundamental constructs in food parenting practices: A content map to guide future research. *Nutr. Rev.* **2016**, *74*, 98–117. [CrossRef]
63. Giel, K.E.; Bulik, C.M.; Fernandez-Aranda, F.; Hay, P.; Keski-Rahkonen, A.; Schag, K.; Schmidt, U.; Zipfel, S. Binge eating disorder. *Nat. Rev. Dis. Prim.* **2022**, *8*, 16. [CrossRef]
64. Kaye, W.H.; Fudge, J.L.; Paulus, M. New insights into symptoms and neurocircuit function of anorexia nervosa. *Nat. Rev. Neurosci.* **2009**, *10*, 573–584. [CrossRef]
65. Tepper, B.J.; Barbarossa, I.T. Taste, Nutrition, and Health. *Nutrients* **2020**, *12*, 155. [CrossRef] [PubMed]
66. Small, D.M.; Prescott, J. Odor/taste integration and the perception of flavor. *Exp. Brain Res.* **2005**, *166*, 345–357. [CrossRef] [PubMed]
67. Rolls, E.T. Taste, olfactory and food texture reward processing in the brain and the control of appetite. *Proc. Nutr. Soc.* **2012**, *71*, 488–501. [CrossRef]
68. Shepherd, G.M. Smell images and the flavour system in the human brain. *Nature* **2006**, *444*, 316–321. [CrossRef] [PubMed]
69. Small, D.M. Taste representation in the human insula. *Brain Struct. Funct.* **2010**, *214*, 551–561. [CrossRef] [PubMed]
70. Chikazoe, J.; Lee, D.H.; Kriegeskorte, N.; Anderson, A.K. Distinct representations of basic taste qualities in human gustatory cortex. *Nat. Commun.* **2019**, *10*, 1048. [CrossRef]
71. Seabrook, L.T.; Borgland, S.L. The orbitofrontal cortex, food intake and obesity. *J. Psychiatry Neurosci.* **2020**, *45*, 304–312. [CrossRef]
72. Dagher, A.; Neseliler, S.; Han, J.E. Appetite as Motivated Choice: Hormonal and Environmental Influences. *Decis. Neurosci. Integr. Perspect.* **2017**, 397–409. [CrossRef]
73. Kaye, W.H.; Wagner, A.; Fudge, J.L.; Paulus, M. Neurocircuity of eating disorders. *Curr. Top. Behav. Neurosci.* **2011**, *6*, 37–57. [CrossRef]
74. Shapiro, A.L.B.; Johnson, S.L.; Sutton, B.; Legget, K.T.; Dabelea, D.; Tregellas, J.R. Eating in the absence of hunger in young children is related to brain reward network hyperactivity and reduced functional connectivity in executive control networks. *Pediatr. Obes.* **2019**, *14*, e12502. [CrossRef] [PubMed]

75. Leenaerts, N.; Jongen, D.; Ceccarini, J.; Van Oudenhove, L.; Vrieze, E. The neurobiological reward system and binge eating: A critical systematic review of neuroimaging studies. *Int. J. Eat. Disord.* **2022**, *55*, 1421–1458. [CrossRef] [PubMed]
76. Monosov, I.E. Anterior cingulate is a source of valence-specific information about value and uncertainty. *Nat. Commun.* **2017**, *8*, 134. [CrossRef] [PubMed]
77. Weafer, J.; Crane, N.A.; Gorka, S.M.; Phan, K.L.; de Wit, H. Neural Correlates of Inhibition and Reward are Negatively Associated. *Neuroimage* **2019**, *196*, 188. [CrossRef]
78. Kelley, A.E.; Baldo, B.A.; Pratt, W.E.; Will, M.J. Corticostriatal-hypothalamic circuitry and food motivation: Integration of energy, action and reward. *Physiol. Behav.* **2005**, *86*, 773–795. [CrossRef]
79. Berridge, K.C. Food reward: Brain substrates of wanting and liking. *Neurosci. Biobehav. Rev.* **1996**, *20*, 1–25. [CrossRef]
80. O'Doherty, J.P.; Deichmann, R.; Critchley, H.D.; Dolan, R.J. Neural responses during anticipation of a primary taste reward. *Neuron* **2002**, *33*, 815–826. [CrossRef]
81. Small, D.M.; Jones-Gotman, M.; Dagher, A. Feeding-induced dopamine release in dorsal striatum correlates with meal pleasantness ratings in healthy human volunteers. *Neuroimage* **2003**, *19*, 1709–1715. [CrossRef]
82. Craig, A.D. How do you feel--now? The anterior insula and human awareness. *Nat. Rev. Neurosci.* **2009**, *10*, 59–70. [CrossRef]
83. Craig, A.D. Interoception: The sense of the physiological condition of the body. *Curr. Opin. Neurobiol.* **2003**, *13*, 500–505. [CrossRef]
84. Li, J.; An, R.; Zhang, Y.; Li, X.; Wang, S. Correlations of macronutrient-induced functional magnetic resonance imaging signal changes in human brain and gut hormone responses. *Am. J. Clin. Nutr.* **2012**, *96*, 275–282. [CrossRef] [PubMed]
85. Simmons, W.K.; Rapuano, K.M.; Kallman, S.J.; Ingeholm, J.E.; Miller, B.; Gotts, S.J.; Avery, J.A.; Hall, K.D.; Martin, A. Category-specific integration of homeostatic signals in caudal but not rostral human insula. *Nat. Neurosci.* **2013**, *16*, 1551–1552. [CrossRef] [PubMed]
86. Frank, S.; Kullmann, S.; Veit, R. Food related processes in the insular cortex. *Front. Hum. Neurosci.* **2013**, *7*, 499. [CrossRef]
87. Romei, A.; Voigt, K.; Verdejo-Garcia, A. A Perspective on Candidate Neural Underpinnings of Binge Eating Disorder: Reward and Homeostatic Systems. *Curr. Pharm. Des.* **2020**, *26*, 2327–2333. [CrossRef]
88. Wang, G.J.; Volkow, N.D.; Telang, F.; Jayne, M.; Ma, J.; Rao, M.; Zhu, W.; Wong, C.T.; Pappas, N.R.; Geliebter, A.; et al. Exposure to appetitive food stimuli markedly activates the human brain. *Neuroimage* **2004**, *21*, 1790–1797. [CrossRef] [PubMed]
89. Pelchat, M.L.; Johnson, A.; Chan, R.; Valdez, J.; Ragland, J.D. Images of desire: Food-craving activation during fMRI. *Neuroimage* **2004**, *23*, 1486–1493. [CrossRef] [PubMed]
90. Contreras-Rodríguez, O.; Cano, M.; Vilar-López, R.; Rio-Valle, J.S.; Verdejo-Román, J.; Navas, J.F.; Martín-Pérez, C.; Fernández-Aranda, F.; Menchón, J.M.; Soriano-Mas, C.; et al. Visceral adiposity and insular networks: Associations with food craving. *Int. J. Obes.* **2019**, *43*, 503–511. [CrossRef]
91. Wonderlich, J.A.; Bershad, M.; Steinglass, J.E. Exploring Neural Mechanisms Related to Cognitive Control, Reward, and Affect in Eating Disorders: A Narrative Review of FMRI Studies. *Neuropsychiatr. Dis. Treat.* **2021**, *17*, 2053–2062. [CrossRef]
92. Contreras-Rodriguez, O.; Escorihuela, R.M. Dissecting ultra—Processed foods and drinks: Do they have a potential to impact the brain? *Rev. Endocr. Metab. Disord.* **2022**, *23*, 697–717. [CrossRef]
93. Berthoud, H.R. Neural control of appetite: Cross-talk between homeostatic and non-homeostatic systems. *Appetite* **2004**, *43*, 315–317. [CrossRef]
94. Berthoud, H.R. Homeostatic and non-homeostatic pathways involved in the control of food intake and energy balance. *Obesity* **2006**, *14* (Suppl. 5), 197S–200S. [CrossRef] [PubMed]
95. Bodell, L.P.; Wildes, J.E.; Goldschmidt, A.B.; Lepage, R.; Keenan, K.E.; Guyer, A.E.; Hipwell, A.E.; Stepp, S.D.; Forbes, E.E. Associations between Neural Reward Processing and Binge Eating among Adolescent Girls. *J. Adolesc. Health* **2018**, *62*, 107–113. [CrossRef] [PubMed]
96. Gross, J.J. The Extended Process Model of Emotion Regulation: Elaborations, Applications, and Future Directions. *Psychol. Inq.* **2015**, *26*, 130–137. [CrossRef]
97. Somerville, L.; Casey, B. Developmental neurobiology of cognitive control and motivational systems. *Curr. Opin. Neurobiol.* **2010**, *20*, 236–241. [CrossRef]
98. Willner, C.J.; Hoffmann, J.D.; Bailey, C.S.; Harrison, A.P.; Garcia, B.; Ng, Z.J.; Cipriano, C.; Brackett, M.A. The Development of Cognitive Reappraisal from Early Childhood through Adolescence: A Systematic Review and Methodological Recommendations. *Front. Psychol.* **2022**, *13*, 875964. [CrossRef]
99. Berner, L.A.; Marsh, R. Frontostriatal circuits and the development of bulimia nervosa. *Front. Behav. Neurosci.* **2014**, *8*, 395. [CrossRef]
100. Ochsner, K.N.; Silvers, J.A.; Buhle, J.T. Review and evolving model of the cognitive control of emotion. *Ann. N. Y. Acad. Sci.* **2012**, *1251*, E1–E24. [CrossRef]
101. McRae, K.; Gross, J.J.; Weber, J.; Robertson, E.R.; Sokol-Hessner, P.; Ray, R.D.; Gabrieli, J.D.E.; Ochsner, K.N. The development of emotion regulation: An fMRI study of cognitive reappraisal in children, adolescents and young adults. *Soc. Cogn. Affect. Neurosci.* **2012**, *7*, 11–22. [CrossRef]
102. Morris, A.S.; Criss, M.M.; Silk, J.S.; Houltberg, B.J. The Impact of Parenting on Emotion Regulation during Childhood and Adolescence. *Child Dev. Perspect.* **2017**, *11*, 233–238. [CrossRef]

103. Cimino, S.; Marzilli, E.; Tafà, M.; Cerniglia, L. Emotional-Behavioral Regulation, Temperament and Parent–Child Interactions Are Associated with Dopamine Transporter Allelic Polymorphism in Early Childhood: A Pilot Study. *Int. J. Environ. Res. Public Health* **2020**, *17*, 8564. [CrossRef]
104. Zalewski, M.; Lengua, L.J.; Wilson, A.C.; Trancik, A.; Bazinet, A. Emotion Regulation Profiles, Temperament, and Adjustment Problems in Preadolescents. *Child Dev.* **2011**, *82*, 951. [CrossRef] [PubMed]
105. Barzman, D.; Geise, C.; Lin, P.-I. Review of the genetic basis of emotion dysregulation in children and adolescents. *World J. Psychiatry* **2015**, *5*, 112. [CrossRef]
106. Zeman, J.; Cassano, M.; Perry-Parrish, C.; Stegall, S. Emotion regulation in children and adolescents. *J. Dev. Behav. Pediatr.* **2006**, *27*, 155–168. [CrossRef]
107. Bartholdy, S.; O'Daly, O.G.; Campbell, I.C.; Banaschewski, T.; Barker, G.; Bokde, A.L.W.; Bromberg, U.; Büchel, C.; Burke Quinlan, E.; Desrivieres, S.; et al. Neural Correlates of Failed Inhibitory Control as an Early Marker of Disordered Eating in Adolescents. *Biol. Psychiatry* **2019**, *85*, 956–965. [CrossRef] [PubMed]
108. Olsavsky, A.K.; Shott, M.E.; Deguzman, M.C.; Frank, G.K.W.W. Neural correlates of taste reward value across eating disorders. *Psychiatry Res. Neuroimaging* **2019**, *288*, 76–84. [CrossRef] [PubMed]
109. Treasure, J.; Duarte, T.A.; Schmidt, U.; Antunes Duarte, T.; Schmidt, U. Eating disorders. *Lancet* **2020**, *395*, 899–911. [CrossRef]
110. Hardee, J.E.; Phaneuf, C.; Cope, L.; Zucker, R.; Gearhardt, A.; Heitzeg, M. Neural correlates of inhibitory control in youth with symptoms of food addiction. *Appetite* **2020**, *148*, 104578. [CrossRef]
111. Jarcho, J.M.; Tanofsky-Kraff, M.; Nelson, E.E.; Engel, S.G.; Vannucci, A.; Field, S.E.; Romer, A.L.; Hannallah, L.; Brady, S.M.; Demidowich, A.P.; et al. Neural activation during anticipated peer evaluation and laboratory meal intake in overweight girls with and without loss of control eating. *Neuroimage* **2015**, *108*, 343–353. [CrossRef]
112. Goldschmidt, A.B.; Dickstein, D.P.; MacNamara, A.E.; Phan, K.L.; O'Brien, S.; Le Grange, D.; Fisher, J.O.; Keedy, S. A pilot study of neural correlates of loss of control eating in children with overweight/obesity: Probing intermittent access to food as a means of eliciting disinhibited eating. *J. Pediatr. Psychol.* **2018**, *43*, 846–855. [CrossRef]
113. ABCD Study. US Department of Health & Human Services (HHS) ABCD Study. Available online: https://abcdstudy.org/ (accessed on 12 April 2023).
114. Schumann, G.; Loth, E.; Banaschewski, T.; Barbot, A.; Barker, G.; Büchel, C.; Conrod, P.J.; Dalley, J.W.; Flor, H.; Gallinat, J.; et al. The IMAGEN study: Reinforcement-related behaviour in normal brain function and psychopathology. *Mol. Psychiatry* **2010**, *15*, 1128–1139. [CrossRef]
115. Frank, G.K.W.; Shott, M.E.; DeGuzman, M.C. The Neurobiology of Eating Disorders. *Child Adolesc. Psychiatr. Clin. N. Am.* **2019**, *28*, 629–640. [CrossRef]
116. Balodis, I.M.; Molina, N.D.; Kober, H.; Worhunsky, P.D.; White, M.A.; Sinha, R.; Grilo, C.M.; Potenza, M.N. Divergent neural substrates of inhibitory control in binge eating disorder relative to other manifestations of obesity. *Obesity* **2013**, *21*, 367–377. [CrossRef] [PubMed]
117. Hege, M.A.; Stingl, K.T.; Kullmann, S.; Schag, K.; Giel, K.E.; Zipfel, S.; Preissl, H. Attentional impulsivity in binge eating disorder modulates response inhibition performance and frontal brain networks. *Int. J. Obes.* **2015**, *39*, 353–360. [CrossRef] [PubMed]
118. Stice, E.; Burger, K. Neural vulnerability factors for obesity. *Clin. Psychol. Rev.* **2019**, *68*, 38–53. [CrossRef] [PubMed]
119. Frank, G.K.W. Altered brain reward circuits in eating disorders: Chicken or egg? *Curr. Psychiatry Rep.* **2013**, *15*, 396. [CrossRef]
120. Hartmann, A.S.; Czaja, J.; Rief, W.; Hilbert, A. Personality and psychopathology in children with and without loss of control over eating. *Compr. Psychiatry* **2010**, *51*, 572–578. [CrossRef]
121. Giel, K.E.; Teufel, M.; Junne, F.; Zipfel, S.; Schag, K. Food-Related Impulsivity in Obesity and Binge Eating Disorder-A Systematic Update of the Evidence. *Nutrients* **2017**, *9*, 1170. [CrossRef]
122. Rapuano, K.M.; Laurent, J.S.; Hagler, D.J.; Hatton, S.N.; Thompson, W.K.; Jernigan, T.L.; Dale, A.M.; Casey, B.J.; Watts, R. Nucleus accumbens cytoarchitecture predicts weight gain in children. *Proc. Natl. Acad. Sci. USA* **2020**, *117*, 26977–26984. [CrossRef]
123. Assari, S.; Boyce, S.; Bazargan, M. Nucleus accumbens functional connectivity with the frontoparietal network predicts subsequent change in body mass index for American children. *Brain Sci.* **2020**, *10*, 703. [CrossRef]
124. Balodis, I.M.; Kober, H.; Worhunsky, P.D.; White, M.A.; Stevens, M.C.; Pearlson, G.D.; Sinha, R.; Grilo, C.M.; Potenza, M.N. Monetary reward processing in obese individuals with and without binge eating disorder. *Biol. Psychiatry* **2013**, *73*, 877–886. [CrossRef]
125. Frank, G.K.W.; Shott, M.E.; Stoddard, J.; Swindle, S.; Pryor, T.L. Association of Brain Reward Response with Body Mass Index and Ventral Striatal-Hypothalamic Circuitry among Young Women with Eating Disorders. *JAMA Psychiatry* **2021**, *78*, 1123–1133. [CrossRef] [PubMed]
126. Hartogsveld, B.; Quaedflieg, C.W.E.M.; van Ruitenbeek, P.; Smeets, T. Decreased putamen activation in balancing goal-directed and habitual behavior in binge eating disorder. *Psychoneuroendocrinology* **2022**, *136*, 105596. [CrossRef] [PubMed]
127. Miranda-Olivos, R.; Steward, T.; Martínez-Zalacaín, I.; Mestre-Bach, G.; Juaneda-Seguí, A.; Jiménez-Murcia, S.; Fernández-Formoso, J.A.; Vilarrasa, N.; Veciana de las Heras, M.; Custal, N.; et al. The neural correlates of delay discounting in obesity and binge eating disorder. *J. Behav. Addict.* **2021**, *10*, 498–507. [CrossRef]
128. Schienle, A.; Schäfer, A.; Hermann, A.; Vaitl, D. Binge-eating disorder: Reward sensitivity and brain activation to images of food. *Biol. Psychiatry* **2009**, *65*, 654–661. [CrossRef]

129. Reiter, A.M.F.; Heinze, H.J.; Schlagenhauf, F.; Deserno, L. Impaired Flexible Reward-Based Decision-Making in Binge Eating Disorder: Evidence from Computational Modeling and Functional Neuroimaging. *Neuropsychopharmacology* **2017**, *42*, 628–637. [CrossRef] [PubMed]
130. Voon, V.; Joutsa, J.; Majuri, J.; Baek, K.; Nord, C.L.; Arponen, E.; Forsback, S.; Kaasinen, V. The neurochemical substrates of habitual and goal-directed control. *Transl. Psychiatry* **2020**, *10*, 84. [CrossRef] [PubMed]
131. Voon, V.; Derbyshire, K.; Rück, C.; Irvine, M.A.; Worbe, Y.; Enander, J.; Schreiber, L.R.N.; Gillan, C.; Fineberg, N.A.; Sahakian, B.J.; et al. Disorders of compulsivity: A common bias towards learning habits. *Mol. Psychiatry* **2015**, *20*, 345–352. [CrossRef] [PubMed]
132. Skandali, N.; Majuri, J.; Joutsa, J.; Baek, K.; Arponen, E.; Forsback, S.; Kaasinen, V.; Voon, V. The neural substrates of risky rewards and losses in healthy volunteers and patient groups: A PET imaging study. *Psychol. Med.* **2022**, *52*, 3280–3288. [CrossRef]
133. Murray, S.B.; Alba, C.; Duval, C.J.; Nagata, J.M.; Cabeen, R.P.; Lee, D.J.; Toga, A.W.; Siegel, S.J.; Jann, K. Aberrant functional connectivity between reward and inhibitory control networks in pre-adolescent binge eating disorder. *Psychol. Med.* **2022**, 1–10. [CrossRef]
134. Simon, J.J.; Skunde, M.; Walther, S.; Bendszus, M.; Herzog, W.; Friederich, H.C. Neural signature of food reward processing in bulimic-type eating disorders. *Soc. Cogn. Affect. Neurosci.* **2016**, *11*, 1393–1401. [CrossRef]
135. Critchley, H.D.; Rolls, E.T. Hunger and satiety modify the responses of olfactory and visual neurons in the primate orbitofrontal cortex. *J. Neurophysiol.* **1996**, *75*, 1673–1686. [CrossRef] [PubMed]
136. Ely, A.V.; Wierenga, C.E.; Bischoff-Grethe, A.; Bailer, U.F.; Berner, L.A.; Fudge, J.L.; Paulus, M.P.; Kaye, W.H. Response in taste circuitry is not modulated by hunger and satiety in women remitted from bulimia nervosa. *J. Abnorm. Psychol.* **2017**, *126*, 519–530. [CrossRef] [PubMed]
137. Goldstein, R.Z.; Volkow, N.D. Drug addiction and its underlying neurobiological basis: Neuroimaging evidence for the involvement of the frontal cortex. *Am. J. Psychiatry* **2002**, *159*, 1642–1652. [CrossRef] [PubMed]
138. Domingo-Rodriguez, L.; Ruiz de Azua, I.; Dominguez, E.; Senabre, E.; Serra, I.; Kummer, S.; Navandar, M.; Baddenhausen, S.; Hofmann, C.; Andero, R.; et al. A specific prelimbic-nucleus accumbens pathway controls resilience versus vulnerability to food addiction. *Nat. Commun.* **2020**, *11*, 782. [CrossRef] [PubMed]
139. Berthoud, H.R.; Morrison, C.D.; Münzberg, H. The obesity epidemic in the face of homeostatic body weight regulation: What went wrong and how can it be fixed? *Physiol. Behav.* **2020**, *222*, 112959. [CrossRef] [PubMed]
140. Sun, X.X.; Kroemer, N.B.; Veldhuizen, M.G.; Babbs, A.E.; De Araujo, I.E.; Gitelman, D.R.; Sherwin, R.S.; Sinha, R.; Small, D.M. Basolateral Amygdala Response to Food Cues in the Absence of Hunger Is Associated with Weight Gain Susceptibility. *J. Neurosci.* **2015**, *35*, 7964–7976. [CrossRef]
141. Martín-Pérez, C.; Contreras-Rodríguez, O.; Vilar-López, R.; Verdejo-García, A. Hypothalamic Networks in Adolescents with Excess Weight: Stress-Related Connectivity and Associations with Emotional Eating. *J. Am. Acad. Child Adolesc. Psychiatry* **2019**, *58*, 211–220.e5. [CrossRef]
142. Naumann, E.; Svaldi, J.; Wyschka, T.; Heinrichs, M.; von Dawans, B. Stress-induced body dissatisfaction in women with binge eating disorder. *J. Abnorm. Psychol.* **2018**, *127*, 548–558. [CrossRef]
143. Phelps, E.A.; Lempert, K.M.; Sokol-Hessner, P. Emotion and Decision Making: Multiple Modulatory Neural Circuits. *Annu. Rev. Neurosci.* **2014**, *37*, 263–287. [CrossRef]
144. Lyu, Z.; Jackson, T. Acute Stressors Reduce Neural Inhibition to Food Cues and Increase Eating among Binge Eating Disorder Symptomatic Women. *Front. Behav. Neurosci.* **2016**, *10*, 188. [CrossRef]
145. Villarejo, C.; Fernández-Aranda, F.; Jiménez-Murcia, S.; Peñas-Lledó, E.; Granero, R.; Penelo, E.; Tinahones, F.J.; Sancho, C.; Vilarrasa, N.; Montserrat-Gil De Bernabé, M.; et al. Lifetime obesity in patients with eating disorders: Increasing prevalence, clinical and personality correlates. *Eur. Eat. Disord. Rev.* **2012**, *20*, 250–254. [CrossRef] [PubMed]
146. Rapuano, K.M.; Zieselman, A.L.; Kelley, W.M.; Sargent, J.D.; Heatherton, T.F.; Gilbert-Diamond, D. Genetic risk for obesity predicts nucleus accumbens size and responsivity to real-world food cues. *Proc. Natl. Acad. Sci. USA* **2017**, *114*, 160–165. [CrossRef]
147. Tomasi, D.; Volkow, N.D. Striatocortical pathway dysfunction in addiction and obesity: Differences and similarities. *Crit. Rev. Biochem. Mol. Biol.* **2013**, *48*, 1–19. [CrossRef]
148. Boutelle, K.N.; Wierenga, C.E.; Bischoff-Grethe, A.; Melrose, A.J.; Grenesko-Stevens, E.; Paulus, M.P.; Kaye, W.H. Increased brain response to appetitive tastes in the insula and amygdala in obese compared with healthy weight children when sated. *Int. J. Obes.* **2015**, *39*, 620–628. [CrossRef]
149. Herbert, B.M.; Pollatos, O. Attenuated interoceptive sensitivity in overweight and obese individuals. *Eat. Behav.* **2014**, *15*, 445–448. [CrossRef]
150. Mata, F.; Verdejo-Roman, J.; Soriano-Mas, C.; Verdejo-Garcia, A. Insula tuning towards external eating versus interoceptive input in adolescents with overweight and obesity. *Appetite* **2015**, *93*, 24–30. [CrossRef] [PubMed]
151. Gupta, S.; Hawk, T.; Aggarwal, A.; Drewnowski, A. Characterizing ultra-processed foods by energy density, nutrient density, and cost. *Front. Nutr.* **2019**, *6*, 70. [CrossRef] [PubMed]
152. Monteiro, C.A.; Cannon, G.; Levy, R.; Moubarac, J.-C. The Food System. NOVA. The star shines bright. *Public Health* **2016**, *7*, 28–38.

153. Monteiro, C.A.; Cannon, G.; Levy, R.B.; Moubarac, J.C.; Louzada, M.L.C.; Rauber, F.; Khandpur, N.; Cediel, G.; Neri, D.; Martinez-Steele, E.; et al. Ultra-processed foods: What they are and how to identify them. *Public Health Nutr.* **2019**, *22*, 936–941. [CrossRef]
154. Martínez Steele, E.; Khandpur, N.; da Costa Louzada, M.L.; Monteiro, C.A. Association between dietary contribution of ultra-processed foods and urinary concentrations of phthalates and bisphenol in a nationally representative sample of the US population aged 6 years and older. *PLoS ONE* **2020**, *15*, e0236738. [CrossRef]
155. Moodie, R.; Stuckler, D.; Monteiro, C.; Sheron, N.; Neal, B.; Thamarangsi, T.; Lincoln, P.; Casswell, S. Profits and pandemics: Prevention of harmful effects of tobacco, alcohol, and ultra-processed food and drink industries. *Lancet* **2013**, *381*, 670–679. [CrossRef] [PubMed]
156. Elizabeth, L.; Machado, P.; Zinöcker, M.; Baker, P.; Lawrence, M. Ultra-processed foods and health outcomes: A narrative review. *Nutrients* **2020**, *12*, 1955. [CrossRef] [PubMed]
157. De Amicis, R.; Mambrini, S.P.; Pellizzari, M.; Foppiani, A.; Bertoli, S.; Battezzati, A.; Leone, A. Ultra-processed foods and obesity and adiposity parameters among children and adolescents: A systematic review. *Eur. J. Nutr.* **2022**, *61*, 2297–2311. [CrossRef] [PubMed]
158. Neri, D.; Steele, E.M.; Khandpur, N.; Cediel, G.; Zapata, M.E.; Rauber, F.; Marrón-Ponce, J.A.; Machado, P.; da Costa Louzada, M.L.; Andrade, G.C.; et al. Ultraprocessed food consumption and dietary nutrient profiles associated with obesity: A multicountry study of children and adolescents. *Obes. Rev.* **2022**, *23*, e13387. [CrossRef] [PubMed]
159. Schulte, E.; Avena, N.; Gerhardt, A. Which foods may be addictive? The roles of processing, fat content, and glycemic load. *PLoS ONE* **2015**, *10*, e0117959.
160. Filgueiras, A.R.; Pires de Almeida, V.B.; Koch Nogueira, P.C.; Alvares Domene, S.M.; Eduardo da Silva, C.; Sesso, R.; Sawaya, A.L. Exploring the consumption of ultra-processed foods and its association with food addiction in overweight children. *Appetite* **2019**, *135*, 137–145. [CrossRef]
161. Pursey, K.M.; Davis, C.; Burrows, T.L. Nutritional Aspects of Food Addiction. *Curr. Addict. Rep.* **2017**, *4*, 142–150. [CrossRef]
162. Faisal-Cury, A.; Leite, M.A.; Loureiro Escuder, M.M.; Levy, R.B.; Fernanda, M.; Peres, T. The relationship between ultra-processed food consumption and internalising symptoms among adolescents from São Paulo city, Southeast Brazil. *Public Health Nutr.* **2022**, *25*, 2498–2506. [CrossRef]
163. Werneck, A.O.; Vancampfort, D.; Oyeyemi, A.L.; Stubbs, B.; Silva, D.R. Joint association of ultra-processed food and sedentary behavior with anxiety-induced sleep disturbance among Brazilian adolescents. *J. Affect. Disord.* **2020**, *266*, 135–142. [CrossRef]
164. Werneck, A.O.; Hoare, E.; Silva, D.R. Do TV viewing and frequency of ultra-processed food consumption share mediators in relation to adolescent anxiety-induced sleep disturbance? *Public Health Nutr.* **2021**, *24*, 5491–5497. [CrossRef]
165. Swartz, J.; Monk, C. The Role of Corticolimbic Circuitry in the Development of Anxiety Disorders in Children and Adolescents. *Curr. Top. Behav. Neurosci.* **2014**, *16*, 133–148. [CrossRef]
166. Bruce, A.S.; Bruce, J.M.; Black, W.R.; Lepping, R.J.; Henry, J.M.; Cherry, J.B.C.; Martin, L.E.; Papa, V.B.; Davis, A.M.; Brooks, W.M.; et al. Branding and a child's brain: An fMRI study of neural responses to logos. *Soc. Cogn. Affect. Neurosci.* **2014**, *9*, 118. [CrossRef]
167. Adise, S.; Geier, C.F.; Roberts, N.J.; White, C.N.; Keller, K.L. Is brain response to food rewards related to overeating? A test of the reward surfeit model of overeating in children. *Appetite* **2018**, *128*, 167–179. [CrossRef] [PubMed]
168. May, C.E.; Dus, M. Confection Confusion: Interplay between Diet, Taste, and Nutrition. *Trends Endocrinol. Metab.* **2021**, *32*, 95–105. [CrossRef] [PubMed]
169. Liu, D.; Archer, N.; Duesing, K.; Hannan, G.; Keast, R. Mechanism of fat taste perception: Association with diet and obesity. *Prog. Lipid Res.* **2016**, *63*, 41–49. [CrossRef]
170. Hall, K.D.; Ayuketah, A.; Brychta, R.; Cai, H.; Cassimatis, T.; Chen, K.Y.; Chung, S.T.; Costa, E.; Courville, A.; Darcey, V.; et al. Ultra-Processed Diets Cause Excess Calorie Intake and Weight Gain: An Inpatient Randomized Controlled Trial of Ad Libitum Food Intake. *Cell Metab.* **2020**, *32*, 690. [CrossRef] [PubMed]
171. Puig-Vallverdú, J.; Romaguera, D.; Fernández-Barrés, S.; Gignac, F.; Ibarluzea, J.; Santa-Maria, L.; Llop, S.; Gonzalez, S.; Vioque, J.; Riaño-Galán, I.; et al. The association between maternal ultra-processed food consumption during pregnancy and child neuropsychological development: A population-based birth cohort study. *Clin. Nutr.* **2022**, *41*, 2275–2283. [CrossRef] [PubMed]
172. Griffiths, S.; Suksasilp, C.; Lucas, L.; Sebastian, C.L.; Norbury, C. Relationship between early language competence and cognitive emotion regulation in adolescence. *R. Soc. Open Sci.* **2021**, *8*, 210742. [CrossRef]
173. Contreras-Rodriguez, O.; Rales-Moreno, M.; Fernández-Barrés, S.; Cimpean, A.; Arnoriaga-Rodríguez, M.; Puig, J.; Biarnés, C.; Motger-Albertí, A.; Cano, M.; José, M.F.-R. Consumption of ultra-processed foods is associated with depression, mesocorticolimbic volume, and inflammation. *J. Affect. Disord.* **2023**, *335*, 340–348. [CrossRef]
174. Yunker, A.G.; Patel, R.; Page, K.A. Effects of Non-nutritive Sweeteners on Sweet Taste Processing and Neuroendocrine Regulation of Eating Behavior. *Curr. Nutr. Rep.* **2020**, *9*, 278–289. [CrossRef]
175. Yeung, A.W.K.; Wong, N.S.M. How does our brain process sugars and non-nutritive sweeteners differently: A systematic review on functional magnetic resonance imaging studies. *Nutrients* **2020**, *12*, 3010. [CrossRef] [PubMed]
176. Pepino, M.Y. Physiology & behavior metabolic effects of non-nutritive sweeteners. *Physiol. Behav.* **2015**, *152*, 450–455. [PubMed]
177. De Graaf, C.; Kok, F.J. Slow food, fast food and the control of food intake. *Nat. Rev. Endocrinol.* **2010**, *6*, 290–293. [CrossRef] [PubMed]

178. Smeets, P.A.M.; De Graaf, C.; Stafleu, A.; Van Osch, M.J.P.; Van Der Grond, J. Functional magnetic resonance imaging of human hypothalamic responses to sweet taste and calories. *Am. J. Clin. Nutr.* **2005**, *82*, 1011–1016. [CrossRef]
179. Van Opstal, A.M.; Kaal, I.; van den Berg-Huysmans, A.A.; Hoeksma, M.; Blonk, C.; Pijl, H.; Rombouts, S.A.R.B.; van der Grond, J. Dietary sugars and non-caloric sweeteners elicit different homeostatic and hedonic responses in the brain. *Nutrition* **2019**, *60*, 80–86. [CrossRef]
180. Van Opstal, A.M.; Hafkemeijer, A.; van den Berg-Huysmans, A.A.; Hoeksma, M.; Mulder, T.P.J.; Pijl, H.; Rombouts, S.A.R.B.; van der Grond, J. Brain activity and connectivity changes in response to nutritive natural sugars, non-nutritive natural sugar replacements and artificial sweeteners. *Nutr. Neurosci.* **2021**, *24*, 395–405. [CrossRef]
181. Crézé, C.; Candal, L.; Cros, J.; Knebel, J.F.; Seyssel, K.; Stefanoni, N.; Schneiter, P.; Murray, M.M.; Tappy, L.; Toepel, U. The impact of caloric and non-caloric sweeteners on food intake and brain responses to food: A randomized crossover controlled trial in healthy humans. *Nutrients* **2018**, *10*, 615. [CrossRef]
182. Bolhuis, D.P.; Forde, C.G.; Cheng, Y.; Xu, H.; Martin, N.; De Graaf, C. Slow food: Sustained impact of harder foods on the reduction in energy intake over the course of the day. *PLoS ONE* **2014**, *9*, e93370. [CrossRef]
183. Krop, E.M.; Hetherington, M.M.; Nekitsing, C.; Miquel, S.; Postelnicu, L.; Sarkar, A. Influence of oral processing on appetite and food intake—A systematic review and meta-analysis. *Appetite* **2018**, *125*, 253–269. [CrossRef]
184. Viskaal-van Dongen, M.; Kok, F.J.; de Graaf, C. Eating rate of commonly consumed foods promotes food and energy intake. *Appetite* **2011**, *56*, 25–31. [CrossRef]
185. Bian, X.; Chi, L.; Gao, B.; Tu, P.; Ru, H.; Lu, K. Gut microbiome response to sucralose and its potential role in inducing liver inflammation in mice. *Front. Physiol.* **2017**, *8*, 487. [CrossRef] [PubMed]
186. Medina-Reyes, E.I.; Rodríguez-Ibarra, C.; Déciga-Alcaraz, A.; Díaz-Urbina, D.; Chirino, Y.I.; Pedraza-Chaverri, J. Food additives containing nanoparticles induce gastrotoxicity, hepatotoxicity and alterations in animal behavior: The unknown role of oxidative stress. *Food Chem. Toxicol.* **2020**, *146*, 111814. [CrossRef]
187. Laster, J.; Frame, L.A. Beyond the Calories—Is the Problem in the Processing? *Curr. Treat. Options Gastroenterol.* **2019**, *17*, 577–586. [CrossRef] [PubMed]
188. Edalati, S.; Bagherzadeh, F.; Asghari Jafarabadi, M.; Ebrahimi-Mamaghani, M. Higher ultra-processed food intake is associated with higher DNA damage in healthy adolescents. *Br. J. Nutr.* **2021**, *125*, 568–576. [CrossRef] [PubMed]
189. Pase, C.S.; Metz, V.G.; Roversi, K.; Roversi, K.; Vey, L.T.; Dias, V.T.; Schons, C.F.; de David Antoniazzi, C.T.; Duarte, T.; Duarte, M.; et al. Trans fat intake during pregnancy or lactation increases anxiety-like behavior and alters proinflammatory cytokines and glucocorticoid receptor levels in the hippocampus of adult offspring. *Brain Res. Bull.* **2021**, *166*, 110–117. [CrossRef] [PubMed]
190. Trevizol, F.; Roversi, K.; Dias, V.T.; Roversi, K.; Pase, C.S.; Barcelos, R.C.S.; Benvegnu, D.M.; Kuhn, F.T.; Dolci, G.S.; Ross, D.H.; et al. Influence of lifelong dietary fats on the brain fatty acids and amphetamine-induced behavioral responses in adult rat. *Prog. Neuro Psychopharmacol. Biol. Psychiatry* **2013**, *45*, 215–222. [CrossRef]
191. Trevizol, F.; Roversi, K.R.; Dias, V.T.; Roversi, K.; Barcelos, R.C.S.; Kuhn, F.T.; Pase, C.S.; Golombieski, R.; Veit, J.C.; Piccolo, J.; et al. Cross-generational trans fat intake facilitates mania-like behavior: Oxidative and molecular markers in brain cortex. *Neuroscience* **2015**, *286*, 353–363. [CrossRef]
192. D'cunha, N.M.; Sergi, D.; Lane, M.M.; Naumovski, N.; Gamage, E.; Rajendran, A.; Kouvari, M.; Gauci, S.; Dissanayka, T.; Marx, W.; et al. The Effects of Dietary Advanced Glycation End-Products on Neurocognitive and Mental Disorders. *Nutrients* **2022**, *14*, 2421. [CrossRef]
193. Butler, M.J.; Perrini, A.A.; Eckel, L.A. The role of the gut microbiome, immunity, and neuroinflammation in the pathophysiology of eating disorders. *Nutrients* **2021**, *13*, 500. [CrossRef]
194. Heidari, Z.; Mohammadipour, A.; Haeri, P.; Ebrahimzadeh-Bideskan, A. The effect of titanium dioxide nanoparticles on mice midbrain substantia nigra. *Iran. J. Basic Med. Sci.* **2019**, *22*, 745–751. [CrossRef]
195. Hu, R.; Gong, X.; Duan, Y.; Li, N.; Che, Y.; Cui, Y.; Zhou, M.; Liu, C.; Wang, H.; Hong, F. Neurotoxicological effects and the impairment of spatial recognition memory in mice caused by exposure to TiO_2 nanoparticles. *Biomaterials* **2010**, *31*, 8043–8050. [CrossRef] [PubMed]
196. Sheng, L.; Ze, Y.; Wang, L.; Yu, X.; Hong, J.; Zhao, X.; Ze, X.; Liu, D.; Xu, B.; Zhu, Y.; et al. Mechanisms of TiO_2 nanoparticle-induced neuronal apoptosis in rat primary cultured hippocampal neurons. *J. Biomed. Mater. Res.* **2015**, *103*, 1141–1149. [CrossRef] [PubMed]
197. Ze, Y.; Sheng, L.; Zhao, X.; Hong, J.; Ze, X.; Yu, X.; Pan, X.; Lin, A.; Zhao, Y.; Zhang, C.; et al. TiO_2 nanoparticles induced hippocampal neuroinflammation in mice. *PLoS ONE* **2014**, *9*, e92230. [CrossRef] [PubMed]
198. Węsierska, M.; Dziendzikowska, K.; Gromadzka-Ostrowska, J.; Dudek, J.; Polkowska-Motrenko, H.; Audinot, J.N.; Gutleb, A.C.; Lankoff, A.; Kruszewski, M. Silver ions are responsible for memory impairment induced by oral administration of silver nanoparticles. *Toxicol. Lett.* **2018**, *290*, 133–144. [CrossRef]
199. Wierenga, C.E.; Ely, A.; Bischoff-Grethe, A.; Bailer, U.F.; Simmons, A.N.; Kaye, W.H. Are Extremes of Consumption in Eating Disorders Related to an Altered Balance between Reward and Inhibition? *Front. Behav. Neurosci.* **2014**, *8*, 410. [CrossRef]

200. Rajjo, T.; Mohammed, K.; Alsawas, M.; Ahmed, A.T.; Farah, W.; Asi, N.; Almasri, J.; Prokop, L.J.; Murad, M.H. Treatment of Pediatric Obesity: An Umbrella Systematic Review. *J. Clin. Endocrinol. Metab.* **2017**, *102*, 763–775. [CrossRef]
201. Fullana, M.A.; Abramovitch, A.; Via, E.; López-Sola, C.; Goldberg, X.; Reina, N.; Fortea, L.; Solanes, A.; Buckley, M.J.; Ramella-Cravaro, V.; et al. Diagnostic biomarkers for obsessive-compulsive disorder: A reasonable quest or ignis fatuus? *Neurosci. Biobehav. Rev.* **2020**, *118*, 504–513. [CrossRef]

Disclaimer/Publisher's Note: The statements, opinions and data contained in all publications are solely those of the individual author(s) and contributor(s) and not of MDPI and/or the editor(s). MDPI and/or the editor(s) disclaim responsibility for any injury to people or property resulting from any ideas, methods, instructions or products referred to in the content.

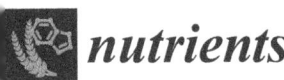

Article

Comparison of the Prevalence of Eating Disorders among Dietetics Students and Students of Other Fields of Study at Selected Universities (Silesia, Poland)

Aneta Matusik [1], Mateusz Grajek [2,*], Patryk Szlacheta [3] and Ilona Korzonek-Szlacheta [1]

1. Department of Prevention of Metabolic Diseases, Faculty of Health Sciences in Bytom, Medical University of Silesia in Katowice, 41902 Bytom, Poland
2. Department of Public Health, Faculty of Health Sciences in Bytom, Medical University of Silesia in Katowice, 41902 Bytom, Poland
3. Department of Toxicology and Health Protection, Faculty of Health Sciences in Bytom, Medical University of Silesia in Katowice, 41902 Bytom, Poland
* Correspondence: mgrajek@sum.edu.pl

Abstract: Background: Over the past few years, an increase in the incidence of eating disorders has been noted. An increase in the pace of life, an increase in the availability of a wide variety of food products, and, to a large extent, the involvement of mass media are cited as reasons for this phenomenon. The promotion of a slim figure by the mass media is equated with achieving success in life, but also the advertising of a wide selection of food products (often highly processed) can have a serious impact on the development of eating disorders. This phenomenon is particularly observed in industrialized Western countries. Objective: Therefore, it was decided to test and compare whether dietetics students are indeed more predisposed to developing eating disorders than students not in the nutrition field. Material and methods: the study included 310 individuals representing two equal groups of fields of study—dietetics and other students. The study used standardized questionnaire—EAT-26. Results: It was found that almost half (46%) of the respondents (both dietetics students and students of other majors) met at least one criterion out of three that could indicate the probable existence or susceptibility to an eating disorder. These individuals should see a specialist for further diagnosis. There was no significant effect of the field of study on the overall EAT-26 test score ($p > 0.05$). When this result was corrected for BMI values for those with the lowest scores on this indicator, the risk of eating disorders was found to be higher among students of majors other than dietetics ($X^2 = 13.572$; $V = 0.831$ $p = 0.001$). Conclusions: Almost half of the respondents in both study groups showed a predisposition to eating disorders based on the EAT-26 test. Despite the presence of a correlation in individual responses that dietetics students are more predisposed to eating disorders, no such relationship was found according to the final EAT-26 test scores. However, it was observed that non-dietetics students who had low BMI values showed higher tendencies toward behaviors indicative of eating disorders.

Keywords: eating disorders; EAT-26; students; dietetics

1. Introduction

Eating disorders are disease entities with underlying psychological factors. They are defined as persistent behaviors associated with food intake leading to changes in consumption, contributing to psychosocial impairment and mental disorders [1,2]. People who struggle with an eating disorder often experience depression. They often become addicted to alcohol, drugs, or sexual activities, for example, and self-harm. The symptoms of eating disorders are closely related to the internal feelings of the patient (e.g., pain, stress, fear, loneliness, low self-esteem). The literature distinguishes several factors that can affect the formation of an abnormal relationship with food. The most commonly cited are psychological, biological, social, behavioral, and cultural factors [3]. In particular, the age of the sufferer may be linked to factors that influenced the development of the disorder. Among the young population, family and environmental factors come first. Among the causes of an appetite disorder in children and adolescents are body fat content in girls, hormonal changes, and the influence of peer groups. In adults, socio-cultural factors can influence the disorder [4]. Appetite disorders have been differentiated according to the criteria outlined in the major mental illness classification systems: International Statistical Classification of Diseases and Related Health Problems ICD-11 in European countries and the American Psychiatric Association's Diagnostic and Statistical Manual of Mental Disorders DSM-5 in the United States [5].

Over the past few years, an increase in the incidence of eating disorders has been noted, yet Poland still has very few epidemiological studies on eating disorders. The most reliable data from 2011 indicate that anorexia nervosa occurs in about 2% of people before the age of 18, and these are 10 times more likely to be female. There are no studies in Poland estimating these values in terms of the elderly population and people belonging to specific groups (physically active people, associated with healthy eating and attention to physical appearance) [6]. However, an increase in the pace of life, an increase in the availability of a wide variety of food products, and, to a large extent, the involvement of mass media are cited as reasons for this phenomenon. The promotion of a slim figure by the mass media is equated with achieving success in life, but also the advertising of a wide selection of food products (often highly processed) can have a serious impact on the development of eating disorders. This phenomenon is particularly observed in industrialized Western countries. Eating disorders mainly (but not exclusively) affect adolescents and young adults. An increase in the incidence of an abnormal relationship with food, especially among people who practice endurance and aesthetic sports, such as running, ballet, gymnastics, or figure skating, has also been observed. What is more, an increase in the prevalence of eating disorders has been noted among those studying courses related to proper nutrition [7,8]. Dietetics students, by their curriculum, are subjected to intensive education on proper nutrition. In addition to the knowledge they acquire in classes, they increase their knowledge of contemporary fashionable diets and nutritional trends. In this way, they want to meet the expectations set by their future patients. They begin to program their lives to look and behave healthily throughout lives, which can in turn trigger a nascent obsession with nutrition and their figure. Society's pressure for them to be impeccable role models in eating and appearance may be the cause of their developing an abnormal relationship with food [9].

Since there is a lack of research on this issue in recent years, especially in Poland, it was decided to check in an in-house study whether dietetics students are indeed more likely to suffer from eating disorders than students of other majors. The group studied in the in-house paper consisted of 310 students: 155 students in dietetics and 155 students in other majors unrelated to nutrition.

Therefore, it was decided to test and compare whether dietetics students are indeed more predisposed to developing eating disorders than students not in the nutrition field. The basis of the study was to address the hypothesis that the prevalence of eating disorders among dietetics students is higher than among students in other fields of study.

2. Materials and Methods

2.1. Study Area and Sample

The survey was conducted from March to April 2022 among dietetics students. The survey was conducted using a mixed survey method, and a questionnaire technique. In this study group, 155 dietetics students participated in the direct survey, including 96% women and 4% men. The survey was also conducted among students of other majors of the selected universities by electronic means, as an indirect survey (CAWI). This group also accounted for 155 students, including 77% women and 23% men. Students of an economic university comprised 51 respondents, students of a general university comprised

52 respondents, and students of a music university comprised 52 respondents. A total of 310 students between the ages of 18 and 25 participated in the research work. They were students at different stages of their studies.

2.2. Research Tool

The prevalence of eating disorders was analyzed using the EAT-26 questionnaire and a metric. The metric included gender, age, university name, and degree. In addition, students were asked about their current body weight and height. Based on this, from the formula: body weight (kg)/height (m^2), BMI (kg/m^2) was calculated, which was interpreted according to the WHO-approved BMI classification for adults [10] (Table 1).

Table 1. BMI classification for adults [10].

BMI (kg/m^2)	Interpretation of BMI
<16.00	Starvation
16.00–16.99	Emaciation
17.00–18.49	Underweight
18.50–24.99	Body weight normal
25.00–29.99	Overweight
30.00–34.99	First-degree obesity
35.00–39.99	Grade II obesity
≥40.00	Grade III obesity

The research study used an eating disorder screening tool, the American Eating Attitudes Test (EAT-26) questionnaire by Garner et al. [11]. The EAT-26 is a standardized questionnaire for detecting risk symptoms of eating disorders. It is designed both for screening individuals with a clinical diagnosis and for screening among those at risk for anorexia, bulimia, or obesity. The EAT-26 is one of the most widely used screening tools in eating disorder prevalence studies worldwide. The test is an abbreviated version of the EAT-40 created by Garner et al. [11] The interpretation of the EAT -26 questionnaire consists of three "referral criteria" that determine whether the respondent should come in for a further assessment of an eating disorder risk. They include:

(1) EAT total actual score consists of 26 questions or statements on attitudes toward nutrition. Items 1–25 are scored as follows: Always = 3; Usually = 2; Often = 1; Other answers = 0. Item 26 is scored in reverse (Never = 3, etc.) The screening test can be scored from 0 to 78. A respondent with a score of 20 or more is at risk of developing an eating disorder and should see a specialist for further diagnosis.

(2) Behavioral questions indicate possible symptoms of an appetite disorder or recent significant weight loss. They concern compensatory behaviors (use of laxatives, weight loss, provoking vomiting, overeating, engaging in excessive physical activity, and significant weight loss in a short period). If the respondent answered affirmatively to any of the behavioral questions, as shown in the table, this may indicate the existence of abnormalities and the need for further diagnosis of eating disorders (Table 2).

Table 2. Scoring on behavioral questions [11].

	Never	1/Month	2–3/Month	1/Week	2–6/Week	1/Day
(A) Overeating	-	-	X	X	X	X
(B) Vomiting	-	X	X	X	X	X
(C) Pharmacology	-	X	X	X	X	X
(D) Exercises	-	-	-	-	-	X
(E) Weight-loss	-	X	-	-	X	-

(3) Low body weight compared to age norms: the questionnaire includes detailed questions about height, weight, and gender. This information was used to calculate the body mass index (BMI) to determine the possible risk of an eating disorder. Below is a table that indicates whether the subject is underweight by age and gender (Table 3).

Table 3. Interpretation of BMI compared to age and gender norms [11].

Age	9	10	11	12	13	14	15	16	17	18	19	20	>20
BMI-female	14.0	14.5	14.5	15.0	15.5	16.0	16.5	17.0	17.5	18.0	18.0	18.5	19.0
BMI-male	14.0	14.5	15.0	15.0	16.0	16.5	17.0	17.5	18.0	18.5	19.0	19.5	20.5

2.3. Eligibility Criteria and Ethical Consent

The criteria for inclusion in the study group were the following two conditions: (1) voluntary participation in the study and complete completion of the questionnaire and (2) student status at the time of the study. In addition, during the initial interview with the respondents, they were asked about previous psychiatric episodes, thus checking their history of using a psychologist or psychiatrist. The fact, of their use was noted as a criterion for exclusion from further study, as those with prior diagnosis and treatment of eating disorders, mood disorders, anxiety disorders, and others could significantly affect the final outcome of the study.

All study participants gave informed consent to participate in the study by completing a questionnaire. The study was approved by the Bioethics Committee of the Medical University of Silesia in Katowice (PCN/0022/KB/211/20) in light of the Act on Medical and Dental Professions (5 December 1996), which includes a definition of medical experimentation. The study participants consciously agreed to participate in the study.

2.4. Statistical Analysis

Statistical analysis was performed using Statistica 13.0. The analysis was performed via the Chi-square test. A $p = 0.05$ was taken as the level of statistical significance. The V-Cramer correlation coefficient was also used to test the strength of the relationship of statistical characteristics. In each case where the symbol NS (non-significance) was placed next to the *p*-value, it indicates a lack of statistical significance.

3. Results

3.1. Sample Characteristics

A total of 310 students participated in the conducted study. The first half of the group ($n = 155$) consisted of medical university dietetics students. The second half of the study group consisted of students from various majors of selected non-dietetics universities ($n = 155$). In total, 51 students participated from the economic university, 52 students participated from the general university, and 52 students participated from the music university. Among the dietetics students surveyed, women accounted for 96% ($n = 149$) and men for 4% ($n = 6$) of the respondents. However, in the second group of respondents, women accounted for 77% ($n = 120$) and men for 23% ($n = 35$) of the respondents. Among dietetics students, 68% of respondents declared that they were in their bachelor's degree program, and 32% of respondents were in their second-degree program. In the second group, 62% of respondents were first-degree students, while 38% were second-degree students.

3.2. BMI of Participants

The calculated BMI of the dietetics students showed that 12% ($n = 19$) of the respondents were overweight, 2% ($n = 3$) were first-degree obese, 8% ($n = 13$) were underweight, and 2% ($n = 3$) were emaciated. Body weight in the normal range was 75% ($n = 117$) of dietetics students. In contrast, among students in other majors, 15% ($n = 23$) of respondents were overweight, 5% ($n = 8$) were first-degree obese, 8% ($n = 12$) were underweight, 4% ($n = 6$) were emaciated, and 1% ($n = 1$) were starved. Normal body weight was 68% ($n = 105$) of the students. Based on the calculated BMI of the respondents and subsequent comparison with age norms, it was found that 14% of dietetics students and 17% of students in other majors had too low body weight compared to age norms. There was no significant effect of the field of study on low body weight compared to age norms ($p > 0.05$-NS).

3.3. Risk of Eating Disorders

Based on the assigned score from the EAT-26, Part A questionnaire, it was estimated that 15% of both dietetics students and students from other majors are at risk for eating disorder-related diseases and should seek evaluation by a specialist for further diagnosis. There was no significant effect of the field of study on the total score of the actual items of the EAT-26, Part A test (≥ 20), which may indicate the risk of developing an eating disorder ($p > 0.05$-NS). According to the accepted scores on behavioral questions from the EAT-26 test, Part B, it was estimated that 33% of dietetics students and 28% of students in other majors met a criterion that could indicate a risk of developing an eating disorder. There was no significant effect of the field of study on the EAT-26 test score on behavioral questions ($p > 0.05$-NS). Based on the overall scores and interpretation of the EAT-26 questionnaire, it was found that almost half (46%) of the respondents (both dietetics students and students of other majors) met at least one criterion out of three that could indicate the probable existence or susceptibility to an eating disorder. These individuals should see a specialist for further diagnosis. There was no significant effect of the field of study on the overall EAT-26 test score ($p > 0.05$-NS). When this result was corrected for BMI values for those with the lowest scores on this indicator, the risk of eating disorders was found to be higher among students of majors other than dietetics ($X^2 = 13.572$; $V = 0.831$ $p = 0.001$). All the results described are summarized in Table 4.

Table 4. Summary of eating disorder risk estimation (EAT-26) ($n = 310$).

EAT-26	Dietetics Students		Other Students		p-Value
	Elevated Risk	No Risk	Elevated Risk	No Risk	
Part A	15%	85%	15%	85%	
Part B	33%	67%	28%	72%	$p > 0.05$
Entire	46%	54%	46%	54%	
All adjusted for BMI	12%	88%	31%	69%	$p = 0.001$

4. Discussion

Nowadays, eating disorders are a common phenomenon. Over the past 50 years, there has been an increase in the incidence of bulimia, anorexia, and compulsive eating syndrome in particular [12]. About 8–9% of the population has been found to struggle with gluttony or mental anorexia [13]. Craving disorders usually begin during adolescence and young adulthood. During this period, individuals are often prone to stressful events including taking exams, making decisions about the future, and moving to college. The result is an accompanying fear of adulthood. Studies have shown that the estimated prevalence of appetite disorders among college students ranges from 8 to 20% [14,15].

It is worrisome that a significant number of students who develop symptoms of eating disorders have not been diagnosed or sought treatment. Screening for this condition appears to be an important need to help sufferers in the early stages of the disease. Inappropriate dietary practices such as vomiting, fasting, restrictive diets, and laxative abuse, among others, can influence the development of disordered eating behavior. Nutritional counseling as part of a multidisciplinary approach plays a special role in the treatment of appetite disorders.

It may seem that dietetics students, thanks to specialized training in healthy eating habits, meal planning, or weight control, are less likely to have eating behavior disorders than those studying non-food-related majors. There is another belief that dietetics students view the start of their studies as a motivation to deal with their problems, which are inappropriate attitudes toward nutrition, as well as a desire to lower their body weight. These behaviors may exist before the start of the study but may also develop during education as a result of excessive preoccupation with healthy eating [14]. Our work confirms that 14% of nutrition students were overweight or obese. What is more, 14% of those surveyed also happened to lose 10 kg or more in the last 6 months. In contrast, among students of other majors, this percentage was only 5%; $p < 0.05$. In addition, 13% of dietetics students declared that they had been treated for eating disorders while, among students of other majors, this percentage was half as much at 6%; $p < 0.05$.

Another international study found that 77% of nutritionists from 14 countries believe that eating disorders are a problem for dietetics students [16]. Some studies suggest that the prevalence of eating disorders in nutrition students is higher than in students in other majors [17,18]. A study comparing eating behaviors between nutrition students and students in other majors in Portugal found that those in the first group showed greater dietary restrictions with subsequent bouts of overeating than students in other majors [17]. Another study conducted in South Africa also observed a higher risk of eating disorders among dietetics students 33.3% compared to other non-nutrition students 16.9%; $p = 0.059$ [19].

One important parameter in diagnosing bulimia or anorexia is an overestimation of body size. Sufferers perceive themselves as obese, despite being of the right weight or even underweight. Characteristically, there is a contradiction between BMI, actual images, and subjective assessment of the sufferer's outward appearance [20]. Even though 85% of dieters were of normal weight or even underweight, as many as 32% of them "always", "usually", or "often" took steps to reduce their weight. In contrast, among students in other majors, 81% were normal weight, underweight, or skinny, and 32% of them chose to take action to lower their weight. The study by Buviora et al. found that most of the students analyzed were of normal weight; meanwhile, only half of the students recognized this fact. The disturbed body image mainly concerned girls, as 17% perceived themselves as overweight, while it was found in half of these respondents [20].

Another factor that predisposes to eating disorders is devoting too much time and thought to food. It is observed that nowadays high-calorie products are being advertised, and there is a trend for eating a variety of foods without limits. In turn, it is also fashionable to have an athletic figure, which is associated with achieving success [9]. These two contradictory trends may influence the public to use various types of diets to lose weight in a short period. In addition, physical activity is observed to burn off excessive calories eaten and thus maintain a slim figure. All these factors can lead to an emerging obsession with food [21]. Especially according to some studies among nutrition students, who experience pressure from society to eat properly and have a slim figure. This can contribute to excessive control over the food they eat [22]. Of the dieters surveyed, 28% marked the answer "always", "usually", or "often" when asked about spending too much time and thoughts about food, while the other group had a lower percentage. at 21%; $p = 0.004$. In contrast, in a study by Taha et al. a similar percentage (33.5%) of students admitted that thoughts about food absorb them a lot [23].

One of the hallmarks of eating disorders is a paralyzing fear of gaining weight. Among the dietetics students surveyed, almost half—43%—are "always", "usually", or "often" terrified at the thought of being obese, and among students in other majors this percentage is slightly lower at 39% ($p > 0.05$-NS). On the other hand, among nutrition students, despite being of normal weight or even underweight, 28% are consumed with the desire to be thinner, and among students in other majors, the percentage is 27%; $p > 0.05$-NS. Furthermore, 27% of normal-weight or underweight dietetics students "always," "usually", or "often" think insistently about fat on their bodies. In contrast, the percentage in the second group is lower at −16%; $p < 0.05$. Contrasting these results with a study of Brazilian adolescents, by far the majority of respondents declared fear of weight gain [24]. In a study by Toral et al., 26.7% of nutrition students were observed to have significant dissatisfaction regarding their body image [25].

For people with eating disorders, especially among anorexia patients, every meal is a certain ritual. Slimming people know the caloric value of the foods they eat. The marker of lifelong success becomes counting the calories of meals every day, as well as those burned during exercise [26]. Among nutrition students, the majority of respondents (79%) are "always," "usually", or "often" aware of the caloric value of the products they eat. In contrast, among non-diet students, almost half as many—41%—know exactly how many calories a product has; $p = 0.000$. Additionally, 39% of nutrition students think about burning calories during exercise. In contrast, 37% of the other group thinks about calories lost during physical activity; $p > 0.05$-NS. In contrast, in a study by other authors, among Mexican nutrition students, almost half of the respondents who had symptoms of an appetite disorder counted the caloric value before meals [27], while among students in Saudi Arabia, 67% of students thought about calories burned during exercise [22]. However, it is worth noting that caloric awareness of products may not represent a real risk of anorexia among dieters, among others, as it may be characteristic of the nutrition students studied due to their field of study.

According to the accepted scores from the EAT-26 test, Part A, of the dietetics students surveyed, 15% scored 20 points or more, which may indicate concern about diet, weight, or problematic behavior. In the second group of subjects, the result was the same —15% of students in other majors also received a positive test result (EAT $\geq$ 20), which may indicate a risk for eating disorders. This percentage was comparable to a previous study in Florida in the United States in which 10% of nutrition students, as well as the same percentage of students in other majors, received a score of −20 or higher on the EAT-26 test. Compared to other countries, this percentage is lower than that of French students (20.5%) [18] and medical students from Pakistan (22.75%) [28].

In Part B of the survey on behavioral questions, 33% of dietetics students met a criterion that could indicate a risk of developing an appetite disorder. These were behaviors, occurring at a certain time of the type: paroxysmal overeating, vomiting, use of diuretics, laxatives, excessive exercise, or loss of 10 kg recently. In the second group of subjects, the result was slightly lower at 28% ($p > 0.05$-NS), suggesting the need for further investigation into eating disorders. In a study by Harris et al., there were also no significant differences between the two groups regarding behavioral questions [29]. In contrast, in a study among students in Palestine using the EAT-26 test, slightly more—46%—of students endorsed at least one of the additional behavioral behaviors associated with an eating disorder [30].

In contrast, according to the BMI thresholds presented in the EAT-26 interpretation, 14% of dietetics students were underweight compared to their age and gender, while among students in other majors this problem affected slightly more—17% of respondents. The study by Zhiping et al. also found no differences in underweight between the two groups. The percentages, however, were slightly smaller, as 4.1% of nutrition students were underweight compared to age norms, while students in other majors were underweight by 5.6% [17].

Based on the overall accepted scores and interpretation of the EAT-26 test, as many as almost half (46%) of dietetics students, and as it turned out, the same percentage of students in other majors, met at least one criterion that could indicate a risk of developing an eating disorder. As can be seen, the study did not find that dietetics students are at higher risk of developing an eating disorder than students in other majors. Other studies have also found similar results. Among Portuguese students aged 18–15, there was no difference in the risk of developing eating disorders between dietetics students and other non-food majors [19]. In a study in Washington, using the EAT-26 test, no such relationship was observed either [31].

It is becoming a common belief that nutrition students are more predisposed to appetite disorders than students in other majors. The implication is that future dietitians may feel pressure from their surroundings to eat healthily and present an impeccable figure at all times. In addition, some patients might not use the services of a dietitian with excessive body weight, which could indicate that person's lack of competence. In addition, nutrition students are "fed" during classes with constant messages about proper nutrition. All of these factors can give rise to an obsession with food, proper eating habits, and outward appearance [32,33]. However, in our work, we did not find a correlation (according to the accepted EAT-26 test scores) that dietetics students are more likely to have eating disorders than non-dietetics students. This may indicate that not only in nutrition students, but also in students of other majors, the problem of an abnormal relationship with food is becoming common. In addition, it is worth noting that the survey among non-nutrition students was conducted electronically, where often the social media group at a given university of 2000 people. The available survey likely attracted the attention of students who observed some abnormal eating behavior in themselves or were interested in this topic.

Although according to the final accepted EAT-26 test scores, there was no correlation that dietetics students were more predisposed to eating disorders, such correlations appeared in individual responses. A significant influence of the type of field of study on too frequent thoughts about body fat, despite being of the right weight or even underweight, preoccupation with food, and devoting too much time and thought to food was noted. These symptoms can predispose to the onset of eating disorders. Moreover, a significant effect of the type of college on losing 10 kg in the past 6 months was noted ($p = 0.006$), as well as past treatment for eating disorders ($p < 0.05$). A significant effect of the type of college was also observed on the caloric awareness of meals eaten ($p = 0.000$), consumption of diet foods ($p = 0.000$), avoidance of sugar-containing products ($p = 0.142$), or eating for longer periods than others ($p = 0.000$). Although eating diet foods or avoiding sweets may indicate a restrictive approach to eating and eating a meal at a longer time than others may be associated with anorexia, these behaviors may not, however, represent a real threat of an eating disorder. They are likely to be characteristic of the dietetics students surveyed due to the type of study and may also be indicative of normal eating habits.

In addition, it should be emphasized that even though a significant proportion of students (46%) were noted to meet at least one criterion in the EAT-26 test that may indicate a risk of developing an appetite disorder, this does not necessarily mean a real risk of bulimia or anorexia among the surveyed students. It is also worth mentioning that the presence of a single symptom characteristic of anorexia nervosa or gluttonousness, even if it appears sporadically in the company of other symptoms of the disease, should not be rigidly associated with the appearance of anorexia or bulimia nervosa in a person. Despite appearances, eating disorders are difficult to diagnose. Some symptoms in different types of eating disorders overlap. This makes it difficult to correctly diagnose the disease. It is important to catch certain tendencies at an early stage that may indicate a risk of developing an eating disorder in the future. Thus, it is urged that as many screening tests as possible be conducted in this direction among young people to detect a possible disease at an early stage and implement appropriate treatment before it is too late.

5. Conclusions

Almost half of the respondents in both study groups showed a predisposition to eating disorders based on the EAT-26 test. Despite the presence of a correlation in individual responses that dietetics students are more predisposed to eating disorders, no such relationship was found according to the final EAT-26 test scores. However, it was observed that non-dietetics students who had low BMI values showed higher tendencies toward behaviors indicative of eating disorders.

Author Contributions: Conceptualization, A.M.; methodology, A.M. and M.G.; validation, P.S.; formal analysis, M.G.; investigation, A.M.; resources, A.M. data curation, M.G.; writing—original draft preparation, A.M. and M.G.; writing—review and editing, P.S.; visualization, M.G.; supervision, I.K.-S.; project administration, M.G. All authors have read and agreed to the published version of the manuscript.

Funding: This research received no external funding.

Institutional Review Board Statement: Not applicable.

Informed Consent Statement: Informed consent was obtained from all subjects involved in the study.

Data Availability Statement: The original contributions presented in the study are included in the article; further inquiries can be directed to the corresponding author.

Acknowledgments: The authors would like to thank all the participants in the study.

Conflicts of Interest: The authors declare that the research was conducted in the absence of any commercial or financial relationships that could be construed as a potential conflict of interest.

References

1. Brytek-Matera, A.; Czepczor, K. Models of eating disorders: A theoretical investigation of an abnormal eating pattern sand body image disturbance. *Arch. Psychiatry Psychother.* **2017**, *19*, 16–26. [CrossRef]
2. American Psychiatric Association. *Diagnostic and Statistical Manual of Mental Disorders*, 5th ed.; American Psych Publishing: Arlington, VA, USA, 2013.
3. Puzio, A.; Biskupek-Wanot, A.; Wanot, B. *Eating Disorders*; American Psychological Association: Washington, DC, USA, 2020. [CrossRef]
4. Sciepuro, A. Psychotherapy of families in clinical practice. In *Psychiatry in General Medical Practices*; 2015; Volume VII, pp. 131–135.
5. WHO. *ICD-11 International Classification of Diseases 11 the Revision. The Global Standard for Diagnostic Health Information*; WHO: Geneva, Switzerland, 2019.
6. Bator, E.; Bronkowska, M.; Ślepecki, D.; Biernat, J. Anoreksja-przyczyny, przebieg, le-czenie. *Now. Lek.* **2011**, *80*, 184–191.
7. Grajek, M.; Krupa-Kotara, K.; Sas-Nowosielski, K.; Misterska, E.; Kobza, J. Prevalence of Orthorexia in Groups of Students with Varied Diets and Physical Activity (Silesia, Poland). *Nutrients* **2022**, *14*, 2816. [CrossRef] [PubMed]
8. Skoracka, K.; Pastusiak, K.; Bogdanski, P. *The Triad of Sportswomen-Nutritional Management*; Via Medical: Abu Dhabi, United Arab Emirates. Available online: https://www.viamedica.pl/ (accessed on 10 February 2022).
9. Nergiz-Unal, R.; Bilgiç, P.; Yabanci, N. High tendency to the substantial concern on body shape and eating disorders risk of the students majoring in Nutrition or Sport Sciences. *Nutr. Res. Prac.* **2014**, *8*, 713–718. [CrossRef]
10. World Health Organization. *Mean Body Mass Index (BMI)*; WHO: Geneva, Switzerland, 2019.
11. Garner, D. The Eating Attitudes Test (EAT-26). Available online: https://www.eat-26.com/interpretation/ and https://www.eat-26.com/scoring/ (accessed on 10 February 2022).
12. Treasure, J.; Duarte, T.A.; Schmidt, U. Eating disorders. *Lancet* **2020**, *395*, 899–911. [CrossRef]
13. Curylo, A. Body image in men with eating disorders—A case report. *Psychotherapy* **2016**, *4*, 57–70.
14. Yu, Z.; Tan, M. Disordered Eating Behaviors and Food Addiction among Nutrition Major College Students. *Nutrients* **2016**, *8*, 673. [CrossRef]
15. Tavolacci, M.P.; Grigioni, S.; Richard, L.; Meyrignac, G.; Déchelotte, P.; Ladner, J. Eating disorders and associated health risks among college students. *J. Nutr. Wyk. Behav.* **2015**, *47*, 412–420. [CrossRef]
16. Drummond, D.; Hare, M.S. Dietitians and eating disorders: An international issue. *Can. J. Diet. Pract. Res.* **2012**, *73*, 86–90. [CrossRef]
17. Poinhos, R.; Alves, D.; Vieira, E.; Pinhao, S.; Oliveira, B.M.; Correia, F. Eating behavior among undergraduate students. Comparing nutrition students with other courses. *Appetite* **2015**, *84*, 28–33. [CrossRef]
18. Kolka, M.; Abayomi, J. Body image dissatisfaction among food-related degree students. *Nutr. Food Sci.* **2012**, *42*, 139–147. [CrossRef]

19. Kassier, S.; Veldman, F. Eating behavior, eating attitude and body mass index of dietetic students versus non-dietetic majors: A South African perspective. *S. Afr. J. Clin. Nutr.* **2014**, *27*, 109–113.
20. Izydorczyk, B. Body image disturbances and personality structure in people with anorexia and bulimia nervosa. *Psychiatry Dipl.* **2017**, *14*, 16–22.
21. Bialokoz-Kalinowska, I.; Kierus, K.; Piotrowska; Jastrzebska, J. Eating disorders in adolescents-initial diagnosis in the primary care physician's office. *Pediatr. Med. Rodz.* **2012**, *8*, 298–303.
22. El-Azeem Taha, A.A.A.; Abu-Zaid, H.A.; El-Sayed Desouky, D. Eating Disorders Among Female Students of Taif University, Saudi Arabia. *Arch. Iran. Med.* **2018**, *21*, 111–117.
23. Jasik, I. Mental bulimia-modern adolescents in the snare of eating disorders. *TYGIEL Sci. Publ. House* **2018**, *5*, 123–140.
24. Brandt, L.M.T.; Fernandes, L.H.F.; Aragãoc, A.S.; Luna, T.P.D.C.; Feliciano, R.M.; Auad, S.M.; Cavalcanti, A.L. Risk Behavior For Bulimia Among Adolescents. *Rev. Paul. Pediatr.* **2019**, *37*, 217–224. [CrossRef]
25. Toral, N.; Gubert, M.B.; Spaniol, A.M.; Monteiro, R.A. Eating disorders and body image satisfaction among Brazilian undergraduate nutrition students and dietitians. *Arch. Latinoam. Nutr.* **2016**, *66*, 129–134.
26. Khalsa, S.S.; Hassanpour, M.S.; Strober, M.; Craske, M.G.; Arevian, A.C.; Feusner, J.D. Interoceptive Anxiety and Body Representation in Anorexia Nervosa. *Front. Psychiatry* **2018**, *9*, 444. [CrossRef]
27. Chávez-Rosales, E.; Camacho Ruíz, E.J.; Maya Martínez, M.D.L.Á.; Márquez Molina, O. Conductas alimentarias y sintomatología de trastornos del comportamiento alimentario en estudiantes de nutrición. *Mex. J. Eat. Disord.* **2012**, *3*, 29–37.
28. Memon, A.A.; Adil, S.E.; Siddiqui, E.U.; Naeem, S.S.; Ali, S.A.; Mehmood, K. Eating disorders in medical students of Karachi, Pakistan-a cross-sectional study. *BMC Res. Notes* **2012**, *5*, 84. [CrossRef]
29. Harris, N.; Gee, D.; d'Acquisto, D.; Ogan, D.; Pritchett, K. Eating disorder risk, exercise dependence and body weight dissatisfaction among female nutrition and exercise science university majors. *J. Behav. Addict.* **2015**, *4*, 206–209. [CrossRef]
30. Saleh, R.N.; Salameh, R.A.; Yhya, H.H.; Sweileh, W.M. Disordered eating attitudes in female students of An-Najah National University: A cross-sectional study. *J. Eat. Disord.* **2018**, *6*, 1–6. [CrossRef]
31. Mealha, V.; Ferreira, C.; Guerra, I.; Ravasco, P. Students of dietetics & nutrition; a high risk group for eating disorders? *Nutr. Hosp.* **2013**, *28*, 1558–1566.
32. Trindade, A.P.; Appolinario, J.C.; Mattos, P.; Treasure, J.; Nazar, B.P. Eating disorder symptoms in Brazilian university students: A systematic review and meta-analysis. *Braz. J. Psychiatry.* **2019**, *41*, 179–187. [CrossRef]
33. Moehlecke, M.; Blume, C.A.; Cureau, F.V.; Kieling, C.; Schaan, B.D. Self-perceived body image, dissatisfaction with body weight and nutritional status of Brazilian adolescents: A nationwide study. *J. Pediatr.* **2020**, *96*, 76–83. [CrossRef]

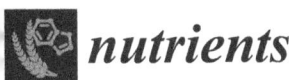

Article

Prevalence of Emotional Eating in Groups of Students with Varied Diets and Physical Activity in Poland

Mateusz Grajek [1,2,*], Karolina Krupa-Kotara [3], Agnieszka Białek-Dratwa [4], Wiktoria Staśkiewicz [5], Mateusz Rozmiarek [6], Ewa Misterska [7] and Krzysztof Sas-Nowosielski [2]

[1] Department of Public Health, Faculty of Health Sciences in Bytom, Medical University of Silesia in Katowice, 41902 Bytom, Poland
[2] Department of Humanistic Foundations of Physical Culture, Faculty of Physical Education, Jerzy Kukuczka Academy of Physical Education in Katowice, 40065 Katowice, Poland
[3] Department of Epidemiology, Faculty of Health Sciences in Bytom, Medical University of Silesia in Katowice, 41902 Bytom, Poland
[4] Department of Human Nutrition, Faculty of Health Sciences in Bytom, Medical University of Silesia in Katowice, 41902 Bytom, Poland
[5] Department of Technology and Food Quality Evaluation, Faculty of Health Sciences in Bytom, Medical University of Silesia in Katowice, 41902 Bytom, Poland
[6] Department of Sports Tourism, Faculty of Physical Culture Sciences, Poznan University of Physical Education, 61871 Poznan, Poland
[7] Department of Pedagogy and Psychology, Faculty of Social Studies in Poznan, Poznan School of Security, 60778 Poznan, Poland
* Correspondence: mgrajek@sum.edu.pl

Citation: Grajek, M.; Krupa-Kotara, K.; Białek-Dratwa, A.; Staśkiewicz, W.; Rozmiarek, M.; Misterska, E.; Sas-Nowosielski, K. Prevalence of Emotional Eating in Groups of Students with Varied Diets and Physical Activity in Poland. *Nutrients* **2022**, *14*, 3289. https://doi.org/10.3390/nu14163289

Academic Editors: Roser Granero, Susana Jiménez-Murcia, Fernando Fernández-Aranda and Paolo Brambilla

Received: 9 July 2022
Accepted: 10 August 2022
Published: 11 August 2022

Publisher's Note: MDPI stays neutral with regard to jurisdictional claims in published maps and institutional affiliations.

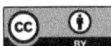

Copyright: © 2022 by the authors. Licensee MDPI, Basel, Switzerland. This article is an open access article distributed under the terms and conditions of the Creative Commons Attribution (CC BY) license (https://creativecommons.org/licenses/by/4.0/).

Abstract: Background: Emotional eating (EE) is not a separate eating disorder, but rather a type of behavior within a group of various eating behaviors that are influenced by habits, stress, emotions, and individual attitudes toward eating. The relationship between eating and emotions can be considered on two parallel levels: psychological and physiological. In the case of the psychological response, stress generates a variety of bodily responses relating to coping with stress. Objective: Therefore, the main objective of this study was to evaluate and compare the prevalence of emotional eating in groups of students in health-related and non-health-related fields in terms of their differential health behaviors—diet and physical activity levels. Material and Methods: The cross-sectional survey study included 300 individuals representing two groups of students distinguished by their fields of study—one group was in health-related fields (HRF) and the other was in non-health-related fields (NRF). The study used standardized questionnaires: the PSS-10 and TFEQ-13. Results: The gender of the subjects was as follows: women, 60.0% (174 subjects) (HRF: 47.1%, n= 82; NRF: 52.9%, n = 92); men, 40.0% (116 subjects) (HRF: 53.4%, n = 62; NRF: 46.6%, n = 54). The age of the subjects was 26 years (±2 years). Based on the results of the TFEQ-13, among 120 subjects (41.4%) there were behaviors consistent with limiting food intake (HRF: 72.4%; NRF: 11.0%), while 64 subjects (20.7%) were characterized by a lack of control over food intake (HRF: 13.8%, 20 subjects; NRF: 27.4%, 20 subjects). Emotional eating was characteristic of 106 students (37.9%), with the NRF group dominating (61.6%, n = 90). It was observed that a high PSS-10 score is mainly characteristic of individuals who exhibit EE. Conclusions: The results obtained in the study indicate that lifestyle can have a real impact on the development of emotional eating problems. Individuals who are characterized by elevated BMI values, unhealthy diets, low rates of physical activity, who underestimate meal size in terms of weight and calories, and have high-stress feelings are more likely to develop emotional eating. These results also indicate that further research in this area should be undertaken to indicate whether the relationships shown can be generalized.

Keywords: emotional eating (EE); diet; physical activity; field of study; stress

1. Introduction

Emotional eating (EE) is not a separate eating disorder, but rather a type of behavior within a group of various eating behaviors that are influenced by habits, stress, emotions, and individual attitudes toward eating [1]. The relationship between eating and emotions can be considered on two parallel levels: psychological and physiological. In the case of the psychological response, stress generates a variety of bodily responses relating to coping with stress; a person under stress seeks to minimize feelings of tension accompanying given situations [2]. In physiological terms, stress, due to activation of the nervous system, causes an increase or decrease in appetite which is the basis for changes in eating behavior [1].

In a stressful situation, a person implements a series of specific activities known as stress coping. These mechanisms are aimed at changing the situation in which the individual finds himself and improving the persistent emotional state [3,4]. These actions are focused on a task-oriented approach to the problem causing stress, its solution, emotional self-regulation regarding tension, and alleviation of negative emotional states [2].

In stressful situations, eating seems to be one of the most common, simplest, and least conscious actions, and it is independent of the body weight or eating behavior of those responding in this way. In a stressful situation, eating becomes a factor in relieving emotional tension. It is used for this purpose for several reasons [3–5]. (1) Food is readily available nowadays, associated with a large number of grocery stores, restaurants, bars, cafes, pastry stores, and outlets where fast-food dishes and sweet and salty snacks (which persons reach for most often in a stressful situation) can be easily obtained. (2) Eating does not require the participation of other persons. The preparation of a full meal as well as a quick snack (candy, chips, crackers) does not have to depend on the presence or skill of other persons, nor on the skill of the person reducing emotional tension with food. (3) Eating is socially acceptable, which means that eating under stress does not elicit negative judgments or comments from others, unlike alcohol, cigarettes or psychoactive substances, the use of which can also stem from a desire to reduce stress. (4) Food has a strong positive connotation, mainly through associations dating back to early childhood; food is associated with the presence of the mother, a sense of security, emotional closeness, and joy.

Emotional eating (EE), unlike specific eating disorders, is not associated with a complete loss of control over the quantity and quality of food consumed. Affected individuals can stop eating at any time while experiencing the relief associated with relieving emotional tension and stress [6]. Unfortunately, because EE is not explicitly recognized as an eating disorder, but rather an eating phenomenon, there are no homogeneous diagnostic criteria, and presumptions about the prevalence of EE are based on psychometric tools popularly used in research [4]. Epidemiological data on stress eating syndrome is unknown, due to the possibly high profile of the problem, but it is known that stress eating is more common in persons with obesity [5]. It is also possible that sociodemographic and psychosocial factors such as gender, age, education, occupation, income level, stress resistance, and emotion regulation strategies have a real impact on the incidence of this condition [3]. The main exposure group, in this case, seems to be young persons who are affected by the modern rush of life and maybe more strongly exposed to stressors due to their work and education [4]. One way to counteract obesity is to expend energy through regular physical activity. In addition to the benefits of weight reduction, those who are physically active may see a reduction in low back and joint pain, improved fitness and performance, as well as improved well-being and increased self-esteem [7]. It is worth noting that physical activity plays an important role in obesity prevention not only among the elderly [8], but above all has a huge impact on shaping individuals already in childhood and adolescence, thus contributing to a reduced risk of obesity in adulthood [9]. Unfortunately, adults, due to their desire for rapid improvements in their health, often engage in risky behavior in terms of physical activity, led by the use and abuse of sports supplements [10] or the practice of unhealthy or even life-threatening diets [11]. Therefore, activities aimed at promoting physical activity among the public in a sustainable manner, for example by local governments [12] or healthcare professionals [13], are extremely important.

The main objective of this study was to evaluate and compare the prevalence of emotional eating in groups students in health related and non-health related fields in terms of their differential health behaviors—diet and physical activity levels.

The following research hypotheses were posed in preparation for the study:

1. Emotional eating is more common among persons who have a non-rational diet.
2. Emotional eating is more common among individuals who represent a low level of physical activity.
3. Emotional eating is more common among persons who underestimate the size and calorie portions of foods.
4. Emotional eating is more common among persons who exhibit high levels of daily life stress.

2. Materials and Methods

2.1. Study Background

The study is a continuation of the research presented in the paper: Grajek, M.; Krupa-Kotara, K.; Sas-Nowosielski, K.; Misterska, E.; Kobza, J. Prevalence of Orthorexia in Groups of Students with Varied Diets and Physical Activity (Silesia, Poland). Nutrients 2022, 14, 2816. https://doi.org/10.3390/nu1414281. Hence, the methodological description of the study, the characteristics of the group, and the description of the main indicators (diet, level of physical activity, ability to estimate portion size, and calorie content of a meal) are the same for both studies.

2.2. Sample Group

The study included 300 individuals representing equally sized groups of students from two fields of study, health-related fields (HRF) and non-health-related fields (NRF). The sample size was estimated based on the minimum sample size formula, and the data substituted from the formula took into account the total number of students of a given year at a given university. This ensured that a representative group of survey participants was achieved. The survey questionnaire was directed to all students of a particular year and field of study. The return rate of the questionnaire was estimated at 82.5%.

All subjects were students in the final year of their master's degree (second year of their sophomore year):

- HRF group (144 subjects): dietetics (Medical University of Silesia in Katowice) was studied by 48.6% of the subjects (n = 80), and physical education (Academy of Physical Education in Katowice) by 51.4% of the subjects (n = 74).
- NRF group (146 subjects): management (University of Economics in Katowice) was studied by 47.3% of the subjects (n = 69), and computer science (Silesian University of Technology) by 52.7% (n = 77).

Based on an abbreviated medical history, it was noted that 5.2% (15 subjects) were diagnosed with chronic diseases; these were seasonal allergies—diseases that do not significantly affect their lifestyles. The main addiction in the surveyed groups was smoking, to which 3.8% of students (11 persons) admitted. No persons compulsively consumed alcohol or took other psychoactive drugs.

2.3. Eligibility Criteria

The HRF group consisted of 150 final-year students with majors in dietetics and physical education. The rationale for selecting this group was the fact that they have in-depth and professional knowledge in the field of rational nutrition and physical activity. The NRF group consisted of 150 students in their final year of second-degree studies with majors in management and computer science. The rationale for selecting this group was the fact that they did not have in-depth and professional knowledge in the field of rational nutrition and physical activity, at least at the university level. The assumption for the selection of these majors was that the gender groups were more or less equal. Such majors as dietetics and management are more often chosen by females, and physical education or computer science by males.

Individuals in the NRF group showing concurrent education (or past education) in a health-related field were excluded from the study. Individuals who had applied knowledge and skills in rational nutrition and physical activity in their professional work were treated similarly. The physiological state of the respondent was also taken into account. Persons suffering from diseases that influence the diet and/or physical activity of the respondent (e.g., allergies, food intolerances, metabolic diseases, tumors, etc.) were excluded from the research. The same was applied to subjects who represented a specific dietary model (elimination diet or pregnancy and puerperium).

The study was limited to students in their final year of study because, in the authors' opinion, they are highly likely to have a broad knowledge of health sciences and physical culture sciences (in the case of health students). In the case of the second group, it was also decided to include students in their final year of study so as not to disrupt the inclusion criteria and to deal with a relatively homogeneous group of students.

The study was approved by the Bioethics Committee of the Medical University of Silesia in Katowice, in light of the Act on Medical and Dental Professions of 5 December 1996, which includes a definition of medical experimentation. The study participants consciously agreed to participate in the study.

2.4. Research Tools

Body mass index was calculated using the formula: BMI (kg/m^2) = body weight (kg)/height (m)^2. The results were then interpreted using a scale [14]: ≥ 30.00 kg/m^2, obesity; 25.00–29.99 kg/m^2, overweight; 18.50–24.99 kg/m^2, normal body weight; 17.00–18.49 kg/m^2, underweight; and ≤ 16.99 kg/m^2, malnutrition.

In the assessment of dietary intake, the author's tool based on nutrition standards for the Polish population [15] was used, which included 20 dietary indices (e.g., frequency of consumption of individual product groups, number of meals during the day, regularity of meals during the day, snacking, fluids consumed). Respondents chose 'yes' or 'no' next to a given question about nutrition. One point was awarded for each correct answer (by the applied standards), so the highest possible total score was 20. To prioritize the results, the following scale was adopted: 18–20 points, very good nutrition; 14–17 points, good; 10–13 points, moderate; ≤ 9 points, poor nutrition. The questionnaire has been used previously by the authors as part of another study [16]. The tool was validated by initially sharing it with a group of 10 topic specialists. These individuals had the opportunity to add suggestions and revisions to the questions. The questions were revised according to the most common suggestions made by the specialists. The questionnaire was then made available twice to a group of 30 adults (two weeks apart). Based on the measurements, π Scott's coefficient was calculated. For questions 1–3, 5–10, 12–15, and 18–20 a relevance of 0.93 (very good) was obtained. For questions 4, 11, 16, and 17 a relevance of 0.72 (good) was obtained.

Based on the physical activity score in the questionnaire, respondents were assigned a physical activity index (PAL) based on current recommendations for physical activity [14]: 1.2, no physical activity; 1.4, low physical activity (approximately 140 min per week); 1.6, medium physical activity (approximately 280 min per week); 1.8, high physical activity (approximately 420 min per week); and 2.0, very high physical activity (approximately 560 min per week).

The PSS-10 is used to assess the intensity of stress related to one's living situation over the past month. The scale is designed mainly for research purposes and can be used in practice, screening, prevention, and assessing the effectiveness of therapeutic interventions. Scores from 0 to 13 are considered low, while scores of 20 and above are considered high. Internal consistency was checked in a study of a 120-person group of adults, yielding a Cronbach's alpha index of 0.86. The correlation of all questions with the overall scale score is satisfactory. Reliability determined by testing a group of 30 students twice at an interval of two days was 0.90, and at an interval of four weeks was 0.72 [17].

With the TFEQ-13, it is possible to assess three behaviors using 13 questions comprising three subscales: five questions relate to eating restriction (questions 1, 9, 10, 12, and 13), five questions relate to lack of control over eating (questions 2, 5–7, and 11), and three questions are directly related to eating under the influence of emotions (EE) (questions 2, 4, and 8). The questionnaire contains standardized answers on a four-point scale ranging from zero to three. The respondent marks the most defining statement next to each sentence: 'definitely yes', 'rather yes', 'rather no', and 'definitely no'. Values are calculated separately for each subscale. The higher the score obtained, the higher the strength of the behavior. Internal consistency alpha Cronbach's coefficient for the entire scale was 0.78, and for the subscales it was 0.78 for eating restriction, 0.76 for lack of control over eating, and 0.72 for eating under the influence of emotions. All subscales correlated with each other significantly positively ($p < 0.001$) [18], of which only the score indicating EE was used in the present study.

2.5. Study Procedure

The study consisted of a survey questionnaire and an album of sample foods and dishes. The study was conducted according to scientific ethics, anonymity rules, and the RODO clause (Polish Law on Respect for Classified Information). The survey was conducted using an online form, which is an acceptable method in psychological research. The link to the questionnaire was distributed to participants using email boxes dedicated by the university. During data collection, methods were used to prevent fake/bot responder phenomenon by checking login times and questionnaire completion times. In addition, the questionnaire was secured with a CAPCHTA key. The questionnaire of the survey consisted of a metric (data of the subject: gender, age, a field of study and occupation, and anthropometric data—declared height and body weight); the author's questionnaire of dietary habits based on the guidelines and standards of the National Institute of Public Health and the National Center for Nutrition Education [15]; questions about physical activity practiced and its level based on WHO guidelines [14]; the Perceived Stress Scale—PSS-10 (polish adaptation) [19]; and the Three-Factor Food Questionnaire (TFEQ-13). The survey questionnaire was available online May–June 2021.

In the second stage of the study, respondents were presented with a scrapbook containing sample foods and dishes. An album of sample foods and dishes was used to verify the ability to estimate the size and calorie content of portions, consisting of 12 photographs consistent with the division of foods into 12 groups (one photograph per group) [18]. The study using the album was conducted with the sensory panel of the Department of Dietetics, Faculty of Health Sciences in Bytom, Silesian Medical University in Katowice, Poland, July–August 2021. Before each study, visual perception (perception of images) was tested using a scrapbook. For this purpose, selected Ishihara boards and optical illusion boards were used. Both tools are commonly used to assess so-called visual daltonism and the perception of objects in pictures (e.g., size, shape, length). To link the results of the questionnaire with the album, each participant of the study was given an individual number while filling in the questionnaire, which was then also entered into the album.

2.6. Statistical Analysis

Tables were prepared for all extracted data from the survey questionnaire, and descriptive statistics (percentages (%), counts (N; n), mean (X), standard deviations (SD)) were calculated. Detailed statistical analyses were conducted, regarding the demonstration of differences between the represented behaviors (pro-health or anti-health) and the occurrence of EE in the sample group. To analyze the above material, the chi-square (χ^2) test and the V-Cramér (V) coefficient of the strength of the relationship (with Yates and Fisher's correction) were used. A probability level of $p = 0.05$ was assumed for the study.

3. Results

The gender of the subjects was as follows: women, 60.0%, 184 subjects (HRF: 30.6%, n = 92; NRF: 30.6%, n = 92); men, 40.0%, 116 subjects (HRF: 20.6%, n = 62; NRF: 18.2%, n = 54). The age of the subjects was 26 years (±2 years). More than 269 persons (89.9%) lived in large cities (defined as more than 100,000 residents), 23 persons (7.5%) lived in smaller cities (defined as less than 100,000 residents), and 8 persons (2.6%) lived in rural areas. Only 13.1% of respondents (38 persons) had permanent employment, i.e., in the telecommunications, service, and administrative/office sectors. Of the surveyed group, 75.6% had an income of an average level, 12.2% had an above-average income, and 12.2% had a below-average income (the minimum wage in Poland in 2021 was PLN 3010—about €630). Statistically, the groups did not differ in the above variables (Table 1).

Table 1. Comparison of the studied groups (N = 300; HRF = 150; NRF = 150).

Group		HRF	NRF	Total	χ^2	p-Value
Gender	Female	92 (30.6%)	92 (30.6%)	184 (61.2%)	21.391	
	Male	62 (20.6%)	54 (18.2%)	116 (38.8%)	29.122	
Age		26 ± 2 *	26 ± 2 *	26 ± 2 *	18.974	
Residence	Large city	139 (46.3%)	130 (43.6%)	269 (89.9%)	32.004	$p > 0.05$
	Small city	12 (4.0%	11 (3.5%)	23 (7.5%)	35.680	
	Rural area	3 (1.0%)	5 (1.6%)	8 (2.6%)	31.404	
Income		PLN 3000 ± 500 * (€600 ± 120) *	PLN 3000 ± 450 * (€600 ± 100) *	PLN 3000 ± 475 * (€600 ± 110) *	28.901	

HRF, health-related field; NRF, non-health-related field; χ^2, chi-square test; * mean ± standard deviation.

Regarding BMI, more than 15.2% of the subjects were characterized as underweight (44 subjects in the HRF group). Normal weight was a characteristic of 178 subjects (61.3%). Overweight and obesity were present only in the NRF group, with a total of 68 subjects (23.4%). Based on the results of the dietary assessment, it was found that the best dietary model was characterized by the HRF group; in this group, 97.2% of students were characterized by a very good and good dietary mode (84.0%, 121 persons; 13.4%, 19 persons, respectively). The NRF group, on the other hand, was dominated by sufficient dietary mode, at 64.4% of all cases in this group (94 persons). Less popular was the dietary model marked as "good", with only 24.6% of this group (36 persons). It should be emphasized that an incorrect dietary pattern was represented only by persons from the HRF group (3.9% of the total number of subjects, 11 persons).

Low physical activity in the PAL index was characteristic for 46.2% of respondents (122 persons), and most often chosen by persons from the NRF group (79.5%, 97 persons). Medium physical activity was observed in 25.7% of the respondents (68 persons); this activity concerned both the HRF group (33.8%, 48 persons) and the NRF group (16.4%, 20 persons). Physical activity at a high and very high level concerned 28.1% of the students (75 persons). These were mainly persons from the HRF group (48.4%, 70 persons). However, two individuals from the HRF and 24 individuals from the NRF group did not engage in any physical exercise daily (1.4% vs. 16.4%).

Taking into account the test of estimating the size and caloric content of portions, it was found that 32.4% (94 persons) overestimated the size of the portions of products and dishes indicated in the photographs. In this group, there were mostly persons studying in health faculties (57.6%, 83 persons); less often, there were persons from other faculties (7.5%, 11 persons). In the case of underestimation (33.8%, n = 98), the situation was reversed—persons from the NRF group mainly underestimated the size of products and dishes (56.2%, n = 82); in the HRF group, much fewer persons underestimated (11.1%, n = 16). The remaining persons correctly indicated the size of the portion (33.8%, 98 persons). Analyzing the results of the test on the ability to estimate the calorie content of portions based on photographs, it was observed that 35.8% (104 persons) overestimated the calorie content of the products and dishes indicated in the photographs. This group included mainly health-related persons (58.3%, 84 persons), and less frequently, non-health-related persons (13.0%, 19 persons). On the other hand, in the case of underestimation of the energy of dishes (35.2%, n = 102), persons from the NRF group mostly underestimated the caloric value of products and dishes presented in the album (55.5%, n = 81); in the HRF group, such cases were much less (15.3%, n = 22). The remaining persons correctly indicated the calorie content of the portion (29.0%, n = 84).

The respondents' level of perceived stress was measured twice—before and after the survey—and since no statistically significant relationship was shown between the measurements, it was decided to average these results ($p > 0.05$). Analysis of the PSS-10 questionnaire showed that 86.7% (130 persons) of the HRF group and 46.7% (70 persons) of the NRF group had low levels of stress. Correspondingly, 23.3% (20 persons) in the HRF and 53.3% (80 persons) in the NRF show elevated levels of stress. One question of the scale concerned the frequency of stressful situations that exceed the body's resilience and result in feelings of discomfort, aggression, and jitteriness. Both the HRF and NRF groups had an average score measuring between two and three points—2.41 for the HRF and 2.56 for the NRF, which indicates that in the frequency of stressful situations in life the group can be considered homogeneous.

Based on the results of the TFEQ-13, among 120 subjects (41.4%) there were behaviors consistent with limiting food intake (HRF, 72.4%; NRF, 11.0%), while 64 subjects (20.7%) were characterized by a lack of control over food intake (HRF: 13.8%, 20 subjects; NRF: 27.4%, 20 subjects). Emotional eating was characteristic of 106 students (37.9%), with the NRF group dominating (61.6%, n = 90). It was observed that a high PSS-10 score is mainly characteristic of individuals who exhibit EE ($\chi^2 = 10.279$; V = 0.731; $p = 0.001$): PSS-10 average score in HRF group was 29 ± 2 and NRF group it was 34 ± 2 ($\chi^2 = 11.893$; V = 0.657; $p = 0.001$). Slightly higher high-stress scores were observed in representatives of the NRF group. These results were compared with those of PSS-10, and details of the analysis are shown in Table 2.

Table 2. Comparison of PSS-10 and TFEQ-13 scores in the study group (N = 300; HRF = 150; NRF = 150).

	Group		HRF		NRF		Total	χ^2	V	p-Value
			All	Only EE Cases (by TFEQ-13)	All	Only EE Cases (by TFEQ-13)				
PSS-10	Low perceived stress	200 (66.67%)	130 (86.70%)	8 (8.48%)	70 (46.70%)	19 (20.14%)	200 (66.67%)	12.113	0.611	0.003 *
	Average score		7 ± 1	9 ± 2	11 ± 1	12 ± 1	10.8 ± 0.9	11.244	0.522	0.002 *
	High perceived stress	100 (33.33%)	20 (23.30%)	8 (8.48%)	80 (53.30%)	71 (75.26%)	100 (33.33%)	10.279	0.731	0.001 *
	Average score		27 ± 1	29 ± 2	32 ± 2	34 ± 2	30.8 ± 1.0	11.893	0.657	0.001 *

HRF, health-related field; NRF, non-health-related field; χ^2, chi-square test; V, V-Cramer; PSS-10, perceived stress scale; EE, emotional eating; TFEQ-13, Three-Factor Eating Questionnaire; * p-value statistical significance.

Another analysis concerns the group in which EE behavior was demonstrated (n = 106). High BMI values were present in the NRF group, indicating a statistically significant relationship between the indicated characteristics ($\chi^2 = 13.238$; V = 0.723; $p = 0.0001$). Similarly, the same was true for diet. Individuals representing a good (27.6%) and very good (16.2%) diet are less likely to belong to the group of those with an increased risk of emotional eating. In this case, there was also a statistically significant correlation associated with NRF group membership ($\chi^2 = 10.984$; V = 0.683; $p = 0.0001$). Next, it was decided to verify the relationship between the occurrence of emotive eating and the level of physical activity represented. Based on the statistical inference performed, it was found that low PAL values were present in NRF subjects, indicating the presence of a statistically significant relationship between the indicated characteristics ($\chi^2 = 8.117$; $V = 0.597$; $p = 0.002$). On the statistical analyses conducted, it should be concluded that both in the case of estimating portion size and caloricity of meals there is a statistical relationship: NRF subjects characterized by emotional eating are more likely to underestimate the size and caloricity of the meal ($\chi^2 = 12.467$; $V = 0.601$; $p = 0.0001/\chi^2 = 11.551$; $V = 0.582$; $p = 0.0001$). The last verification concerned the relationship between the occurrence of emotional eating in the study group and the level of perceived stress. Higher levels of stress have been shown to occur in NRF individuals ($\chi^2 = 9.963$; $V = 0.699$; $p = 0.015$)—Table 3.

Table 3. Scores of subscales on emotional eating by selected indicators (N = 106; HRF = 16; NRF = 90).

	Group	HRF	NRF	Total	χ^2	V	p-Value
BMI	Malnutrition	0	0	0	13.238	0.723	0.0001 *
	Underweight	0	0	0			
	Normoweight	10 (10.60%)	22 (23.32%)	38 (40.28%)			
	Overweight	6 (6.36%)	55 (58.30%)	61 (64.66%)			
	Obesity	0	7 (7.42%)	7 (7.42%)			
Diet quality	Poor	0	3 (3.18%)	3 (3.18%)	10.984	0.683	0.0001 *
	Moderate	2 (2.12%)	72 (76.32%)	74 (78.44%)			
	Good	14 (14.84%)	15 (15.90%)	29 (30.74%)			
	Very Good	0	0	0			
PAL	PAL 1.4	4 (4.24%)	34 (36.04%)	3 (3.18%)	8.117	0.597	0.002 *
	PAL 1.6	12 (12.72%)	31 (32.86%)	43 (45.58%)			
	PAL 1.8	0	25 (26.50%)	25 (26.50%)			
	PAL 2.0	0	0	0			
Portion size	Underestimation	0	56 (59.36%)	56 (59.36%)	12.467	0.601	0.0001 *
	Estimate	16 (16.96%)	34 (36.04%)	50 (53.00%)			
	Revaluation	0	0	0			
Caloric size	Underestimation	6 (6.36%)	45 (47.70%)	51 (54.06%)	11.551		0.0001 *
	Estimate	10 (10.60%)	34 (36.04%)	44 (46.64%)			
	Revaluation	0	11 (11.66%)	11 (11.66%)			
PSS-10	Low	8 (8.48%)	19 (20.14%)	37 (39.22%)	9.963	0.699	0.015 *
	High	8 (8.48%)	71 (75.26%)	79 (83.74%)			

HRF, health-related field; NRF, non-health-related field; χ^2, chi-square test; V, V-Cramer; BMI, Body Mass Index; PAL, physical activity level; PSS-10, perceived stress scale; * p-value statistical significance.

4. Discussion

Under conditions of prolonged negative emotions, vulnerable people take action to change a given situation and improve their mental state. Often these actions are not taken consciously but are only performed intuitively. One way to intuitively cope with stress is to reach for food, as hunger is often mistaken for feelings of stress. Stress is closely linked to nutrition, not least because the elevated cortisol levels in this state trigger feelings of hunger [20]. In addition, stress increases the demand for serotonin (5-hydroxytryptamine), which in turn results in an increased demand for carbohydrates, which affect the release of endorphins and increase serotonin synthesis [21].

According to Kosicka-Gębska et al., 22% of the Polish population reaches for sweets in situations that cause stress [22]. The reason that sweets are the most common choice of food during stress is related to several factors. One of them is the increased need for carbohydrates [21,23,24]. Stress accelerates the breakdown of serotonin, so it is more common to feel the urge to introduce sugars into the body to make up for serotonin deficiencies. However, the soothing effect of serotonin is temporary, lasting about three hours, and once its levels are reduced again, the desire for sweet foods is restored [25]. Carbohydrates activate insulin, which in turn stimulates the brain to produce tryptophan, a precursor to serotonin. When the body's serotonin levels drop, people may feel depressed or stressed. Therefore, they reach for sugary foods, which will again cause serotonin to be secreted and reduce feelings of stress [26]. The effect of serotonin is that people feel calmer and sleepier; people stop thinking about stress after a meal rich in carbohydrates and scant protein [27].

The author of the term 'emotional eating', Hilda Bruch [28,29], as well as many modern researchers [30–32], assume that excessive food intake under the influence of emotions is the result of a failure to adequately distinguish between physiological hunger signals and emotional hunger. This results in excessive food intake (to reduce negative emotions) and weight gain [33,34]. Another explanation is the vicious cycle mechanism of food-mediated emotion regulation, according to which negative emotions are the source of physiological stimulation misidentified as feelings of hunger. This stimulus contributes to the immediate consumption of food, which consequently leads to a temporary reduction in negative emotions. Subsequently, the level of negative emotions increases again, which is associated with further food intake and progressive weight gain [35,36].

Van Strien et al. studied the relationship between emotions (joy and sadness) and eating, with highly emotional participants eating significantly more in a sad mood than in a joyful mood [37]. Macht et al. found that before the exam, participants in the stress group reported higher ratings of negative emotions (tension, fear, or emotional distress) and lower ratings of positive emotions (happiness, relaxation, or positive mood), with a corresponding higher tendency to eat to distract from the stress. These findings underscore the importance of capturing positive and negative emotions when examining associations with eating behavior [38]. Not only can positive emotions be associated with eating, but also how the absence of pleasant emotions when experiencing unpleasant emotions can have an impact [37]. The finding that positive emotions can influence eating makes intuitive sense when considering the use of food as part of social rituals (such as birthdays, weddings, and religious events) [39]. The implication is that while individuals do not necessarily use food to regulate positive emotions, positive emotions can trigger increased consumption through associative learning. Alternatively, a positive emotional state can divert attention from the source of positive emotions, interfering with the conscious reduction of food intake [40].

Stress is the most commonly studied emotion in assessing eating behavior. Both chronic stress and temporary stress have been associated with higher food intake, with people eating more during periods of stress [41–44]. However, depression and sadness have also been reported as antecedents of eating behavior [45]. Boredom and emotional eating showed strong positive correlations [46], and people who were ashamed ate more in a taste test experiment, with no effect on guilt [47]. Aggression and anger were positively correlated with emotional eating [48].

Emotions were also found to influence the type of food eaten. Feelings of stress influenced food choices toward more palatable and less healthy meals [49,50], while motivation to eat to regulate negativity was associated with an unhealthy eating pattern [51]. These findings suggest that negative emotions can trigger unhealthy eating behaviors, and poor food choices, and food is used to regulate stressful or negative emotions in healthy and overweight individuals. If we consider the demands of daily life, using unhealthy foods to regulate negative emotional states can contribute to a steady increase in weight over time.

Individual differences also appear to be highly significant. For example, people with higher dietary restriction scores feel a greater desire to eat when asked to accept or suppress their emotions [52]. Sleep quality also requires attention. The combination of sleep deprivation and a propensity for emotional eating has been associated with increased food consumption [53]. Short sleep is thought to increase hunger and appetite through the effects it has on leptin and ghrelin, and sleep deprivation itself may act as an additional stressor [54,55]. Thus, poor sleep can potentially undermine or cancel out the effects of any intervention. Conversely, it is possible that adopting a good sleep pattern is part of an intervention that may enhance the effect of other interventions [56].

The study by Bennett et al. determined the relationship between emotional eating behaviors and the tendency to eat palatable foods among college students aged 19.6 ± 1.0 years. The mean BMI of the subjects was 24.1 ± 1.2 kg/m^2. There was a positive correlation between BMI and negative emotions and negative situations ($p < 0.01$). A one-unit increase in BMI resulted in a 0.293-unit increase in negative situation scores and a 0.626-unit increase in negative emotions scores [57].

Greene et al. found that college students who scored high on emotional eating had higher BMIs than students who scored lower on emotional eating. Therefore, understanding the importance of emotional eating may be particularly important in preventing weight gain during college, which can lead to obesity in adulthood [58]. Students frequently cited happiness and stress as the two most frequently experienced emotions. The main source of stress cited by students was school [59]. In particular, studying for exams, completing school assignments, and time management were cited as sources of stress.

Stress affected the eating behavior of men and women, but in opposite ways. Women increased consumption when they were stressed about school—as many as 62% of the women surveyed gave this answer. Under normal conditions, 80% reported making healthy food choices, but in a stressful situation, only 33% ate healthily [60]. A study conducted on a group of Australian students by Papier et al. found that more than half (52.9%) of the students suffered from stress, with relatively more women (57.4%) than men (47.4%). Female students who experienced mild to moderate stress were 2.22 times less likely to eat processed foods ($p < 0.01$) than non-stressed female students. Men who experienced mild to moderate levels of stress tended to eat more highly processed foods ($p < 0.05$) and drink more alcohol ($p < 0.05$) than non-stressed male students [61]. This may suggest a decrease in healthy food intake and an increase in unhealthy food intake during periods of emotional stress-eating.

A study by Lazarevich et al. examined the relationship between depressive symptoms, emotional eating, and BMI in Mexican college students. They found that depressive symptoms were associated with emotional eating in both men ($p < 0.001$) and women ($p < 0.001$), while emotional eating was associated with BMI and men ($p < 0.001$) and women ($p < 0.001$). The indirect effect of depression through emotional eating on BMI accounted for a significant portion of the total effect in both men (23.1%) and women (25%) [62].

Students are a high-risk group for the development of emotional eating disorders due to their exposure to numerous factors, i.e., stressful situations, peer pressure, and lack of time for physical activity. Fields of study related to 'health' in the broadest sense shape behavioral patterns that influence the maintenance of mental as well as physical health. Therefore, the results obtained in our study indicate better indicators in the aspect of emotional nutrition in this group.

5. Strengths and Limitations

The research on the prevalence of emotional eating among students of different majors allowed us to understand the basic mechanisms, cause–effect relationships, and determinants of the occurrence of the indicated disorders. Conducting the research required much work and preparation in the form of developing research tools and becoming familiar with existing psychometric tools measuring the risk of emotional eating. Of course, the paper does not suggest that it is the field of study that influences the development of the disorder, but rather that individuals who choose it are characterized by certain traits that predispose them to it. This should be understood in the way that, thanks to the results of the study, it is possible to detect groups of persons who should be included in the observation in

Childhood and adolescent obesity are associated with multi-organ system morbidity, which includes metabolic and musculoskeletal disturbances, cardiovascular comorbidities, and pulmonary complications, in addition to greater risk of premature death [4]. Accordingly, childhood/adolescent obesity is associated with a greater prevalence of cardiometabolic risk factors and with changes in the heart, including enlarged heart chambers, increased left ventricular mass, and decreased left ventricle ejection fraction [5,6]. In addition to physical comorbidities, children with excess weight are more prone to psychosocial distress than children of a healthy weight; this may be further impacted by bullying/teasing and the stigma of childhood obesity [7]. Childhood obesity increases the risk of obesity in adolescence, which then leads to a greater risk of obesity in adulthood [5]. Approximately 80% of those with obesity during adolescence will have obesity when they become adults, which decreases to around 70% when only considering adults aged >30 years [8]. Childhood and adolescent obesity are associated with a greater risk of obesity-related morbidities in adulthood, including cardiovascular disease, diabetes, and some cancers, as well as a greater risk of cardiovascular death [5,9,10].

Intervention at younger ages is associated with greater long-term decreases in body mass index (BMI) and larger reductions in the risk of future diseases, including cardiovascular conditions, type 2 diabetes, and certain cancers [4,11]. Consequently, the timely diagnosis/treatment of obesity in children and adolescents should be prioritized. Although there is now a better understanding of the complexities of obesity, treatment outcomes for childhood and adolescent obesity remain suboptimal [4,12]. Despite this, studies analyzing underlying obstacles to effective obesity management in adolescents living with obesity (ALwO) are scarce, and there are key evidence gaps in terms of the lived experiences, unmet needs, and challenges of ALwO, their caregivers, and their healthcare professionals (HCPs). A survey study in 11 countries that evaluated behaviors, attitudes, and perceptions of adults with obesity and HCPs reported a propensity for HCPs to delay the initiation of weight management conversations until complications develop [13]. As such, there remains a need to start conversations about weight at an early stage of patient management, before the development of obesity-related complications.

The Awareness, Care, and Treatment In Obesity maNagement (ACTION) Teens study was a global, cross-sectional survey study in 10 countries that aimed to identify behaviors, attitudes, perceptions, and barriers to effective obesity care among ALwO, caregivers of ALwO, and HCPs who treat ALwO [14]. ACTION Teens reported misalignment between the three groups, including a lack of understanding of the effect of obesity on ALwO by caregivers and misperception by HCPs of the motivators and barriers for their patients to lose weight [14]. Herein, we present ACTION Teens data from Spain and discuss the similarities and differences to the global ACTION Teens study. Identifying country-specific behaviors, attitudes, perceptions, and obstacles to obesity care will provide input for strategies with which to improve management of ALwO in Spain.

2. Materials and Methods

2.1. Study Design and Participants

ACTION Teens (ClinicalTrials.gov identifier: NCT05013359) was a cross-sectional, online survey study that collated data from three groups of respondents (ALwO, caregivers, and HCPs) in 10 countries/regions (Australia, Colombia, Italy, Mexico, Saudi Arabia, South Korea, Spain, Taiwan, Turkey, and the United Kingdom). The full methods for ACTION Teens have been published previously [14]. Participants from Spain were surveyed between August and December 2021 (ALwO and caregivers) or between August and September 2021 (HCPs).

For the Spanish cohort, the recruited ALwO were 12 to <18 years old and living in Spain. Obesity was defined as a BMI (calculated from self-reported height, weight, sex, and age) ≥95th percentile for sex and age based on World Health Organization charts (2007) [15]. The recruited caregivers were ≥25 years old, resided (≥50% of the time) with an ALwO in Spain, and participated in healthcare decisions for the ALwO. The recruited

HCPs were required to be practicing in Spain and to have been in clinical practice for 2 or more years. They were also required to spend ≥50% of their time directly caring for patients and to see 10 or more ALwO per month.

2.2. Survey Development

Three distinct but overlapping surveys (one each for ALwO, caregivers, and HCPs) were developed. A steering committee comprising content experts and HCPs co-developed and approved all survey materials. Translation and back-translation from the English version were conducted and accuracy was fulfilled. The questionnaires have been published previously in the Online Supporting Information section of the global ACTION Teens study manuscript [14].

2.3. Procedures

KJT Group Inc. (Rochester, NY, USA) oversaw data acquisition and reporting. An online survey utilizing Decipher Survey software (FocusVision Worldwide Inc., Stamford, CT, USA) was used for data collection. Online panels/databases were used to recruit caregivers and ALwO by targeting and screening adults from a stratified general population sample to identify caregivers of an ALwO. "Matched pairs" of ALwO and caregivers were maximized by asking verified caregivers for permission to enroll their ALwO. Following the maximization of the matched pairs, additional ALwO and caregivers were recruited to obtain the target sample size. HCPs were recruited from online physician panels/databases. Surveys were provided in Spanish and completed online by respondents or via in-person interviews (caregivers and ALwO only).

2.4. Outcomes

As described previously [14], the primary outcome measures included the following: attitudes about people with obesity and obesity, and beliefs related to the impact of obesity; attempts to lose weight in the last year, barriers/motivations to losing weight, and definition of successful weight loss/management; frequency/history of weight conversations including the initiator, and responsibility for starting conversations about weight between HCPs and ALwO/caregivers; interactions between HCPs, ALwO, and caregivers, frequency of diagnosing obesity, reasons for not discussing obesity, and follow-up appointments; and information sources for learning about healthy lifestyles, weight loss/management, and obesity. Five-point Likert scales, yes/no responses, numeric responses, and single/multiple item selection were used to assess outcome measures, as appropriate.

2.5. Sample Size

The target number of completed surveys for Spain was 650 for ALwO, 650 for caregivers, and 250 for HCPs. These sample sizes were chosen to ensure statistical power while maintaining recruitment feasibility.

2.6. Statistical Analysis

As described previously [14], the full analysis set comprised all those who answered the survey in its entirety. KJT Group Inc. analyzed de-identified data using Stata (version IC 14.2; StataCorp LLC, College Station, TX, USA), SPSS (version 23.0; IBM, Armonk, NY, USA) and Excel (Microsoft). Univariate descriptive statistics (proportions, medians, and means) were used to summarize data. For continuous variables, where appropriate, outliers were truncated to the median. For generalizability and mitigation of selection bias, caregiver data were weighted to demographic targets representative for Spain for region, sex, age, household income, and education. Demographic targets were aligned with Spanish census data and were based on data from the United States Census Bureau–International Data Base, World Education News and Reviews (WENR), and Instituto Nacional de Estadística (INE). The target adult general population sample was stratified to match these general population targets to ensure that the qualifying sample was largely representative of the adult population in Spain. The final incoming sample for the adult general population (i.e., the final caregiver sample), which included those failing to qualify for the survey, was then weighted to match the demographic targets. To obtain the nearest possible target and sample balance, weights were calculated using a raking technique; individual respondent weights were capped at 0.5 and 5.00 to avoid extreme design effects.

3. Results

3.1. Participant Characteristics

A total of 648 ALwO, 644 caregivers, and 251 HCPs were surveyed in Spain (Figure S1). The HCP response rate was 16.8%. Due to the recruitment methods, calculation of ALwO and caregiver response rates was not possible [14].

Table 1 shows the demographics and characteristics of the participants. Just over one-third (36%) of the ALwO were female, while almost half of the caregivers (45%) and HCPs (46%) were female. Approximately half (53%) of the ALwO and just over one-third (36%) of the caregivers indicated that the mother or father of the ALwO had overweight. Approximately 60% of the caregivers who answered the survey had overweight/obesity, and HCPs reported that 68% of their ALwO patients had family members with obesity in the household. HCPs' primary medical specialty and professional experience are reported in Table S1.

Table 1. Demographics and clinical characteristics of the ACTION Teens participants from Spain.

Demographic/Characteristic	Spain ALwO	Spain Caregivers	Spain HCPs
Full-country sample, n	648	644	251
Matched pair (ALwO and caregiver), n (%)	55 (8)	55 (9)	N/A
Unmatched, n (%)	593 (92)	589 (91)	N/A
Age in years, mean (SD)	15.0 (1.8)	40.7 (8.9)	43.2 (11.2)
Female, n (%) [a]	231 (36)	289 (45)	116 (46)
Male, n (%) [a]	417 (64)	355 (55)	135 (54)
BMI classification of ALwO [b]			
Obesity Class I	83% (n = 538)	80% (n = 517)	62% (SD: 19.9)
Obesity Class II	8% (n = 51)	13% (n = 85)	26% (SD: 12.3)
Obesity Class III	9% (n = 59)	7% (n = 42)	13% (SD: 11.1)
BMI classification of caregivers and HCPs, n (%) [c]			
Underweight (<18.5 kg/m^2)	N/A	7 (1)	5 (2)
Healthy weight (18.5–24.9 kg/m^2)	N/A	257 (40)	147 (67)
Overweight (25.0–29.9 kg/m^2)	N/A	251 (39)	53 (24)
Obesity Class I–III (≥30 kg/m^2)	N/A	129 (20)	14 (6)

[a] Percentage of male and female participants is based on ALwO/caregiver Q5 (were you born a male or female?) and HCP Q905 (are you male, female, or other?). [b] BMI classification for surveyed ALwO, the ALwO of surveyed caregivers, and the ALwO treated by surveyed HCPs. Obesity Class I = BMI ≥95th percentile for age and sex; Obesity Class II = BMI ≥120% of 95th percentile for age and sex; Obesity Class III = BMI ≥140% of 95th percentile for age and sex. ALwO and caregiver data consist of the percentage (number) of ALwO in each BMI category; HCP data consist of the mean percentage (SD) of their ALwO patients in each BMI category. [c] BMI classification of surveyed caregivers and HCPs (n = 219 for HCPs). ALwO, adolescents living with obesity; BMI, body mass index; HCP, healthcare professional; N/A, not applicable; SD, standard deviation. Table adapted from [14].

3.2. Information Sources

The information sources most commonly used by ALwO to learn about weight loss, healthy lifestyles, and weight management were YouTube, family and friends, information from a doctor, and social media, while for caregivers, they were information from a doctor, family and friends, YouTube, and dietitian/nutritionist (non-doctor) (Figure S2). For HCPs, the most commonly used sources of information were medical education/continuing medical education programs, journal articles, and conferences (Figure S2).

3.3. Perceptions of Obesity

HCPs were more likely than caregivers or ALwO to believe that obesity has a strong/very strong impact on overall health and wellbeing (Figure 1). When evaluating the respondents' perceptions of the impact of obesity compared with other comorbidities, most respondents in the ALwO, caregiver, and HCP groups considered obesity to be as impactful or more impactful than several other health conditions, including diabetes, heart disease, and depression (Figure 1).

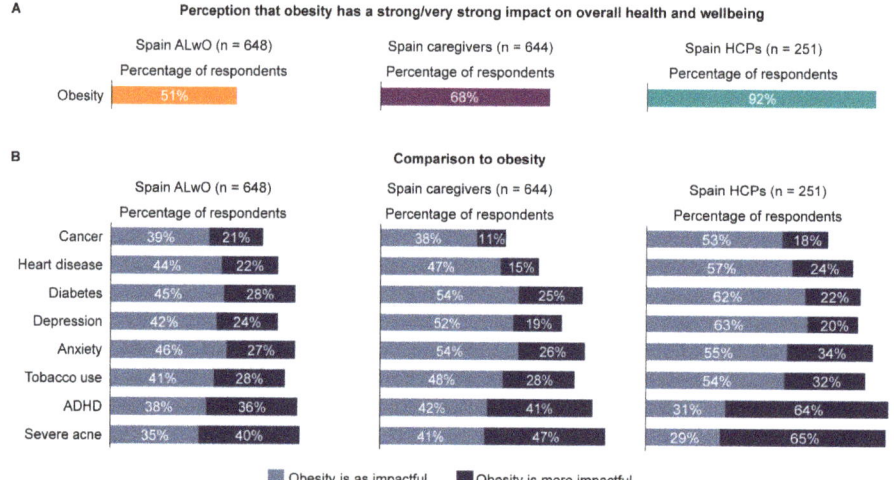

Figure 1. Perceived impact of obesity on overall health and wellbeing among ALwO, caregivers, and HCPs: (**A**) impact of obesity; (**B**) impact of obesity compared with other health conditions. Participants were asked how much of an impact they thought various health conditions had on a person's overall health and wellbeing using the following scale: 1 = no impact, 2 = slight impact, 3 = moderate impact, 4 = strong impact, and 5 = very strong impact (ALwO/caregiver Q510; HCP Q305). Panel A represents the proportion of respondents who indicated that obesity has a strong/very strong impact. Data were recoded to compare each participant's response regarding the impact of obesity with their response regarding the impact of other health conditions, and are shown in panel B; if the response was higher for obesity than for another health condition, it was coded as "Obesity is more impactful"; if equal, it was coded as "Obesity is as impactful". ADHD, attention deficit hyperactivity disorder; ALwO, adolescents living with obesity; HCP, healthcare professional. Figure adapted from [14].

3.4. Impact of Obesity

Most ALwO (53%) considered their weight to be slightly above normal (overweight), while 25% of ALwO thought their weight was normal (Figure 2). However, caregivers were more likely to think that the weight of their ALwO was normal (43%) (Figure 2). Considering their overall health, 59% of ALwO believed it to be at least good. In contrast, 95% of caregivers believed that their ALwO's health was at least good (Figure 2). Only 1% or fewer ALwO and caregivers considered their/their child's health to be poor (Figure 2).

Regarding how much the ALwO worried about their weight, 25% were very or extremely worried and 76% were at least somewhat worried (Figure 2). A similar percentage of caregivers reported that their ALwO was very or extremely worried about their weight (22%), but fewer reported that their ALwO was at least somewhat worried (56%) (Figure 2). More ALwO than caregivers worried a lot or a little about the ALwO's weight affecting their future health (Figure 2).

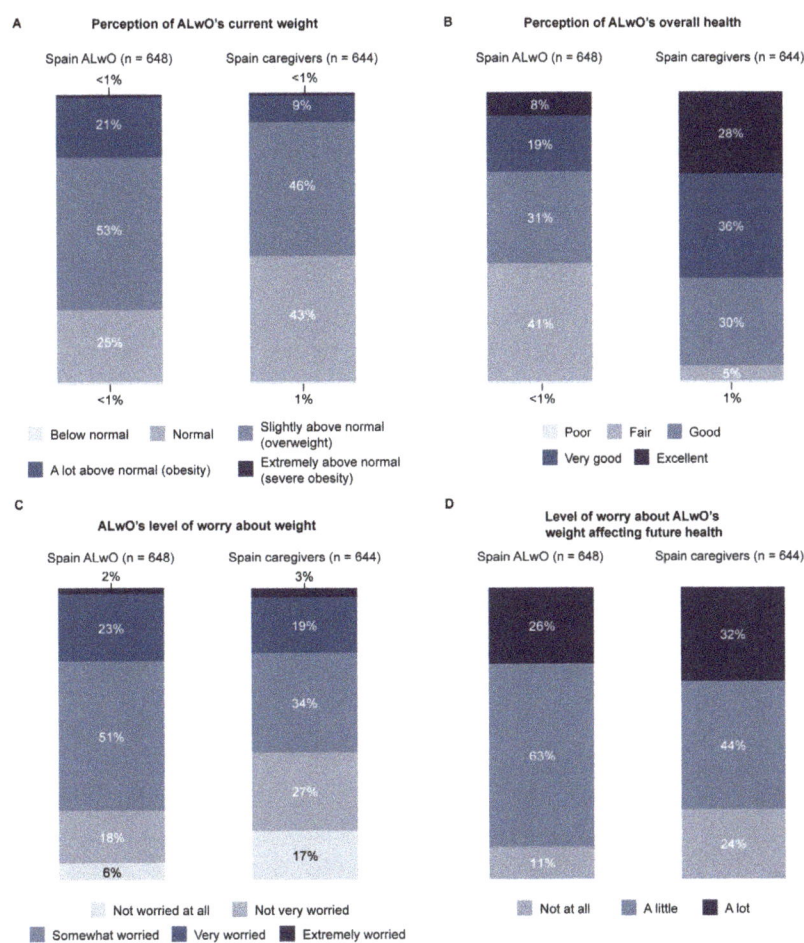

Figure 2. Perceptions of the impact of obesity on ALwO: (**A**) ALwO and caregiver perception of ALwO's current weight; (**B**) ALwO and caregiver perception of ALwO's overall health; (**C**) ALwO and caregiver perception of ALwO's level of worry about weight; (**D**) ALwO and caregiver level of worry about ALwO's weight affecting future health. Percentages represent the proportions of participants who selected each prespecified response option among all recruited ALwO (left bars) and caregivers (right bars). Percentages may not sum to 100% due to rounding. ALwO data are based on responses to ALwO Q106, Q101, Q108, and Q512, and caregiver data are based on responses to caregivers Q106, Q101, Q112, and Q515. ALwO, adolescents living with obesity. Figure adapted from [14].

3.5. Weight Loss

Overall, 39% of caregivers believed that their child will naturally slim down as they grow older, compared with 29% of HCPs (Figure S3). A greater proportion of caregivers than ALwO agreed that the ALwO could lose weight if he/she set their mind to it (Figure 3). More ALwO (48%) than caregivers (28%) felt that weight loss was completely the responsibility of the ALwO (Figure 3), while 21% of HCPs thought that losing weight was completely their patient's responsibility (Figure S3). Similar proportions of ALwO (36%) and caregivers (41%) indicated that they or their child had attempted to lose weight in the past year, but more ALwO (71%) reported they were somewhat or very likely to try to lose weight within 6 months than caregivers (57%) reported for their ALwO (Figure 3).

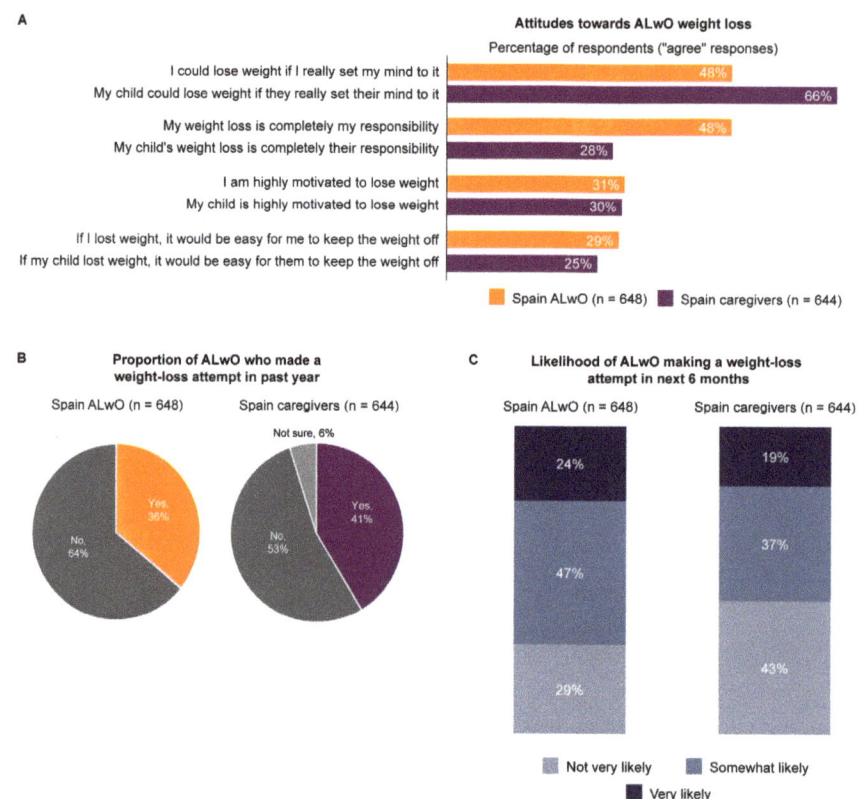

Figure 3. Weight loss attitudes and ALwO weight loss attempts: (**A**) ALwO and caregiver attitudes towards ALwO weight loss; (**B**) proportion of ALwO who attempted to lose weight in the previous year, according to the ALwO and caregivers; (**C**) likelihood of a weight loss attempt by ALwO in the coming 6 months, according to the ALwO and caregivers. Percentages are proportions of participants among all recruited ALwO or caregivers. ALwO data are based on responses to ALwO Q113, Q108a, and Q109, and caregiver data are based on responses to caregivers Q113, Q110a, and Q111. For each question, response options were prespecified, and only one option could be selected. Panel A presents the proportion of participants who indicated that they "strongly agree" or "somewhat agree" with each statement. For panel C, the "not very likely" category includes the response options "not likely at all" and "not very likely", and the "very likely" category includes the response options "very likely" and "extremely likely". Percentages may not sum to 100% due to rounding. ALwO, adolescents living with obesity. Figure adapted from [14].

For ALwO and caregivers, the most frequently reported reason why ALwO wanted to lose weight was to be more fit/in better shape, while for HCPs, it was a desire to improve popularity and social life (Figure 4).

The barriers to ALwO weight loss reported by ALwO and caregivers were similar (Figure S4); the most frequently reported barriers were an inability to control hunger, liking to eat unhealthy food, and lack of motivation. HCPs most commonly agreed that unhealthy eating habits, preference for unhealthy food, and insufficient exercise were barriers to ALwO losing weight, while inability to control hunger ranked 8th (Figure S4). The definitions of success for ALwO weight loss according to ALwO, caregivers, and HCPs are reported in Figure S5.

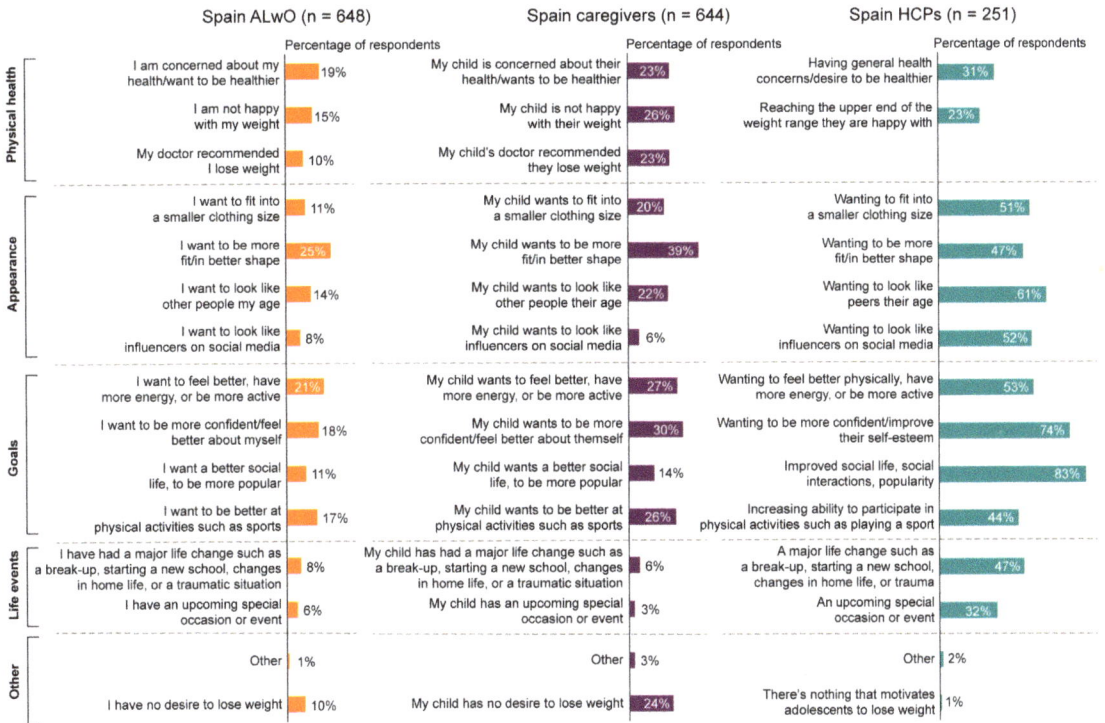

Figure 4. Motivators for ALwO weight loss, as defined by ALwO, caregivers, and HCPs. Response options selected by ALwO and caregivers when asked why they/their child has wanted to lose weight (ALwO/caregiver Q208) are presented in the first two columns. The prespecified response options selected by HCPs when asked what most motivates adolescents to lose weight (HCP Q205) are presented in the third column. ALwO, adolescents living with obesity; HCPs, healthcare professionals. Figure adapted from [14].

3.6. Conversations about Weight

Over half (54%) of ALwO felt they could talk honestly about their weight with their mother or father, but only 23% felt this way about conversations with their HCP. The most common ALwO- and caregiver-reported barriers to conversations about weight with an HCP were not seeing their/their child's weight as a significant medical issue and the ALwO already knowing how to manage their weight (Figure S6). The most frequently reported barrier for ALwO to initiating conversations about their weight, as perceived by HCPs, was the ALwO not feeling comfortable bringing up the topic (65%) (Figure S6).

Approximately half (51%) of caregivers had talked to their child's doctor about their child's weight in the course of the last year. Both ALwO and caregivers (who had talked with an HCP about their/their child's weight in the past year) most frequently reported that the parent/caregiver usually started the conversation (Figure S7); contrary to this, HCPs reported that they initiated weight discussions the majority of the time, but only 29% of HCPs felt they are responsible for starting the conversation (Figure S7).

A greater proportion of ALwO (53%) than caregivers (9%) had been informed about their/their child's obesity diagnosis by their doctor. HCPs reported that they inform, on average, 87% of ALwO or their caregivers about the adolescent's obesity diagnosis. Furthermore, 50% of the HCPs reported they always recorded an obesity diagnosis in the medical record, and 37% recorded it most of the time.

Among ALwO (n = 488) and caregivers (n = 419) who had talked with an HCP about their/their child's weight in the past year, 40% of ALwO and 71% of caregivers reported feeling comfortable doing so, while 26% and 9%, respectively, were not comfortable participating in these discussions. Most ALwO (63%) and caregivers (83%) reported at least one positive feeling following the latest discussion with an HCP, with the most common feelings reported to be "motivated", "supported", and "hopeful" (Figure 5). Among ALwO ($n = 160$) and caregivers ($n = 225$) who had not talked with an HCP about the ALwO's weight, 44% of ALwO and 55% of caregivers would feel comfortable discussing it.

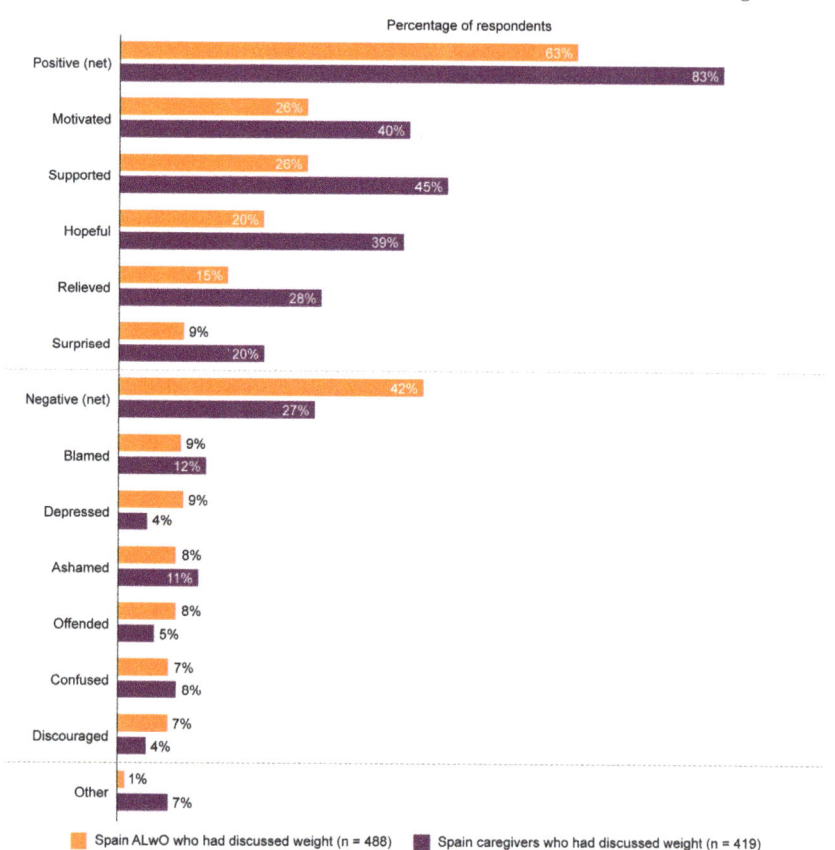

Figure 5. The feelings of ALwO and caregivers following their latest weight discussion with an HCP. Percentages represent the proportions of respondents who selected each of the prespecified response options for ALwO/caregiver Q410, among the subset of ALwO who had discussed weight with an HCP in the past year or the subset of caregivers who had discussed their child's weight with an HCP in the past year (per ALwO/caregiver Q201). The responses of caregivers represent their own feelings rather than their perception of their child's feelings. The net positive category is the proportion of participants who selected at least one positive answer (i.e., motivated, supported, hopeful, relieved, and/or surprised); the net negative category is the proportion of participants who selected at least one negative answer (i.e., blamed, depressed, ashamed, offended, confused, and/or discouraged). ALwO, adolescents living with obesity; HCP, healthcare professional. Figure adapted from [14].

3.7. Weight Management

Most HCPs (87%) believed obesity to be a chronic disease (Figure S8). As reported by ALwO and caregivers, the methods most commonly used by ALwO for managing weight in the past year were becoming more physically active and improving eating habits (Figure S9). The most effective methods for managing weight according to HCPs were becoming more physically active, improving eating habits, and reducing screen time (Figure S9).

4. Discussion

This analysis of the Spanish cohort from the ACTION Teens survey study provides key insights regarding the attitudes, perceptions, and behaviors of ALwO, caregivers, and HCPs, as well as possible obstacles to effective obesity care and Spanish culture-specific factors. There was misalignment between ALwO, caregivers, and HCPs, notably around the perception and impact of obesity and regarding conversations about weight. The findings of this study may change the strategy for interacting with caregivers and adolescents with obesity. The study also highlights the importance of training HCPs not only in biological problems related to obesity, but also in the perceptions, attitudes, and motivations of the people involved.

One-quarter of ALwO and almost half of caregivers considered their/their child's weight to be normal. The lack of recognition of the ALwO's obesity status may reflect the relatively small proportion of ALwO (53%) and caregivers (9%) who had been informed of their/their child's obesity diagnosis by their HCP. In contrast, HCPs stated that they informed the majority (87%) of ALwO/caregivers about the ALwO's diagnosis of obesity, with almost all reporting that they record obesity diagnoses in medical records most or all of the time. This aligns with the global ACTION Teens study, in which a greater proportion of HCPs reported informing ALwO/caregivers of the ALwO's obesity diagnosis compared with reports from ALwO/caregivers themselves [14]. This indicates a miscommunication, both in Spain and globally, between HCPs, ALwO, and caregivers with regard to obesity diagnoses, highlighting the importance of education and communicating weight status to ALwO and caregivers.

Compared with the global cohort, more Spanish caregivers tended to misperceive their child's health/weight, with a greater proportion perceiving the overall health of their ALwO to be at least good (95% vs. 80%, respectively) and believing the weight of their ALwO to be normal (43% vs. 32%) [14]. This result aligns with a cross-sectional analysis of Spanish school children that reported parental underestimation of the weight category of children with obesity in 94% of cases [16]. The tendency for parents/caregivers to underestimate the overweight status of their children has been reported in other studies worldwide that included Spanish participants [17,18]. The greater propensity among Spanish caregivers, compared with those in the ACTION Teens global cohort, to believe their child's weight was normal may be related to greater indulgence towards pediatric obesity and failure to recognize the detrimental impact of obesity in Spain. The high proportion of caregivers with overweight or obesity may also have impacted how they perceive the weight of their child. Visual normalization of obesity has been shown to contribute to the perceptions of caregivers, whereby increased exposure to larger body sizes leads caregivers to shift their perception of normal weight in children, leading to an underestimation of the weight of their child [19,20]. Previous data indicate that the lack of perception of obesity by the family is a determining factor in the development or worsening of childhood obesity [21]. Hence, family involvement is considered fundamental to the prevention of childhood obesity [22].

Considering attitudes towards weight loss, many caregivers (39%) thought that their child would slim down with age. This could indicate a misunderstanding of obesity in adolescence and may be an important barrier to seeking support from their HCP for management of their child's weight. Delayed initiation of medical management may be compounded by views among ALwO and caregivers regarding personal responsibility for weight loss. Approximately one-half of ALwO and one-quarter of caregivers felt that losing weight was solely the ALwO's responsibility. Feelings of personal responsibility for weight loss among individuals with obesity are not uncommon, arising from a narrative that positions obesity as a choice and/or lack of willpower [23]. Furthermore, when analyzing barriers to weight loss, there was discordance between HCPs and ALwO/caregivers on the importance of the inability to control hunger, with ALwO/caregivers, but not HCPs, reporting this as one of their top three barriers. This may indicate a misunderstanding around the biology of obesity, even among HCPs, and calls for improved education on this topic that can be further communicated to patients.

There were no remarkable differences between Spanish and global caregivers in terms of key motivators or barriers to weight loss. Key motivators in all respondent groups in Spain and globally included those related to appearance (e.g., being fit and looking like their peers), improved social status (i.e., their social life, interactions, and popularity), and improved self-confidence [14]. The barriers to weight loss most frequently reported by ALwO and caregivers, both in Spain and globally, were the inability to control hunger, lack of motivation, and a preference for unhealthy foods, while HCPs most often reported poor diet and insufficient physical activity [14].

Although 88% of Spanish ALwO reported barriers to weight loss in the present study, almost three-quarters of ALwO and over one-half of caregivers indicated that they/their child would be somewhat or very likely to try to lose weight within 6 months. Similar proportions of ALwO (75%) and caregivers (63%) were reported in the global study [14]. As such, HCPs should feel encouraged to initiate conversations about weight with ALwO and caregivers.

Guidance from the American Academy of Pediatrics (AAP) highlights the importance of communicating weight status to a child with obesity and their family in order to guide the subsequent evaluation and treatment [24]. However, this first step can be challenging for ALwO, caregivers, and HCPs alike, and can present an initial barrier to the advancement of obesity management. Only a small proportion of HCPs believed that they are responsible for initiating conversations about weight. Furthermore, approximately two-thirds of HCPs reported discomfort among ALwO in bringing up the topic of weight. In contrast, only 26% of ALwO who had discussed weight reported a lack of comfort with the conversation. Moreover, most ALwO and caregivers (63% and 83%, respectively) felt positive about previous weight-related discussions with an HCP. Across those who had not previously had a discussion about weight with an HCP, around half of ALwO and caregivers would feel comfortable with the conversation. As such, HCPs should feel confident in raising the topic of weight in order to facilitate effective treatment strategies. Interestingly, while 51% of Spanish caregivers reported having spoken with their child's doctor about their weight within the last year (compared with 36% of caregivers in the global analysis), less than 10% reported being informed of a diagnosis of obesity (vs. 29% in the global group) [14]. This indicates a miscommunication between HCPs and caregivers that is particularly prominent in Spain compared with other world regions. This may reflect a lack of understanding among Spanish caregivers or an unwillingness of HCPs to engage in challenging discussions.

The recommendations for the prevention and treatment of childhood obesity in Spain are mainly focused on changes in diet and increased exercise, paying little to no attention to the attitudes, behaviors, and motivations of the family and the adolescent, and the importance of these in ensuring successful management of the child's obesity [25–27]. It will be important to integrate the results of this study at the primary care level to facilitate early detection of childhood obesity and provide information about obesity to the family. In Spain, children are checked by the primary pediatrician on numerous occasions during the first years of their lives. As contact with the family is frequent during this time, recommendations related to obesity may have a substantial impact.

The strengths and limitations of this analysis of the Spanish cohort are comparable to those of the overall ACTION Teens study [14]. This was the first evaluation and comparison of the lived experiences of three parties (ALwO, caregivers, and HCPs) involved in obesity management in Spain. This analysis provides valuable information that may be used to align and achieve the objectives of all participating groups. The main limitations of the study include the risk of selection bias and the potential for measurement error due to use of online surveys, the self-reported weight and height data that may have led to underestimation or overestimation of ALwOs' BMI, the cross-sectional study design, and lack of information on body composition and pubertal stage. Furthermore, only 36% of ALwO in the Spanish cohort were female, and so results may be biased towards male ALwO attitudes, perspectives, and behaviors; subgroup analyses based on sex are outside the scope of this manuscript. The majority of ALwO and caregivers (more than 90%) were not matched. In addition, HCP respondents did not directly care for the surveyed ALwO; therefore, it was not possible to carry out paired studies.

Overall, our findings should be generalizable to the wider population of ALwO, caregivers of ALwO, and HCPs treating ALwO in Spain. Although online surveys typically have poor response rates, broad inclusion and exclusion criteria were used to ensure that respondents were representative of ALwO and HCPs treating ALwO in Spain. Furthermore, stratified sampling and demographic weighting of caregiver data were used to ensure that the sample was as representative as possible. Additionally, while there is potential for selection bias with online surveys, this risk was mitigated by not specifying the topic of the survey in adolescent/caregiver email invitations and carefully designing screening questions to ensure that adolescents and caregivers did not know the purpose of the study until they had met the qualification criteria.

5. Conclusions

This analysis of the Spanish cohort of the cross-sectional ACTION Teens survey study highlights existing barriers to effective obesity management of ALwO in Spain, as well as Spanish culture-specific factors. It revealed misperceptions of weight status in a high proportion of ALwO and caregivers of ALwO, and suggested that ALwO are more likely to worry about their weight than their caregivers. Both ALwO and caregivers reported not being able to control hunger as an important barrier to weight loss, while HCPs were more likely to report a poor diet or a lack of physical activity. In addition, communication difficulties and misalignments exist between HCPs, ALwO, and caregivers. HCPs assume that ALwO will not feel comfortable starting conversations about their weight, and a minority of HCPs perceive themselves as being responsible for initiating weight-related discussions. Meanwhile, there is a willingness among both ALwO and caregivers to talk with an HCP about the ALwO's weight; they feel comfortable discussing it and feel positive after having the conversation. Improved communication between ALwO, caregivers, and HCPs is required, alongside a better understanding of the existing barriers to weight loss.

Supplementary Materials: The following supporting information can be downloaded at: https://www.mdpi.com/article/10.3390/nu15133005/s1, Table S1: HCP primary medical specialty and professional experience. Figure S1: Disposition of survey participants from Spain: (A) ALwO and caregivers; (B) HCPs. Figure S2: Sources for information about obesity, healthy lifestyles, weight loss, and weight management: (A) sources used by ALwO and caregivers (≥5% of participants); (B) most important information sources according to ALwO and caregivers (≥5% of participants); (C) sources used by HCPs. Figure S3: HCPs' attitudes towards weight loss in ALwO. Figure S4: ALwO weight loss barriers according to: (A) ALwO and caregivers; (B) HCPs. Figure S5: Definitions of weight loss success among ALwO, caregivers, and HCPs. Figure S6: Barriers to conversations about weight with HCPs: (A) ALwO- and caregiver-reported barriers; (B) HCP-reported barriers; (C) HCPs' perception of ALwO barriers. Figure S7: Perceptions of conversations about weight between ALwO and HCPs: (A) who initiated discussions; (B) who should initiate discussions. Figure S8: HCPs' attitudes towards obesity and ALwO weight management. Figure S9: Weight management methods and recommendations: (A) methods used by ALwO in the past year according to ALwO and caregivers; (B) methods recommended by HCPs; (C) most effective methods for weight management, as perceived by HCPs.

Author Contributions: Conceptualization, J.P.L.S. and F.F.-A.; writing—original draft preparation, J.P.L.S. and C.A.B.; writing—review and editing, all authors. All authors have read and agreed to the published version of the manuscript.

Funding: This research was funded by Novo Nordisk A/S. The article processing charge was funded by Novo Nordisk.

Institutional Review Board Statement: The study was conducted according to the guidelines of the Declaration of Helsinki and approved for Spain by the Institutional Review Board of WCG, Puyallup, WA, USA (IRB tracking number: 20212733; approved 27 July 2021).

Informed Consent Statement: Informed consent was obtained from all subjects (and the parent/legal guardians of the ALwO) involved in the study.

Data Availability Statement: Data will be shared with bona fide researchers submitting a research proposal approved by the independent review board. Individual participant data will be shared in data sets in a de-identified and anonymized format. Data will be made available after research completion. Information about data access request proposals can be found at novonordisk-trials.com.

Acknowledgments: We thank all the study participants and personnel involved. We also thank Andrea Stoltz, Lynn Clement, Peg Jaynes, Rebecca Hahn, and Nick Henderson of KJT Group Inc. for the data collection and analysis. Medical writing support was provided by Jane Murphy, of Apollo, OPEN Health Communications, and funded by Novo Nordisk, in accordance with Good Publication Practice (GPP) guidelines (www.ismpp.org/gpp-2022).

Conflicts of Interest: As described previously [14], two employees of Novo Nordisk were members of the ACTION Teens Steering Committee and thus participated in the design of the study and interpretation of the data. An employee of Novo Nordisk Spain (C.A.B.) is an author of the current manuscript and was involved, alongside the other authors, in interpretation of the data, drafting the manuscript, and approval of the final version. Novo Nordisk also funded medical writing assistance. J.P.L.S. and F.F.-A. received consultancy fees from Novo Nordisk for their role as members of the ACTION Teens Steering Committee during the conduct of the study. J.P.L.S. reports honoraria (for lectures) from Merck, Novo Nordisk, and Sandoz, and participation in advisory boards for Merck and Novo Nordisk, all outside the submitted work. M.R.K. reports honoraria (for lectures) from Novo Nordisk, Pfizer, and Sandoz, and participation in advisory boards for Merck, Novo Nordisk, Pfizer, and Sandoz, all outside of the submitted work. G.P.L. reports honoraria (for lectures) from Novo Nordisk. M.V.B.F. declares no conflicts of interest. C.A.B. is an employee of Novo Nordisk. F.F.-A. reports grants from Novo Nordisk, lecture fees from the organizers of the International Congress on Obesity and MEtabolic Syndrome (ICOMES) conference, support for attending meetings and travel from Novo Nordisk, Editor-in-Chief honorarium from Wiley, and participation in a Data Safety Monitoring Board for the Sustain Project—Germany, all outside of the submitted work; he is also past-president of the Eating Disorders Research Society and Co-Chair of the Eating Disorders Section of the World Psychiatric Association.

References

1. NCD Risk Factor Collaboration (NCD-RisC). Worldwide trends in body-mass index, underweight, overweight, and obesity from 1975 to 2016: A pooled analysis of 2416 population-based measurement studies in 128·9 million children, adolescents, and adults. *Lancet* **2017**, *390*, 2627–2642. [CrossRef] [PubMed]
2. Bravo-Saquicela, D.M.; Sabag, A.; Rezende, L.F.M.; Rey-Lopez, J.P. Has the prevalence of childhood obesity in Spain plateaued? A systematic review and meta-analysis. *Int. J. Environ. Res. Public Health* **2022**, *19*, 5240. [CrossRef] [PubMed]
3. PASOS. Physical Activity, Sedentarism, Lifestyles and Obesity in Spanish Youth. Estudio PASOS 2022—Resultados Preliminares. Available online: https://gasolfoundation.org/wp-content/uploads/2023/01/GF-PASOS-informe-2022-WEB.pdf (accessed on 9 March 2023).
4. Marcus, C.; Danielsson, P.; Hagman, E. Pediatric obesity—Long-term consequences and effect of weight loss. *J. Intern. Med.* **2022**, *292*, 870–891. [CrossRef] [PubMed]
5. Nicolucci, A.; Maffeis, C. The adolescent with obesity: What perspectives for treatment? *Ital. J. Pediatr.* **2022**, *48*, 9. [CrossRef]
6. Cabeza, J.F.; Aristizábal-Duque, C.H.; Sánchez, I.M.B.; Ortiz, M.R.; Almodóvar, A.R.; Ortega, M.D.; Martínez, F.E.; Saldaña, M.R.; Del Pozo, F.J.F.; Álvarez-Ossorio, M.P.; et al. Relationship between overweight and obesity and cardiac dimensions and function in a paediatric population. *Eur. J. Pediatr.* **2022**, *181*, 1943–1949. [CrossRef]
7. Rankin, J.; Matthews, L.; Cobley, S.; Han, A.; Sanders, R.; Wiltshire, H.D.; Baker, J.S. Psychological consequences of childhood obesity: Psychiatric comorbidity and prevention. *Adolesc. Health Med. Ther.* **2016**, *7*, 125–146. [CrossRef]
8. Simmonds, M.; Burch, J.; Llewellyn, A.; Griffiths, C.; Yang, H.; Owen, C.; Duffy, S.; Woolacott, N. The use of measures of obesity in childhood for predicting obesity and the development of obesity-related diseases in adulthood: A systematic review and meta-analysis. *Health Technol. Assess.* **2015**, *19*, 1–336. [CrossRef]

9. Llewellyn, A.; Simmonds, M.; Owen, C.G.; Woolacott, N. Childhood obesity as a predictor of morbidity in adulthood: A systematic review and meta-analysis. *Obes. Rev.* **2016**, *17*, 56–67. [CrossRef]
10. Twig, G.; Yaniv, G.; Levine, H.; Leiba, A.; Goldberger, N.; Derazne, E.; Ben-Ami Shor, D.; Tzur, D.; Afek, A.; Shamiss, A.; et al. Body-mass index in 2.3 million adolescents and cardiovascular death in adulthood. *N. Engl. J. Med.* **2016**, *374*, 2430–2440. [CrossRef]
11. Reinehr, T.; Kleber, M.; Lass, N.; Toschke, A.M. Body mass index patterns over 5 y in obese children motivated to participate in a 1-y lifestyle intervention: Age as a predictor of long-term success. *Am. J. Clin. Nutr.* **2010**, *91*, 1165–1171. [CrossRef]
12. Hagman, E.; Danielsson, P.; Lindberg, L.; Marcus, C.; BORIS Steering Committee. Paediatric obesity treatment during 14 years in Sweden: Lessons from the Swedish Childhood Obesity Treatment Register-BORIS. *Pediatr. Obes.* **2020**, *15*, e12626. [CrossRef]
13. Caterson, I.D.; Alfadda, A.A.; Auerbach, P.; Coutinho, W.; Cuevas, A.; Dicker, D.; Hughes, C.; Iwabu, M.; Kang, J.H.; Nawar, R.; et al. Gaps to bridge: Misalignment between perception, reality and actions in obesity. *Diabetes Obes. Metab.* **2019**, *21*, 1914–1924. [CrossRef]
14. Halford, J.C.G.; Bereket, A.; Bin-Abbas, B.; Chen, W.; Fernández-Aranda, F.; Garibay Nieto, N.; López Siguero, J.P.; Maffeis, C.; Mooney, V.; Osorto, C.K.; et al. Misalignment among adolescents living with obesity, caregivers, and healthcare professionals: ACTION Teens global survey study. *Pediatr. Obes.* **2022**, *17*, e12957. [CrossRef]
15. World Health Organization: Growth Reference Data—BMI-For-Age (5–19 Years). 2007. Available online: https://www.who.int/tools/growth-reference-data-for-5to19-years/indicators/bmi-for-age (accessed on 15 June 2023).
16. Inclán-López, P.; Bartolomé-Gutiérrez, R.; Martínez-Castillo, D.; Rabanales-Sotos, J.; Guisado-Requena, I.M.; Martínez-Andrés, M. Parental perception of weight and feeding practices in schoolchildren: A cross-sectional study. *Int. J. Environ. Res. Public Health* **2021**, *18*, 4014. [CrossRef]
17. Ramos Salas, X.; Buoncristiano, M.; Williams, J.; Kebbe, M.; Spinelli, A.; Nardone, P.; Rito, A.; Duleva, V.; Musić Milanović, S.; Kunesova, M.; et al. Parental Perceptions of Children's Weight Status in 22 Countries: The WHO European Childhood Obesity Surveillance Initiative: COSI 2015/2017. *Obes. Facts* **2021**, *14*, 658–674. [CrossRef]
18. Regber, S.; Novak, M.; Eiben, G.; Bammann, K.; De Henauw, S.; Fernández-Alvira, J.M.; Gwozdz, W.; Kourides, Y.; Moreno, L.A.; Molnár, D.; et al. Parental perceptions of and concerns about child's body weight in eight European countries—The IDEFICS study. *Pediatr. Obes.* **2013**, *8*, 118–129. [CrossRef]
19. Wang, J.; Winkley, K.; Wei, X.; Cao, Y.; Chang, Y.S. The relationships between caregivers' self-reported and visual perception of child weight and their non-responsive feeding practices: A systematic review and meta-analysis. *Appetite* **2023**, *180*, 106343. [CrossRef]
20. Robinson, E. Overweight but unseen: A review of the underestimation of weight status and a visual normalization theory. *Obes. Rev.* **2017**, *18*, 1200–1209. [CrossRef]
21. Martínez, M.; Rico, S.; Rodríguez, F.J.; Guadalupe, G.; Calderón, J.F. Influence of family environment on the development of childhood overweight and obesity in Valverde de Leganes. *Eur. J. Child Dev. Educ. Psychopathol.* **2016**, *4*, 17–29. [CrossRef]
22. Ariza, C.; Ortega-Rodríguez, E.; Sánchez-Martínez, F.; Valmayor, S.; Juárez, O.; Pasarín, M.I. Childhood obesity prevention from a community view. *Aten. Primaria* **2015**, *47*, 246–255. [CrossRef]
23. Grannell, A.; Fallon, F.; Al-Najim, W.; le Roux, C. Obesity and responsibility: Is it time to rethink agency? *Obes. Rev.* **2021**, *22*, e13270. [CrossRef] [PubMed]
24. Hampl, S.E.; Hassink, S.G.; Skinner, A.C.; Armstrong, S.C.; Barlow, S.E.; Bolling, C.F.; Avila Edwards, K.C.; Eneli, I.; Hamre, R.; Joseph, M.M.; et al. Clinical practice guideline for the evaluation and treatment of children and adolescents with obesity. *Pediatrics* **2023**, *151*, e2022060640. [CrossRef] [PubMed]
25. Lechuga Sancho, A.; Palomo Atance, E.; Rivero Martin, M.J.; Gil-Campos, M.; Leis Trabazo, R.; Bahíllo Curieses, M.P.; Bueno Lozano, G. Spanish collaborative study: Description of usual clinical practice in infant obesity. *An. Pediatr.* **2018**, *88*, 340–349. [CrossRef] [PubMed]
26. Ministerio de Sanidad y Política Social. Clinical Practice Guideline on the Prevention and Treatment of Obesity in Children and Adolescents. Ministerio de Ciencia e Innovación. 2009. Available online: https://portal.guiasalud.es/wp-content/uploads/2018/12/GPC_452_obes_infantojuv_AATRM_compl.pdf (accessed on 22 June 2023).
27. Alto Comisionado Para la Lucha contra la Pobreza Infantil. National Strategic Plan to Reduce Childhood Obesity (2022–2030). 2022. Available online: https://www.comisionadopobrezainfantil.gob.es/sites/default/files/Plan_obesidad_Completo_DIGITAL_paginas_1.pdf (accessed on 22 June 2023).

Disclaimer/Publisher's Note: The statements, opinions and data contained in all publications are solely those of the individual author(s) and contributor(s) and not of MDPI and/or the editor(s). MDPI and/or the editor(s) disclaim responsibility for any injury to people or property resulting from any ideas, methods, instructions or products referred to in the content.

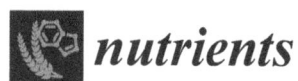

Article

Athletes with Eating Disorders: Analysis of Their Clinical Characteristics, Psychopathology and Response to Treatment

Ana Ibáñez-Caparrós [1,2,3], Isabel Sánchez [4,5,6], Roser Granero [5,6,7], Susana Jiménez-Murcia [4,5,6,8], Magda Rosinska [9], Ansgar Thiel [10], Stephan Zipfel [11,12,13], Joan de Pablo [1,2,3], Lucia Camacho-Barcia [4,5,6,*] and Fernando Fernandez-Aranda [4,5,6,8,*]

[1] Department of Psychiatry, University Hospital Germans Trias i Pujol, 08916 Badalona, Spain; aibanezc.germanstrias@gencat.cat (A.I.-C.); jdepablo.germanstrias@gencat.cat (J.d.P.)
[2] Institut Recerca Germans Trias i Pujol (IGTP), 08916 Badalona, Spain
[3] Department of Psychiatrics and Legal Medicine, School of Medicine, Autonomous University of Barcelona, 08193 Barcelona, Spain
[4] Clinical Psychology Unit, Bellvitge University Hospital, 08907 Barcelona, Spain; isasanchez@bellvitgehospital.cat (I.S.); sjimenez@bellvitgehospital.cat (S.J.-M.)
[5] Psychoneurobiology of Eating and Addictive Behaviors Group, Neurosciences Programme, Bellvitge Biomedical Research Institute (IDIBELL), 08908 Barcelona, Spain; roser.granero@uab.cat
[6] Ciber Fisiopatología Obesidad y Nutrición (CIBERObn), Instituto de Salud Carlos III, 28029 Madrid, Spain
[7] Departament de Psicobiologia i Metodologia de les Ciències de la Salut, Universitat Autònoma de Barcelona, 08193 Barcelona, Spain
[8] Department of Clinical Sciences, School of Medicine and Health Sciences, University of Barcelona, 08907 Barcelona, Spain
[9] Body Image Assessment and Intervention Unit, Department of Clinical Psychology and Health, Autonomous University of Barcelona, 08193 Barcelona, Spain; rosinska.mj@gmail.com
[10] Interfaculty Research Institute for Sport and Physical Activity, University of Tübingen, 72074 Tübingen, Germany; ansgar.thiel@uni-tuebingen.de
[11] Department of Psychosomatic Medicine, University of Tübingen, 72074 Tübingen, Germany; stephan.zipfel@med.uni-tuebingen.de
[12] Centre of Excellence for Eating Disorders (KOMET), University of Tübingen, 72076 Tübingen, Germany
[13] German Centre of Mental Health (DZPG), University of Tübingen, 72076 Tübingen, Germany
* Correspondence: lcamacho@idibell.cat (L.C.-B.); ffernandez@bellvitgehospital.cat (F.F.-A.); Tel.: +34-932607227 (L.-C.-B. & F.F.-A.)

Abstract: Eating disorders (ED) have frequently been described among athletes. However, their specific features and therapy responses are lacking in the literature. The aims of this article were to compare clinical, psychopathological and personality traits between ED patients who were professional athletes (ED-A) with those who were not (ED-NA) and to explore differences in response to treatment. The sample comprised $n = 104$ patients with ED ($n = 52$ ED-A and $n = 52$ matched ED-NA) diagnosed according to DSM-5 criteria. Evaluation consisted of a semi-structured face-to-face clinical interview conducted by expert clinicians and a psychometric battery. Treatment outcome was evaluated when the treatment program ended. ED-A patients showed less body dissatisfaction and psychological distress. No differences were found in treatment outcome among the groups. Within the ED-A group, those participants who performed individual sport activities and aesthetic sports presented higher eating psychopathology, more general psychopathology, differential personality traits and poor therapy outcome. Individual and aesthetic sports presented more severity and worse prognosis. Although usual treatment for ED might be similarly effective in ED-A and ED-NA, it might be important to develop preventive and early detection programs involving sports physicians and psychologists, coaches and family throughout the entire athletic career and afterwards.

Keywords: eating disorders; professional athletes; treatment outcome; physical activity

1. Introduction

Eating disorders (ED) are severe mental illnesses, characterized by disturbances in eating behavior and food intake often accompanied by feelings of distress and concerns about weight or body shape [1]. Lifetime prevalence is approximately 5% considering the different diagnoses: anorexia nervosa (AN), bulimia nervosa (BN), binge eating disorder (BED) and other specified feeding and eating disorders (OSFED) [2]. It is well known that ED produce profound and protracted physical and psychosocial morbidity [2]. Furthermore, in recent years, research has widely documented that the COVID-19 pandemic has had pernicious effects on people diagnosed, or at risk, of suffering from ED, both in eating symptoms (restriction, lower weight, purging) and in general psychopathology (anxiety, depression, obsessive–compulsive symptoms) [3,4]. Disturbingly, mortality risk in AN and BN is five or more times higher when compared with the general population; the main causes of death being suicide and somatic complications [5]. A matter of concern is that ED are frequently undertreated and that there are scarce advances in treatment, especially in adults [6].

High levels of physical activity have been largely associated with ED and their comorbidities [7–9]. This is observed especially in AN, where excessive exercise occurs in 31–80% of patients [10] and has been associated with longer hospital duration, poor treatment outcome, increased likelihood of dropout and risk of relapse and chronicity [11–14]. In other ED, such as BN and OSFED, a high exercise load has been associated with both higher general psychopathology and eating disorder symptomatology [15].

Professional athletes, being at a higher risk of developing ED than the general population [16], constitute a special group that must be considered when evaluating the effects of high levels of physical activity in clinical outcomes. Athletes do not only have extremely high training loads due to sport specific performance requirements, but many athletes fall into an "identity tunnel" [17] by fully focusing their life on elite sports, often leading to an excessive adherence to the norms and values of the elite sports system due to a lack of influences from outside the sporting realm [18,19]. They internalize a mechanistic view of their bodies, perceiving them purely as functional tools for delivering sports performances [20], disregarding non-sport specific aspects of well-being [20,21]. Pain and injuries become normalized and rationalized as a necessity of pushing the limits [22], but also illnesses and mental and physical overload are often ignored, as athletes commonly push through feelings of discomfort [23].

Results of a recent study reported that, in a sample of competitive athletes, over 86% met criteria for an ED/subthreshold ED [24]. Furthermore, when looking at clinical variables, athletes who reported ED pathology showed higher levels of depression and anxiety than athletes without ED pathology [25], but, compared with non-athlete ED patients, research has found mixed results. However, due to their usual high training volume [26], it was difficult to define the term "excessive exercise" in this group and it remained unclear the role it played.

When comparing the type of sport practiced, research has found a higher likelihood of ED in those sports that depend on pressure to lose and/or maintain weight, as in aesthetic sports such as artistic gymnastics, figure skating or classical ballet [27,28]. Regarding individual or team sports, it seems that symptoms of ED are less associated with team sports [29,30].

Thus, even though the practice of a professional sport has been considered a risk factor for a diagnosis of ED, especially in individual and aesthetic sports, there is a lack of research concerning predictors of therapy and treatment outcome in clinical samples of athletes with ED.

The main goals of this study were threefold: (1) to compare clinical, psychopathological and personality traits between professional athletes with ED (ED-A) and non-athletes with ED (ED-NA); (2) to analyze the differences in response to treatment and dropouts between ED-A and ED-NA and whether the type of professional sport performed might be relevant;

(3) to identify the predictive factors of therapeutic success or failure, as well as dropout among both groups.

We hypothesized that ED-related severity, general psychopathology and personality traits would be important determinants of the ED-A sample and would be reflected as poorer treatment outcomes in this group. Additionally, based on the type of sport performed (aesthetic vs. non-aesthetic/group vs. individual), we expected to observe a more dysfunctional profile in individual sports and aesthetic athletes that would be reflected in poorer treatment outcomes.

2. Materials and Methods

2.1. Sample

The total sample comprised $n = 104$ patients with a diagnosis of ED ($n = 38$ AN, $n = 36$ BN, $n = 4$ BED and $n = 26$ OSFED), divided into two matched groups of $n = 52$ participants each. One group of professional athletes was diagnosed with ED (ED-A) and another group of non-athlete patients was diagnosed with ED (ED-NA). Both groups were matched by diagnosis ($n = 19$ AN, $n = 18$ BN, $n = 2$ BED, $n = 13$ OSFED), age, duration of the ED and sex ($n = 39$ women and $n = 13$ men) taken from a larger pool of non-athlete ED cases using propensity scores. Participants were diagnosed according to the DSM-5 criteria [1] following a face-to-face semi-structured interview by expert clinicians specialized in ED. Regarding the OSFED group composition, patients with atypical anorexia nervosa (OSFED-AN), purging disorder (OSFED-P), subthreshold bulimia nervosa and subthreshold binge eating disorder (OSFED-BN) were included. The distribution in our sample was: (OSFED-AN 38.5%, OSFED-BN 26.9% and OSFEC-P 34.6%). Exclusion criteria were: (1) being under 16 years of age; (2) having a learning or intellectual disability; (3) providing incomplete questionnaires; (4) not signing the informed consent form.

2.2. Assessment

Sociodemographic information including sex, civil status, education, employment, socioeconomic status, clinically relevant features regarding ED and psychopathological symptoms were assessed by a structured clinical interview [31]. Athletes were specifically asked about the type of sport practiced. Interviews were conducted by experienced psychologists in ED.

To explore symptoms of ED, general psychopathology and personality traits, we administered a battery of questionnaires regularly applied when treating ED.

Eating disorders inventory-2 (EDI-2) [32] is a 91-item self-report questionnaire used frequently to assess cognitive and behavioral characteristics of ED. This instrument measures 11 subscales: drive for thinness, body dissatisfaction, bulimia, ineffectiveness, perfectionism, interpersonal distrust, interoceptive awareness, maturity fears, asceticism, impulse regulation and social insecurity. The EDI-2 total score provides a global measure of ED severity. The validation for the Spanish population [33] had a mean internal consistency of 0.63 (Cronbach's α). The internal consistency for the current sample was between acceptable (Cronbach-alpha $\alpha = 0.638$ for "ascetic") and excellent ($\alpha = 0.961$ for "total score").

The symptom checklist-90-revised (SCL-90) [34] is a self-reported 90-item questionnaire that explores general psychopathology. It measures nine primary symptom dimensions: somatization, obsession–compulsion, inter-personal sensitivity, depression, anxiety, hostility, phobic anxiety, paranoid ideation and psychoticism. Three global indices are also present: the global severity index (GSI), which evaluates overall distress; the positive symptom distress index (PSDI), which indicates the intensity of the symptoms; the positive symptom total (PST), which assesses self-reported symptoms. Validation for the Spanish population [35] obtained a mean internal consistency of 0.75 (Cronbach's α). The internal consistency for this study was between adequate ($\alpha = 0.725$ for "paranoia") and excellent ($\alpha = 0.977$ for "global indexes").

Temperament and character inventory-revised (TCI-R) [36] is a 240-item questionnaire based on the Cloninger model of personality. It measures four temperaments (harm avoidance, novelty seeking, reward dependence and persistence) and three character (self-directedness, cooperativeness and self-transcendence) dimensions of personality. It has been validated in a Spanish adult population [37]. Cronbach's alpha for the current sample was between adequate ($\alpha = 0.804$ for "novelty seeking") to excellent ($\alpha = 0.926$ for "harm avoidance").

2.3. Procedures

The threshold for the professional level was defined by experienced clinical psychologists during an in-depth interview. The group of professional athletes comprised individuals who lived off their sport, those who received payment for their performance through government grants or sports clubs and those who were in national or autonomic federations and competed at the professional level. In the sample, 16 sports were represented ($n = 52$): football, basketball, korfball, volleyball, canoeing, swimming, fitness, cycling, running, karate, bodybuilding, climbing, figure skating, rhythmic gymnastics, triathlon and snowboarding. Finally, ballet was included in the sample because, although it is not strictly considered a sport, due to its very particular characteristics in the literature, it has been equated to aesthetic sports [28].

For the ED-A analysis, the sample was separated into two subgroups: (1) Individual sports ($n = 42$) vs. team sports ($n = 10$). Defining team sports as having a set of players who interact as a block with a common goal (e.g., football, basketball and volleyball) [37]. (2) Aesthetic ($n = 27$) vs. non aesthetic ($n = 25$). Aesthetic sports include sports where body shape is of great importance in the performance, e.g., rhythmic gymnastics, synchronized swimming and figure skating [37].

2.4. Treatment

As previously described [38], each patient with AN received same-day inpatient treatment addressing nutritional dietary patterns and psychological and psychiatric aspects, based on a CBT program previously described elsewhere [39] with proven efficacy [40]. Patients attended the hospital during the day from 9 AM to 3 PM, 5 days a week (Monday to Friday), for a period of 15 weeks. Food intake was monitored twice a day during breakfast and lunch (the main food intakes of the day). Treatment for the other diagnostic types, such as BN, BED and OSFED, consisted of 16 weekly manualized outpatient group therapy sessions, each lasting 90 min, led by experienced psychologists. This program was published in Spanish and has demonstrated efficacy [41,42]. The common goals of the treatment were training in problem-solving strategies, cognitive restructuring, emotional regulation, improvement of self-esteem and body image and relapse prevention. In addition, therapy addressed eating-related symptomatology through psychoeducation, dietary monitoring and normalization of nutritional patterns.

2.5. Outcome Measures

Patients were assessed again upon discharge and grouped into three categories: "complete remission", "partial remission" and "no remission". Complete remission was defined according to the DSM-5 criteria [1] as the complete absence of symptoms meeting diagnostic criteria for a minimum of 4 consecutive weeks. Partial remission referred to significant symptomatic improvement but with residual symptoms, while patients with poor outcomes were classified as non-remission. These categories were determined by senior clinical staff who considered various factors related to the patients' treatment outcome. They included normalization of dietary patterns, frequency of binge eating episodes and compensatory behaviors (such as self-induced vomiting or abuse of laxatives and diuretics), weight regain and improvement in attitudes towards weight and shape, as well as cognitive aspects related to eating disorders. Objective measures, such as weight status and the number of daily binge-eating and purging episodes, were obtained from food diaries and weight control records. Discontinuation of treatment without medical advice was categorized as "drop-out" (i.e., not attending treatment for three consecutive sessions). The study was approved by the Bellvitge University Hospital and written informed consent was obtained from all participants.

2.6. Statistical Analysis

Stata17 for Windows was used for the statistical procedure. The comparison between the groups was performed with chi-square tests for categorical variables (χ^2) and with analysis of variance (ANOVA) for quantitative variables. The effect size of the relationships was estimated with Cramer's-V coefficient for χ^2 and Cohen's-d for ANOVA, considering mild/moderate for V > 0.20 or |d| > 0.50 and high/large for V > 0.40 or |d| > 0.80 [43]. Regarding the use of the ANOVA in this work, it must be outlined that results obtained in current statistical studies (most of them simulation analyses conducting Monte Carlo modeling) provide empirical evidence for the robustness of the procedure under a wide variety of conditions involving non-normal distributions and heteroscedasticity (therefore, the conditions of outcome variable normally and independently distributed with equal variances among the group have not been evaluated) [44]. For the χ^2 tests, the significance level was obtained with the exact method. In addition, all the univariable analyses carried out with the χ^2 and the ANOVA tests included the Finner's correction procedure to avoid increases in the type-I error due to the multiple statistical comparisons [45].

Logistic regression was used to identify the variables with a significant contribution on the risk of dropout (yes versus no) and bad outcome (yes versus no) during treatment. In this study, bad outcome was considered as the presence of dropout or non-remission. The backwards stepwise method was used, with the list of predictors as: sociodemographic variables (sex, age, marital status, education level, employment status and social position index), eating disorder severity (EDI-2 total), global psychopathological distress (SCL-90R GSI) and personality profile (TCI-R scale scores). The goodness of fit of the logistic regression was tested with the Hosmer–Lemeshow test; the predictive capacity was tested with the pseudo Nagelkerke's-R coefficient.

The Kaplan–Meier (product limit) method estimated the cumulative survival function for the rate of dropout. Survival analysis provided the probability of patients "living" (surviving without the presence of the outcome, in this study, without dropping out during the treatment) for a certain amount of time after beginning therapy [46].

3. Results

3.1. Characteristics of the Sample

Most participants in this study were women (75%), single (81.7%), with a secondary education level (53.8%), either employed or student (74.0%) and pertained to mean low to low social indexes (85.6%). Mean age was 25.4 years-old (SD = 6.8), mean age of onset of the problematic eating behavior was 19.0 years-old (SD = 6.1) and mean duration of the eating related problems was 6.4 years (SD = 5.8). The distribution of the ED subtype was: 36.5% AN, 34.6% BN, 3.8% BED and 25.0% OSFED. No statistical differences between the groups based on sports were observed (see Table 1).

3.2. Comparison between the Groups at Baseline

Considering the clinical variables at baseline (ED symptom severity (EDI-2) and psychopathology (SCL-90R)) and the personality profile (TCI-R), participants within the ED-A sample reported a lower mean in EDI-2 body dissatisfaction and SCL-90R global psychological distress (as measured with the PSDI) (see Table 2).

Table 1. Descriptive of the sample.

		Total (n = 104)		ED-NA (n = 52)		ED-A (n = 52)			
		n	%	n	%	n	%	p	C-V
Sex	Women	78	75.0%	39	75.0%	39	75.0%	1.000	0.000
	Men	26	25.0%	13	25.0%	13	25.0%		
Civil status	Single	85	81.7%	40	76.9%	45	86.5%	0.219	0.171
	Married	13	12.5%	7	13.5%	6	11.5%		
	Divorced	6	5.8%	5	9.6%	1	1.9%		
Education	Primary	28	26.9%	14	26.9%	14	26.9%	0.873	0.051
	Secondary	56	53.8%	27	51.9%	29	55.8%		
	University	20	19.2%	11	21.2%	9	17.3%		
Employment	Employed/student	77	74.0%	35	67.3%	42	80.8%	0.117	0.154
	Unemployed	27	26.0%	17	32.7%	10	19.2%		
Social index	High	1	1.0%	0	0.0%	1	1.9%	0.397	0.198
	Mean high	4	3.8%	3	5.8%	1	1.9%		
	Mean	10	9.6%	5	9.6%	5	9.6%		
	Mean low	35	33.7%	14	26.9%	21	40.4%		
	Low	54	51.9%	30	57.7%	24	46.2%		
		Mean	SD	Mean	SD	Mean	SD	p	|d|
Age (years)		25.37	6.83	25.42	5.89	25.31	7.71	0.932	0.02
Age of onset of ED (years)		19.03	6.12	19.54	4.86	18.52	7.17	0.398	0.17
Duration of ED (years)		6.42	5.84	6.01	5.54	6.82	6.16	0.483	0.14
BMI (kg/m^2)		21.62	6.15	22.51	7.16	20.72	4.84	0.138	0.29
		n	%	n	%	n	%	p	C-V
ED subtype	AN	38	36.5%	19	36.5%	19	36.5%	1.000	0.000
	BN	36	34.6%	18	34.6%	18	34.6%		
	BED	4	3.8%	2	3.8%	2	3.8%		
	OSFED	26	25.0%	13	25.0%	13	25.0%		

Note: ED-NA—eating disorder, non-athlete. ED-A—eating disorder, athlete. AN—anorexia nervosa. BN—bulimia nervosa. BED—binge eating disorder. OSFED—other specified feeding and eating disorder. SD—standard deviation. C-V—Cramer's-V coefficient.

Table 2. Comparison at baseline: ANOVA.

	ED-NA (n = 52)		ED-A (n = 52)			
	Mean	SD	Mean	SD	p	|d|
EDI-2 Drive for thinness	14.33	5.60	12.62	7.16	0.178	0.27
EDI-2 Body dissatisfaction	17.25	8.52	13.06	9.46	**0.019 ***	0.47
EDI-2 Interoceptive awareness	10.08	6.69	9.25	7.16	0.544	0.12
EDI-2 Bulimia	5.37	5.21	5.31	5.23	0.955	0.01
EDI-2 Interpersonal distrust	5.04	4.43	4.87	4.40	0.842	0.04
EDI-2 Ineffectiveness	9.40	7.02	8.48	7.50	0.518	0.13
EDI-2 Maturity fears	7.96	6.03	7.12	5.54	0.458	0.15
EDI-2 Perfectionism	5.75	4.58	6.38	5.58	0.527	0.12
EDI-2 Impulse regulation	6.37	5.70	4.87	5.66	0.181	0.26
EDI-2 Ascetic	7.29	4.03	6.87	4.97	0.634	0.09
EDI-2 Social Insecurity	6.85	4.99	6.52	5.83	0.759	0.06
EDI-2 Total scale	95.63	40.56	85.33	53.82	0.273	0.22
SCL-90R Somatization	1.69	0.85	1.36	0.94	0.060	0.37
SCL-90R Obsessive–compulsive	1.82	0.79	1.52	0.90	0.069	0.36
SCL-90R Interpersonal sensitivity	2.04	0.92	1.69	1.05	0.068	0.36
SCL-90R Depression	2.16	0.82	1.89	1.04	0.155	0.28
SCL-90R Anxiety	1.62	0.86	1.44	0.93	0.306	0.20
SCL-90R Hostility	1.47	1.06	1.15	0.87	0.097	0.33
SCL-90R Phobic anxiety	1.06	0.87	0.89	1.01	0.370	0.18

Table 2. Cont.

	ED-NA (n = 52)		ED-A (n = 52)			
	Mean	SD	Mean	SD	p	|d|
SCL-90R Paranoia ideation	1.50	0.82	1.27	0.88	0.175	0.27
SCL-90R Psychotic ideation	1.41	0.77	1.18	0.76	0.130	0.30
SCL-90R GSI	1.73	0.69	1.47	0.82	0.075	0.35
SCL-90R PST	64.67	15.11	57.27	22.80	0.054	0.38
SCL-90R PSDI	2.35	0.58	2.10	0.65	**0.046 ***	0.40
TCI-R Novelty seeking	101.73	15.17	98.27	16.11	0.262	0.22
TCI-R Harm avoidance	111.92	21.13	107.21	23.27	0.282	0.21
TCI-R Reward dependence	100.94	15.47	100.02	16.02	0.766	0.06
TCI-R Persistence	115.29	21.38	120.04	19.85	0.243	0.23
TCI-R Self-directedness	119.90	20.99	124.73	24.32	0.281	0.21
TCI-R Cooperativeness	132.42	15.88	131.33	18.74	0.748	0.06
TCI-R Self-transcendence	65.67	17.27	65.63	15.14	0.990	0.00

Note: ED-NA—eating disorder, non-athlete. ED-A—eating disorder, athlete. SD—standard deviation. * Bold is significant comparison (0.05).

3.3. Treatment Outcomes

No differences in the risk of dropout and bad outcome during the treatment were obtained comparing the ED-NA versus the ED-A groups (see Table 3).

Table 3. Comparison of the cognitive behavioral therapy (CBT) outcomes: chi-square tests.

		ED-NA (n = 52)		ED-A (n = 52)			
		n	%	n	%	p	C-V
Outcome	Dropout	17	32.7%	15	28.8%	0.596	0.135
	Non-remission	5	9.6%	9	17.3%		
	Partial remission	9	17.3%	11	21.2%		
	Full remission	21	40.4%	17	32.7%		
Dropout	No	35	67.3%	37	71.2%	0.671	0.042
	Yes	17	32.7%	15	28.8%		
Bad outcome	No	30	57.7%	28	53.8%	0.693	0.039
	Yes	22	42.3%	24	46.2%		

Note: ED-NA—eating disorder, non-athlete. ED-A—eating disorder, athlete. C-V—Cramer's-V coefficient.

In the logistic regression models, the predictors indicating higher likelihood of dropout during treatment were the SCL-90R somatic score among ED-NA group and the SCL-90R obsessive–compulsive score among the ED-A group. The odds of a bad outcome were also higher for ED-NA patients with a higher SCL-90R score, while higher levels in SCL-90R obsessive–compulsive, TCI-R self-directedness and self-transcendence were predictors of worse treatment outcome among the ED-A group (see Table 4).

Table 4. Predictive models for the risk of dropout and bad outcome.

Group	Criteria	Subsample: ED-NA	B	SE	p	OR	95% CI (OR)		H-L	N-R2
ED-NA	Dropout	SCL-90R Somatic	0.847	0.399	0.034	2.333	1.067	5.100	0.147	0.130
	Bad outcome	SCL-90R Somatic	0.842	0.380	0.027	2.321	1.102	4.889	0.202	0.137
ED-A	Dropout	SCL-90R Obsessive–comp.	2.008	0.910	0.027	7.452	1.252	44.36	0.052	0.155
	Bad outcome	SCL-90R Obsessive–comp.	1.117	0.573	0.040	3.056	1.000	9.403	0.222	0.223
		TCI-R Self-directedness	0.043	0.022	0.035	1.044	1.000	1.090		
		TCI-R Self-transcendence	0.047	0.024	0.032	1.049	1.000	1.100		

Note: ED-NA—eating disorder, non-athlete. ED-A—eating disorder, athlete. Bad outcome—dropout or non-remission. HL—Hosmer–Lemeshow (p-value). N-R2—Nagelkerke's pseudo-R2. List of predictors: sociodemographic, ED severity (EDI-2 total score), psychopathology distress (SCL-90R GSI) and personality traits (TCI-R).

3.4. Comparison Based on the Sport Type

The first block in Table 5 displays the comparison between ED-A patients who reported individual versus group sports. Individual sport was characterized by a higher mean in the ED symptom severity measures (concretely in the EDI-2 drive for thinness, body dissatisfaction, ineffectiveness and total score), worse psychopathological state (SCL-90R somatic and hostility scales), higher self-transcendence and lower cooperativeness. ED-A also registered a longer duration of the ED and a different distribution of the treatment outcome (lower risk of dropout and partial remission; higher risk of non-remission). No differences in the cumulative survival curves comparing individual versus group sports were found (Figure 1).

Table 5. Comparison based on the sport type.

		Individual (n = 42)		Group (n = 10)				Non-Aesthetic (n = 25)		Aesthetic (n = 27)			
Measures at Baseline		Mean	SD	Mean	SD	p	|d|	Mean	SD	Mean	SD	p	|d|
Age (years)		25.93	6.95	22.70	10.38	0.238	0.37	26.80	7.11	23.93	8.12	0.182	0.38
Age of onset of ED (years)		18.12	6.32	20.20	10.27	0.415	0.24	20.12	6.78	17.04	7.32	0.122	0.44
Duration of ED (years)		7.85	6.41	2.50	1.43	**0.012 ***	**1.15 †**	6.71	6.51	6.93	5.93	0.901	0.03
EDI-2 Drive for thinness		13.76	6.80	7.80	6.94	**0.016 ***	**0.87 †**	10.48	7.63	14.59	6.19	**0.037 ***	**0.59 †**
EDI-2 Body dissatisfaction		13.90	9.88	9.50	6.69	0.188	**0.52 †**	10.36	9.05	15.56	9.30	**0.047 ***	**0.57 †**
EDI-2 Interoceptive awareness		9.86	7.40	6.70	5.70	0.214	0.48	7.60	6.65	10.78	7.41	0.111	0.45
EDI-2 Bulimia		5.83	5.38	3.10	4.04	0.139	**0.57 †**	4.32	4.36	6.22	5.86	0.193	0.37
EDI-2 Interpersonal distrust		5.07	4.65	4.00	3.20	0.494	0.27	4.48	4.35	5.22	4.49	0.548	0.17
EDI-2 Ineffectiveness		9.19	7.62	5.50	6.45	0.164	**0.52 †**	6.64	6.21	10.19	8.27	0.088	**0.51 †**
EDI-2 Maturity fears		7.19	5.80	6.80	4.54	0.844	0.07	7.12	4.30	7.11	6.57	0.995	0.00
EDI-2 Perfectionism		6.83	5.57	4.50	5.46	0.238	0.42	4.84	4.93	7.81	5.84	0.054	**0.55 †**
EDI-2 Impulse regulation		5.29	6.03	3.10	3.41	0.277	0.45	4.20	4.60	5.48	6.52	0.420	0.23
EDI-2 Ascetic		7.19	4.88	5.50	5.36	0.338	0.33	5.72	4.54	7.93	5.19	0.110	0.45
EDI-2 Social Insecurity		6.81	6.18	5.30	4.06	0.467	0.29	5.20	4.92	7.74	6.41	0.117	0.44
EDI-2 Total scale		90.93	54.69	61.80	45.01	0.125	**0.58 †**	70.96	50.05	98.63	54.66	0.063	**0.53 †**
SCL-90R Somatization		1.46	0.95	0.92	0.83	0.106	**0.60 †**	1.37	0.95	1.35	0.95	0.928	0.03
SCL-90R Obsessive–compulsive		1.58	0.88	1.26	1.00	0.322	0.34	1.36	0.99	1.66	0.80	0.233	0.33
SCL-90R Interpersonal sensitivity		1.73	1.05	1.52	1.13	0.588	0.19	1.55	1.09	1.81	1.03	0.379	0.25
SCL-90R Depression		1.95	1.03	1.63	1.09	0.381	0.31	1.78	1.07	2.00	1.03	0.441	0.22
SCL-90R Anxiety		1.48	0.91	1.25	1.02	0.477	0.24	1.31	0.95	1.56	0.91	0.345	0.26
SCL-90R Hostility		1.26	0.90	0.70	0.59	0.069	**0.73 †**	1.15	0.90	1.15	0.86	0.978	0.01
SCL-90R Phobic anxiety		0.94	1.05	0.67	0.81	0.451	0.29	0.83	0.97	0.94	1.06	0.704	0.11
SCL-90R Paranoia ideation		1.35	0.89	0.95	0.81	0.202	0.47	1.17	0.88	1.36	0.89	0.448	0.21
SCL-90R Psychotic ideation		1.25	0.76	0.91	0.75	0.210	0.45	1.03	0.74	1.32	0.76	0.171	0.39
SCL-90R GSI		1.53	0.81	1.19	0.86	0.232	0.42	1.38	0.85	1.55	0.80	0.476	0.20
SCL-90R PST		59.10	22.41	49.60	24.06	0.240	0.41	54.36	25.01	59.96	20.66	0.381	0.24
SCL-90R PSDI		2.15	0.66	1.91	0.64	0.294	0.38	2.02	0.72	2.18	0.59	0.385	0.24
TCI-R Novelty seeking		98.88	17.03	95.70	11.83	0.580	0.22	101.72	18.59	95.07	12.97	0.139	0.41
TCI-R Harm avoidance		105.93	24.18	112.60	19.09	0.421	0.31	101.44	19.87	112.56	25.22	0.085	**0.52 †**
TCI-R Reward dependence		98.90	16.12	104.70	15.49	0.308	0.37	100.32	16.46	99.74	15.90	0.898	0.04
TCI-R Persistence		120.62	20.53	117.60	17.45	0.670	0.16	119.96	12.74	120.11	24.96	0.978	0.01
TCI-R Self-directedness		123.00	25.32	132.00	18.88	0.297	0.40	130.72	23.21	119.19	24.42	0.088	**0.51 †**
TCI-R Cooperativeness		128.55	19.29	143.00	10.39	**0.027 ***	**0.93 †**	134.56	12.57	128.33	22.89	0.235	0.34
TCI-R Self-transcendence		67.05	16.02	59.70	8.99	0.170	**0.57 †**	62.40	15.27	68.63	14.66	0.140	0.42
Treatment outcome		n	%	n	%	p	C-V	n	%	n	%	p	C-V
Outcome	Dropout	11	26.2%	4	40.0%	0.376	**0.247 †**	3	12.0%	12	44.4%	**0.050 ***	**0.387 †**
	Non-remission	9	21.4%	0	0.0%			5	20.0%	4	14.8%		
	Partial remission	8	19.0%	3	30.0%			8	32.0%	3	11.1%		
	Full remission	14	33.3%	3	30.0%			9	36.0%	8	29.6%		
Dropout	No	31	73.8%	6	60.0%	0.448	0.120	22	88.0%	15	55.6%	**0.014 ***	**0.358 †**
	Yes	11	26.2%	4	40.0%			3	12.0%	12	44.4%		
Bad outcome	No	22	52.4%	6	60.0%	0.736	0.060	17	68.0%	11	40.7%	0.058	**0.273 †**
	Yes	20	47.6%	4	40.0%			8	32.0%	16	59.3%		

Note: SD—standard deviation. C-V—Cramer's-V coefficient. * Bold signifies significant comparison (0.05). † Bold signifies effect size into the ranges mild/moderate to high/large.

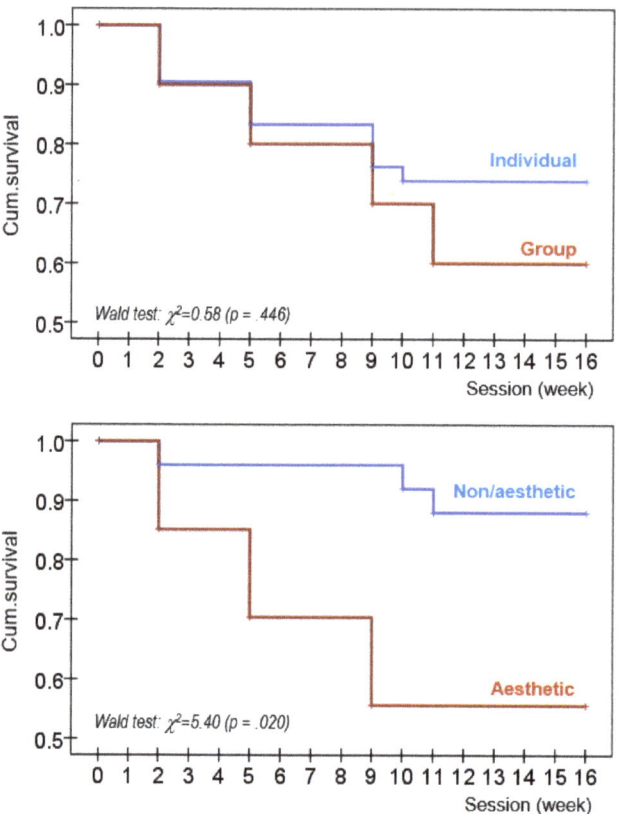

Figure 1. Survival function for the rate of dropout based on the sport type (Cox regression).

The second block in Table 5 shows the comparison between individual non-aesthetic sports versus individual-aesthetic sports. The aesthetic sports group was characterized by a higher mean in the EDI-2 drive for thinness, body dissatisfaction, ineffectiveness, perfectionism and total scale, as well as by a higher score in harm avoidance and a lower score in self-directedness. Differences in the treatment outcomes were also identified, such that aesthetic sports related to worse results during therapy (higher risk and rate of dropout, see Figure 1).

4. Discussion

This present study aimed to examine differences between patients with ED who were professional athletes (ED-A) and those who were not (ED-NA) regarding clinical features, personality traits and treatment outcomes. As a secondary goal, our research intended to give a better understanding of the role that sport plays in professional athletes with an ED and to provide a framework for future research involving these patients. To our knowledge, this is one of the first studies that attempts to analyze therapy outcome in this specific population.

4.1. Clinical Features and Personality Traits

Although we hypothesized that we would find differences in clinical features and personality traits between the ED-A and ED-NA groups, when analyzing the data, no relevant statistical differences were found. These findings were in line with previous results [47,48] and suggest that, due to the clinical similarities between the athlete and non-athlete groups, similar clinical approaches may be appropriate.

When examining clinical symptoms of ED, we found differences in body dissatisfaction, where lower mean values in the ED-A group were reported. It has been suggested that, while professional sports imply high physical demands, becoming involved in sports practice could be linked with a better perception of body shape [49,50]. Some underlined potential reasons for this difference could be due to the fact that the athlete's figure may be closer to society's ideal body [51] and that athletes may have increased appreciation for the functionality of the body but not so much for its shape [52].

Regarding psychopathology, the ED-A group showed less global psychological discomfort. In our sample, sports practice seemed to play a protective role in terms of psychopathology and, whereas some authors have considered that even elite sport can act as a protective factor in mental health [53,54], others have considered that the need for high performance could act as a trigger for psychological discomfort with elevated anxiety and depression, as well as obsessive symptoms [55–59] and substance addiction [9,27].

Similarly, when analyzing the personality profile, personality traits did not differ between our clinical samples of athletes and non-athletes. However, special attention should be paid to traits, which have been largely associated with predisposing personality traits to ED [60,61] but could be considered as beneficial for athletic performance, referred to as "the good athlete" [47] or "athletic personality" [62], such as perfectionism, obsession, overcompliance and harm avoidance. This is especially true in light of previous studies on the normalization of pain, injury and mental overload, as well as the prevalence of presentism in elite athletes [20–23].

Within the analysis performed in the ED-A group, some differences emerged between the type of sport. Individual sports presented a higher severity in ED symptoms, more psychopathology and higher self-transcendence and lower cooperativeness as personality traits. Interestingly, the cooperativeness mean score in the team sports group was within normal values for the general population, which may suggest a positive effect of the collaborative teamwork associated with these sports. These findings were consistent with previous research that showed that, in individual sports, athletes were more individualistic and sought their own goals more than having fun when practicing the sports [63]. The aesthetic sports group in this study, and according to the literature [26,64–66], showed the most dysfunctional profile, with higher rates in ED symptoms and maladaptive personality traits, as higher scores in harm avoidance and lower scores in self-directedness were identified; this added to their greater concern about body shape and could determine why it took longer for them to seek help [25]. Therefore, in this group of patients, prevention and early diagnosis may be the most important aspects, as, once the disorder is established, it could be difficult to adhere to treatment since, on many occasions, they experience the ED symptoms in an ego-syntonic way with their personality and sport values and goals.

4.2. Response to Treatment

When comparing ED-A and ED-NA, no differences were observed regarding the treatment outcome or dropouts. These results were expected, considering the lack of differences in clinical and personality features between these groups. This reaffirmed the idea that no differential treatments are needed and that similar clinical approaches may be appropriate. However, special attention should be paid to athletes who, as part of an outpatient program, would be reluctant to undergo treatment because of the impact it may have on their sporting goals [24,67].

As we expected, the subgroup of aesthetic sports showed higher rates of dropouts and bad outcome than the non-aesthetic sports. These results were in accordance with the fact that these patients experienced more severity in clinical ED symptoms [26] and maladaptive personality features [68] that could condition worse prognoses and risks of chronicity. Additionally, in individual sports, especially aesthetic ones, body shape and leanness were associated with the misconception of maximizing performance and therefore it probably took longer to seek help and increased the risk of chronicity; thus, prevention and early intervention in this subgroup would be especially necessary.

4.3. Predictive Factors of Therapeutic Success

In our analysis, for the athletes' subgroup, the predictors of worse treatment outcome had higher levels in the obsessive–compulsive, self-directedness and self-transcendence scales. The presence of obsession compulsiveness could imply difficulty in modifying cognitions and, thus, could hinder adherence to treatment. High rates of self-directedness, which is the ability to adapt behavior to achieve personal goals, and self-transcendence, which includes idealism, could predict worse treatment outcomes in this group of patients due to the aims and values of their sports practice and not with the disease. In ED, some predictors of bad outcome have been related to premorbid depression, obsessive–compulsive symptoms and long duration of disease [69–71]. Furthermore, different studies have suggested the importance of personality traits in treatment outcomes of ED. TCI dimensions [36], such as low self-directedness and low cooperativeness, have been related to more likelihood in not finishing treatment [72,73], while persistence was associated with dropouts [74] and self-transcendence was predictive of premature termination of hospitalization in an inpatient sample [75].

Our analysis of predictor factors seemed consistent with the fact that there are no clinically relevant differences between ED-A and ED-NA. As similar treatment approaches seem to be appropriate, it is necessary to individually evaluate a correct way to implement exercise programs in the ED population. Even though in the professional athlete population it is important to pay special attention at the beginning of their career in order to recognize early ED symptomatology, it is imperative to follow the evolution during their careers, principally once they finish their professional activity. Our results showed a wide variability in the age of onset of ED, displaying that the pathology in some athletes may start when the professional activity is over. Some evidence suggests that retired professional athletes may be at high risk of mental health problems, including anxiety and depression symptoms [68]. Further studies are needed to understand what happens regarding the ED symptoms once the professional athlete retires.

The benefits of physical activity for mental health have been widely demonstrated, both for mental health symptoms and for the prevention of mental disorders [76,77]. However, due to the high incidence of dysfunctional exercise in patients with ED, some specialists prefer to limit physical activity during treatment [78]. Nevertheless, a growing number of studies have shown that incorporating physical activity into the routine care of these patients can improve ED symptomatology and can be an effective intervention for the management of these disorders [79–84]. Experienced clinicians have reaffirmed the need to incorporate physical activity into ED treatment protocols within a psychotherapeutic approach, not only for the physical and mental health benefits but also to help patients learn how to engage in exercise in an adaptive manner [85].

Some limitations of our study should be noted. The retrospective and self-reported data collection could limit the validity and the reliability of our findings. The sample of this study was collected in a specialized eating disorders' unit; this could imply more severity of the disease and comorbidities in this group of patients. The small sample size was another limitation. We performed a power analysis for the mean comparisons between the ED-NA group versus the ED-A group (sample sizes equal to 52 per group), with the assumption of comparing T-standardized measures (which are common in clinical areas and are generated on the basis of reference population-based samples with a mean equal to 50 and a standard deviation equal to 10) and potential differences delta of at least 10 points between the conditions. This analysis provided a power equal to 0.71 (close to, but below, the reference threshold in the scientific area, $1 - \beta = 0.80$). A second analysis was performed, also considering two independent mean-comparisons, but for sample sizes of 42 and 10 (the most disadvantaged situation in the study). This new calculation provided a power equal to 0.42 (well below the 0.80 threshold). Contrariwise, a strength of this study was the clinical sample of professional athletes with ED that was analyzed. There are scarce amounts of studies examining clinical samples of patients with proper eating disorder diagnosis who go through a protocolized standardized treatment, compared with non-athlete eating-disorder patients. However, in this study, we were not able to consider some important variables, such as excessive training or body composition, which would have been valuable variables to include. It would be interesting for future studies to include this information when analyzing these populations.

5. Conclusions

In conclusion, no major clinical differences were observed between athletes and non-athletes with ED, so similar treatment strategies could be appropriate for both groups. Nevertheless, some differences emerged regarding seeking treatment that should be considered. Therefore, investigating the role of professional sport performance in these outcomes may help to better understand these interactions and introduce new interventions based on the development of strategies that include exercise supervised by mental health exercise prescription specialists to improve body image concerns and psychological symptoms. We believe that physical activity needs to be included in ED guidelines and further research should be conducted to elucidate this paradigm shift in ED, especially in some types of AN and BN.

On the other hand, individual and aesthetic sports have shown a higher risk of worse prognosis and chronicity for athletes. Therefore, an effort should be made to develop preventive and early detection programs involving sports doctors, coaches and family, as well as sports psychologists, who should not only be concerned with performance and motivation but also with prevention and detection of early mental diseases. These programs must be carried out throughout athletes' sporting lives, from the beginning of sports practice to after retirement.

Author Contributions: Conceptualization, F.F.-A., I.S. and A.I.-C.; methodology, R.G.; formal analysis, R.G.; writing—original draft preparation, A.I.-C., L.C.-B. and I.S.; writing—review and editing, L.C.-B., I.S, M.R., A.T., S.Z., J.d.P., F.F.-A. and S.J.-M.; supervision, F.F.-A. and S.J.-M.; funding acquisition, F.F.-A. and S.J.-M. All authors have read and agreed to the published version of the manuscript.

Funding: This research was funded by Instituto de Salud Carlos III (ISCIII) (FIS PI20/00132) and co-funded by FEDER funds/European Regional Development Fund (ERDF), a way to build Europe. CIBERobn is an initiative of ISCIII. This study was also funded by European Union's Horizon 2020 research and innovation program under grant agreement no. 847879 (PRIME/H2020, Prevention and Remediation of Insulin Multimorbidity in Europe). Additional funding was received from AGAUR-Generalitat de Catalunya (2021-SGR-00824). LCB was supported by Sara Borrell fellowship -CD22/00171- Instituto de Salud Carlos III (ISCIII) and co-funded by the European Union. RG was supported by the Catalan Institution for Research and Advanced Studies (ICREA-Academia, 2021-Programme). MR was supported by an FI grant from the Catalan Agency for the Management of Grants for University-AGAUR (2020 FISDU 00579).

Institutional Review Board Statement: The study was conducted in accordance with the Declaration of Helsinki and approved by the Ethics Committee of BELLVITGE UNIVERSITY HOSPITALNAME OF INSTITUTE (protocol code 2021/2613, date of approval 2 September 2021).

Informed Consent Statement: Informed consent was obtained from all subjects involved in the study.

Data Availability Statement: All inquiries regarding availability of the data should be referred to the corresponding author (FFA), as there are ongoing studies using the data and to preserve patient confidentiality. Requests will be considered on a case-by-case basis.

Acknowledgments: We thank CERCA Programme/Generalitat de Catalunya for institutional support. We also thank Instituto de Salud Carlos III (ISCIII), CIBERobn (an initiative of ISCIII), FEDER funds/European Regional Development Fund (ERDF), a way to build Europe and European Social Fund (ESF, investing in your future).

Conflicts of Interest: F.F.-A. and S.J.-M. received consultancy honoraria from Novo Nordisk and F.F.-A. editorial honoraria as EIC from Wiley. The rest of the authors declare no conflict of interest. The funders had no role in the design of the study; in the collection, analyses, or interpretation of data; in the writing of the manuscript or in the decision to publish the results.

References

1. American Psychiatric Association. *Diagnostic and Statistical Manual of Mental Disorders DSM-5*; American Psychiatric Publishing: Washington, DC, USA, 2013.
2. Treasure, J.; Claudino, A.M.; Zucker, N. Eating disorders. *Lancet* **2010**, *375*, 583. [CrossRef]
3. Fernández-Aranda, F.; Casas, M.; Claes, L.; Bryan, D.C.; Favaro, A.; Granero, R.; Gudiol, C.; Jiménez-Murcia, S.; Karwautz, A.; Le Grange, D.; et al. COVID-19 and implications for eating disorders. *Eur. Eat. Disord. Rev.* **2020**, *28*, 239–245. [CrossRef] [PubMed]
4. Devoe, D.J.; Han, A.; Anderson, A.; Katzman, D.K.; Patten, S.B.; Soumbasis, A.; Flanagan, J.; Paslakis, G.; Vyver, E.; Marcoux, G.; et al. The impact of the COVID-19 pandemic on eating disorders: A systematic review. *Int. J. Eat. Disord.* **2023**, *56*, 5–25. [CrossRef] [PubMed]
5. Smink, F.R.E.; Van Hoeken, D.; Hoek, H.W. Epidemiology of eating disorders: Incidence, prevalence and mortality rates. *Curr. Psychiatry Rep.* **2012**, *14*, 406–414. [CrossRef] [PubMed]
6. Hay, P. Current approach to eating disorders: A clinical update. *Intern. Med. J.* **2020**, *50*, 24–29. [CrossRef]
7. Kron, L.; Katz, J.L.; Gorzynski, G.; Weiner, H. Hyperactivity in anorexia nervosa: A fundamental clinical feature. *Compr. Psychiatry* **1978**, *19*, 433–440. [CrossRef]
8. Hebebrand, J.; Exner, C.; Hebebrand, K.; Holtkamp, C.; Casper, R.C.; Remschmidt, H.; Herpertz-Dahlmann, B.; Klingenspor, M. Hyperactivity in patients with anorexia nervosa and in semistarved rats: Evidence for a pivotal role of hypoleptinemia. *Physiol. Behav.* **2003**, *79*, 25–37. [CrossRef]
9. Gunnarsson, B.; Entezarjou, A.; Fernández-Aranda, F.; Jiménez-Murcia, S.; Kenttä, G.; Håkansson, A. Understanding exercise addiction, psychiatric characteristics and use of anabolic androgenic steroids among recreational athletes—An online survey study. *Front. Sport. Act. Living* **2022**, *4*, 903777. [CrossRef]
10. Rizk, M.; Mattar, L.; Kern, L.; Berthoz, S.; Duclos, J.; Viltart, O.; Godart, N. Physical Activity in Eating Disorders: A Systematic Review. *Nutrients* **2020**, *12*, 183. [CrossRef]
11. Solenberger, S.E. Exercise and eating disorders: A 3-year inpatient hospital record analysis. *Eat. Behav.* **2001**, *2*, 151–168. [CrossRef]
12. Dalle Grave, R.; Calugi, S.; Marchesini, G. Compulsive exercise to control shape or weight in eating disorders: Prevalence, associated features, and treatment outcome. *Compr. Psychiatry* **2008**, *49*, 346–352. [CrossRef]
13. El Ghoch, M.; Calugi, S.; Pellegrini, M.; Milanese, C.; Busacchi, M.; Battistini, N.C.; Bernabè, J.; Dalle Grave, R. Measured physical activity in anorexia nervosa: Features and treatment outcome. *Int. J. Eat. Disord.* **2013**, *46*, 709–712. [CrossRef]
14. Strober, M.; Freeman, R.; Morrell, W. The long-term course of severe anorexia nervosa in adolescents: Survival analysis of recovery, relapse, and outcome predictors over 10–15 years in a prospective study. *Int. J. Eat. Disord.* **1997**, *22*, 339–360. [CrossRef]
15. Sauchelli, S.; Arcelus, J.; Granero, R.; Jiménez-Murcia, S.; Agüera, Z.; Del Pino-Gutiérrez, A.; Fernández-Aranda, F. Dimensions of compulsive exercise across eating disorder diagnostic subtypes and the validation of the spanish version of the compulsive exercise test. *Front. Psychol.* **2016**, *7*, 1852. [CrossRef]
16. Torstveit, M.K.; Rosenvinge, J.H.; Sundgot-Borgen, J. Prevalence of eating disorders and the predictive power of risk models in female elite athletes: A controlled study. *Scand. J. Med. Sci. Sports* **2008**, *18*, 108–118. [CrossRef]
17. Curry, T.J. A Little Pain Never Hurt Anyone: Athletic Career Socialization and the Normalization of Sports Injury. *Symb. Interact.* **1993**, *16*, 273–290. [CrossRef]
18. Hughes, R.; Coakley, J. Positive Deviance among Athletes: The Implications of Overconformity to the Sport Ethic. *Sociol. Sport J.* **2016**, *8*, 307–325. [CrossRef]
19. Schnell, A.; Mayer, J.; Diehl, K.; Zipfel, S.; Thiel, A. Giving everything for athletic success!—Sports-specific risk acceptance of elite adolescent athletes. *Psychol. Sport Exerc.* **2014**, *15*, 165–172. [CrossRef]
20. Theberge, N. "Just a Normal Bad Part of What I Do": Elite Athletes' accounts of the relationship between health and sport. *Sociol. Sport J.* **2008**, *25*, 206–222. [CrossRef]
21. Thiel, A.; Schubring, A.; Schneider, S.; Zipfel, S.; Mayer, J. Health in Elite Sports—A "Bio-Psycho-Social" Perspective. *Dtsch. Z. Sportmed.* **2015**, *66*, 241–247. [CrossRef]
22. Nixon, H.L. Cultural, structural and status dimensions of pain and injury experiences in sport. In *Sporting Bodies, Damaged Selves: Sociological Studies of Sports-Related Injury*; Young, K., Ed.; Elsevier Ltd.: Oxford, UK, 2004; pp. 81–98.
23. Mayer, J.; Giel, K.E.; Malcolm, D.; Schneider, S.; Diehl, K.; Zipfel, S.; Thiel, A. Compete or rest? Willingness to compete hurt among adolescent elite athletes. *Psychol. Sport Exerc.* **2018**, *35*, 143–150. [CrossRef]
24. Flatt, R.E.; Thornton, L.M.; Fitzsimmons-Craft, E.E.; Balantekin, K.N.; Smolar, L.; Mysko, C.; Wilfley, D.E.; Taylor, C.B.; DeFreese, J.D.; Bardone-Cone, A.M.; et al. Comparing eating disorder characteristics and treatment in self-identified competitive athletes and non-athletes from the National Eating Disorders Association online screening tool. *Int. J. Eat. Disord.* **2021**, *54*, 365–375. [CrossRef] [PubMed]
25. Landkammer, F.; Winter, K.; Thiel, A.; Sassenberg, K. Team Sports Off the Field: Competing Excludes Cooperating for Individual but Not for Team Athletes. *Front. Psychol.* **2019**, *10*, 2470. [CrossRef] [PubMed]
26. Krentz, E.M.; Warschburger, P. A longitudinal investigation of sports-related risk factors for disordered eating in aesthetic sports. *Scand. J. Med. Sci. Sports* **2013**, *23*, 303–310. [CrossRef]
27. Sundgot-Borgen, J. Risk and trigger factors for the development of eating disorders in female elite athletes. *Med. Sci. Sports Exerc.* **1994**, *26*, 414–419. [CrossRef]

28. Arcelus, J.; Witcomb, G.L.; Mitchell, A. Prevalence of eating disorders amongst dancers: A systemic review and meta-analysis. *Eur. Eat. Disord. Rev.* **2014**, *22*, 92–101. [CrossRef]
29. Heradstveit, O.; Hysing, M.; Nilsen, S.A.; Bøe, T. Symptoms of disordered eating and participation in individual- and team sports: A population-based study of adolescents. *Eat. Behav.* **2020**, *39*, 101434. [CrossRef]
30. Giel, K.E.; Hermann-Werner, A.; Mayer, J.; Diehl, K.; Schneider, S.; Thiel, A.; Zipfel, S. Eating disorder pathology in elite adolescent athletes. *Int. J. Eat. Disord.* **2016**, *49*, 553–562. [CrossRef]
31. Salkind, N. Structured Clinical Interview for DSM-IV. In *Encyclopedia of Measurement and Statistics*; American Psychiatric Association: Arlington, VA, USA, 2015; pp. 1–94.
32. Garner, D.M. *EDI-2: Professional Manual*; Psychological Assessment Resources: Odessa, FL, USA, 1991.
33. Garner, D.M. *EDI 2: Inventario de Trastornos de la Conducta Alimentaria*; TEA Ediciones: Madrid, Spain, 1998; Volume 267, ISBN 84-7174-536-4.
34. Derogatis, L.R.; Unger, R. *SCL-90-R: Symptom Checklist-90-Revised: Administration, Scoring and Procedures Manual*; Clinical Psychometric Research: Baltimore, MD, USA, 1996.
35. Gonzales de Rivera, J.L.; de Las Cuevas, C. *SCL-90-R Cuestionario de 90 Sintomas*; TEA Editorial: Madrid, Spain, 2002.
36. Cloninger, C.R. *The Temperament and Character Inventory-Revised*; Center for Psychobiology of Personality: Sant Louis, MO, USA, 1999.
37. Sundgot-Borgen, J.; Larsen, S. Pathogenic weight-control methods and self-reported eating disorders in female elite athletes and controls. *Scand. J. Med. Sci. Sports* **1993**, *3*, 150–155. [CrossRef]
38. Fernández-Aranda, F.; Treasure, J.; Paslakis, G.; Agüera, Z.; Giménez, M.; Granero, R.; Sánchez, I.; Serrano-Troncoso, E.; Gorwood, P.; Herpertz-Dahlmann, B.; et al. The impact of duration of illness on treatment nonresponse and drop-out: Exploring the relevance of enduring eating disorder concept. *Eur. Eat. Disord. Rev.* **2021**, *29*, 499–513. [CrossRef]
39. Fernandez-Aranda, F.; Turon, V. *Trastornos Alimentarios. Guia Basica de Tratamiento en Anorexia y Bulimia*; Masson: Barcelona, Spain, 1998; Volume 1, ISBN 84-458-0746-3.
40. Agüera, Z.; Romero, X.; Arcelus, J.; Sánchez, I.; Riesco, N.; Jiménez-Murcia, S.; González-Gómez, J.; Granero, R.; Custal, N.; De Bernabé, M.M.G.; et al. Changes in body composition in anorexia nervosa: Predictors of recovery and treatment outcome. *PLoS ONE* **2015**, *10*, e0143012. [CrossRef]
41. Agüera, Z.; Riesco, N.; Jiménez-Murcia, S.; Islam, M.A.; Granero, R.; Vicente, E.; Peñas-Lledó, E.; Arcelus, J.; Sánchez, I.; Menchon, J.M.; et al. Cognitive behaviour therapy response and dropout rate across purging and nonpurging bulimia nervosa and binge eating disorder: DSM-5 implications. *BMC Psychiatry* **2013**, *13*, 285. [CrossRef]
42. Agüera, Z.; Sánchez, I.; Granero, R.; Riesco, N.; Steward, T.; Martín-Romera, V.; Jiménez-Murcia, S.; Romero, X.; Caroleo, M.; Segura-García, C.; et al. Short-Term Treatment Outcomes and Dropout Risk in Men and Women with Eating Disorders. *Eur. Eat. Disord. Rev.* **2017**, *25*, 293–301. [CrossRef]
43. Kelley, K.; Preacher, K.J. On effect size. *Psychol. Methods* **2012**, *17*, 137–152. [CrossRef]
44. Blanca, M.J.; Alarcón, R.; Arnau, J.; Bono, R.; Bendayan, R. Non-normal data: Is ANOVA still a valid option? *Psicothema* **2017**, *29*, 552–557. [CrossRef]
45. Finner, H.; Roters, M. On the False Discovery Rate and Expected Type I Errors. *Biom. J.* **2001**, *43*, 985. [CrossRef]
46. Aalen, O.O.; Borgan, Ø.; Gjessing, H.K. *Survival and Event History Analysis: A Process Point of View*; Statistics for Biology and Health; Springer: New York, NY, USA, 2008; ISBN 978-0-387-20287-7.
47. Thompson, R.A.; Sherman, R.T. "Good athlete" traits and characteristics of anorexia nervosa: Are they similar? *Eat. Disord.* **1999**, *7*, 181–190. [CrossRef]
48. Sundgot-Borgen, J. Eating Disorders in Female Athletes. *Sports Med.* **1994**, *17*, 176–188. [CrossRef]
49. Karrer, Y.; Halioua, R.; Mötteli, S.; Iff, S.; Seifritz, E.; Jäger, M.; Claussen, M.C. Disordered eating and eating disorders in male elite athletes: A scoping review. *BMJ Open Sport Exerc. Med.* **2020**, *6*, e000801. [CrossRef]
50. Zhan, C.; Heatherington, L.; Klingenberg, B. Disordered eating- and exercise-related behaviors and cognitions during the first year college transition. *J. Am. Coll. Health* **2022**, *70*, 852–863. [CrossRef]
51. Brownell, K.D. Dieting and the search for the perfect body: Where physiology and culture collide. *Behav. Ther.* **1991**, *22*, 1–12. [CrossRef]
52. Chapa, D.A.N.; Johnson, S.N.; Richson, B.N.; Bjorlie, K.; Won, Y.Q.; Nelson, S.V.; Ayres, J.; Jun, D.; Forbush, K.T.; Christensen, K.A.; et al. Eating-disorder psychopathology in female athletes and non-athletes: A meta-analysis. *Int. J. Eat. Disord.* **2022**, *55*, 861–885. [CrossRef] [PubMed]
53. Smolak, L.; Murnen, S.K.; Ruble, A.E. Female athletes and eating problems: A meta-analysis. *Int. J. Eat. Disord.* **2000**, *27*, 371–380. [CrossRef]
54. Grasdalsmoen, M.; Clarsen, B.; Sivertsen, B. Mental Health in Elite Student Athletes: Exploring the Link between Training Volume and Mental Health Problems in Norwegian College and University Students. *Front. Sports Act. Living* **2022**, *4*, 817757. [CrossRef]
55. Rice, S.M.; Purcell, R.; De Silva, S.; Mawren, D.; McGorry, P.D.; Parker, A.G. The Mental Health of Elite Athletes: A Narrative Systematic Review. *Sports Med.* **2016**, *46*, 1333–1353. [CrossRef]
56. Rice, S.M.; Gwyther, K.; Santesteban-Echarri, O.; Baron, D.; Gorczynski, P.; Gouttebarge, V.; Reardon, C.L.; Hitchcock, M.E.; Hainline, B.; Purcell, R. Determinants of anxiety in elite athletes: A systematic review and meta-analysis. *Br. J. Sports Med.* **2019**, *53*, 722–730. [CrossRef]

57. Forys, W.J.; Tokuhama-Espinosa, T. The Athlete's Paradox: Adaptable Depression. *Sports* **2022**, *10*, 105. [CrossRef]
58. Weber, S.; Puta, C.; Lesinski, M.; Gabriel, B.; Steidten, T.; Bär, K.J.; Herbsleb, M.; Granacher, U.; Gabriel, H.H.W. Symptoms of anxiety and depression in young athletes using the hospital anxiety and depression scale. *Front. Physiol.* **2018**, *9*, 182. [CrossRef]
59. Marazziti, D.; Parra, E.; Amadori, S.; Arone, A.; Palermo, S.; Massa, L.; Simoncini, M.; Carbone, M.G.; Dell'osso, L. Obsessive-compulsive and depressive symptoms in professional tennis players. *Clin. Neuropsychiatry* **2021**, *18*, 304–311. [CrossRef]
60. Barakat, S.; McLean, S.A.; Bryant, E.; Le, A.; Marks, P.; Aouad, P.; Barakat, S.; Boakes, R.; Brennan, L.; Bryant, E.; et al. Risk factors for eating disorders: Findings from a rapid review. *J. Eat. Disord.* **2023**, *11*, 8. [CrossRef]
61. Culbert, K.M.; Racine, S.E.; Klump, K.L. Research Review: What we have learned about the causes of eating disorders—A synthesis of sociocultural, psychological, and biological research. *J. Child Psychol. Psychiatry Allied Discip.* **2015**, *56*, 1141–1164. [CrossRef]
62. Hauck, E.R.; Blumenthal, J.A. Obsessive and Compulsive Traits in Athletes. *Sport. Med.* **1992**, *14*, 215–227. [CrossRef]
63. Pluhar, E.; McCracken, C.; Griffith, K.L.; Christino, M.A.; Sugimoto, D.; Meehan, W.P. Team sport athletes may be less likely to suffer anxiety or depression than individual sport athletes. *J. Sports Sci. Med.* **2019**, *18*, 490–496.
64. Martinsen, M.; Sundgot-Borgen, J. Higher prevalence of eating disorders among adolescent elite athletes than controls. *Med. Sci. Sports Exerc.* **2013**, *45*, 1188–1197. [CrossRef]
65. Sundgot-Borgen, J. Weight and eating disorders in elite athletes. *Scand. J. Med. Sci. Sports* **2002**, *12*, 259–260. [CrossRef]
66. Werner, A.; Thiel, A.; Schneider, S.; Mayer, J.; Giel, K.E.; Zipfel, S. Weight-control behaviour and weight-concerns in young elite athletes—A systematic review. *J. Eat. Disord.* **2013**, *1*, 18. [CrossRef]
67. Sundgot-Borgen, J.; Torstveit, M.K. Aspects of disordered eating continuum in elite high-intensity sports. *Scand. J. Med. Sci. Sports* **2010**, *20*, 112–121. [CrossRef]
68. Kemarat, S.; Theanthong, A.; Yeemin, W.; Suwankan, S. Personality characteristics and competitive anxiety in individual and team athletes. *PLoS ONE* **2022**, *17*, e0262486. [CrossRef]
69. Keski-Rahkonen, A.; Raevuori, A.; Bulik, C.M.; Hoek, H.W.; Rissanen, A.; Kaprio, J. Factors associated with recovery from anorexia nervosa: A population-based study. *Int. J. Eat. Disord.* **2014**, *47*, 117–123. [CrossRef]
70. Bossert, S.; Schmölz, U.; Wiegand, M.; Junker, M.; Krieg, J.C. Predictors of short-term treatment outcome in bulimia nervosa inpatients. *Behav. Res. Ther.* **1992**, *30*, 193–199. [CrossRef]
71. Schoemaker, C. Does early intervention improve the prognosis in anorexia nervosa? A systematic review of the treatment-outcome literature. *Int. J. Eat. Disord.* **1997**, *21*, 1–15. [CrossRef]
72. Fassino, S.; Abbate Daga, G.; Pierò, A.; Rovera, G.G. Dropout from brief psychotherapy in anorexia nervosa. *Psychother. Psychosom.* **2002**, *71*, 200–206. [CrossRef] [PubMed]
73. Fassino, S.; Pierò, A.; Tomba, E.; Abbate-Daga, G. Factors associated with dropout from treatment for eating disorders: A comprehensive literature review. *BMC Psychiatry* **2009**, *9*, 67. [CrossRef] [PubMed]
74. Dalle Grave, R.; Calugi, S.; Brambilla, F.; Abbate-Daga, G.; Fassino, S.; Marchesini, G. The effect of inpatient cognitive-behavioral therapy for eating disorders on temperament and character. *Behav. Res. Ther.* **2007**, *45*, 1335–1344. [CrossRef] [PubMed]
75. Pham-Scottez, A.; Huas, C.; Perez-Diaz, F.; Nordon, C.; Divac, S.; Dardennes, R.; Speranza, M.; Rouillon, F. Why do people with eating disorders drop out from inpatient treatment?: The role of personality factors. *J. Nerv. Ment. Dis.* **2012**, *200*, 807–813. [CrossRef]
76. Schuch, F.B.; Vancampfort, D. Physical activity, exercise, and mental disorders: It is time to move on. *Trends Psychiatry Psychother.* **2021**, *43*, 177–184. [CrossRef]
77. Smith, P.J.; Merwin, R.M. The Role of Exercise in Management of Mental Health Disorders: An Integrative Review. *Annu. Rev. Med.* **2021**, *72*, 45–62. [CrossRef]
78. Quesnel, D.A.; Cooper, M.; Fernandez-del-Valle, M.; Reilly, A.; Calogero, R.M. Medical and physiological complications of exercise for individuals with an eating disorder: A narrative review. *J. Eat. Disord.* **2023**, *11*, 3. [CrossRef]
79. Raisi, A.; Zerbini, V.; Piva, T.; Belvederi Murri, M.; Menegatti, E.; Caruso, L.; Masotti, S.; Grazzi, G.; Mazzoni, G.; Mandini, S. Treating Binge Eating Disorder with Physical Exercise: A Systematic Review and Meta-analysis. *J. Nutr. Educ. Behav.* **2023**. [CrossRef]
80. Toutain, M.; Gauthier, A.; Leconte, P. Exercise therapy in the treatment of anorexia nervosa: Its effects depending on the type of physical exercise—A systematic review. *Front. Psychiatry* **2022**, *13*, 939856. [CrossRef]
81. Diers, L.; Rydell, S.A.; Watts, A.; Neumark-Sztainer, D. A yoga-based therapy program designed to improve body image among an outpatient eating disordered population: Program description and results from a mixed-methods pilot study. *Eat. Disord.* **2020**, *28*, 476–493. [CrossRef]
82. Kern, L.; Morvan, Y.; Mattar, L.; Molina, E.; Tailhardat, L.; Peguet, A.; De Tournemire, R.; Hirot, F.; Rizk, M.; Godart, N.; et al. Development and evaluation of an adapted physical activity program in anorexia nervosa inpatients: A pilot study. *Eur. Eat. Disord. Rev.* **2020**, *28*, 687–700. [CrossRef]
83. Carei, T.R.; Fyfe-Johnson, A.L.; Breuner, C.C.; Brown, M.A. Randomized Controlled Clinical Trial of Yoga in the Treatment of Eating Disorders. *J. Adolesc. Health* **2010**, *46*, 346–351. [CrossRef]

84. Martínez-Sánchez, S.M.; Martínez-García, T.E.; Bueno-Antequera, J.; Munguía-Izquierdo, D. Feasibility and effect of a Pilates program on the clinical, physical and sleep parameters of adolescents with anorexia nervosa. *Complement. Ther. Clin. Pract.* **2020**, *39*, 101161. [CrossRef]
85. Danielsen, M.; Rø, Ø.; Bjørnelv, S. How to integrate physical activity and exercise approaches into inpatient treatment for eating disorders: Fifteen years of clinical experience and research. *J. Eat. Disord.* **2018**, *6*, 34. [CrossRef]

Disclaimer/Publisher's Note: The statements, opinions and data contained in all publications are solely those of the individual author(s) and contributor(s) and not of MDPI and/or the editor(s). MDPI and/or the editor(s) disclaim responsibility for any injury to people or property resulting from any ideas, methods, instructions or products referred to in the content.

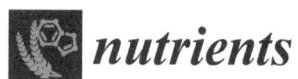

Article

Eating Disorders and Intimate Partner Violence: The Influence of Fear of Loneliness and Social Withdrawal

Janire Momeñe [1], Ana Estévez [1], Mark D. Griffiths [2], Patricia Macía [3], Marta Herrero [1], Leticia Olave [4] and Itziar Iruarrizaga [4,*]

[1] Psychology Department, School of Health Sciences, University of Deusto, 48080 Bilbao, Spain; janiremomene@deusto.es (J.M.); aestevez@deusto.es (A.E.); m.herrero@deusto.es (M.H.)
[2] International Gaming Research Unit, Psychology Department, Nottingham Trent University, Nottingham NG1 4FQ, UK; mark.griffiths@ntu.ac.uk
[3] Department of Basic Psychological Processes and Their Development, University of the Basque Country/Euskal Herriko Unibertsitatea (UPV/EHU), 20018 Donostia-San Sebastián, Spain; patricia.macia@ehu.eus
[4] Department of Experimental Psychology, Cognitive Processes and Speech Therapy, Faculty of Social Work, Complutense University of Madrid, Pozuelo de Alarcón, 28223 Madrid, Spain; leticiaolave@ucm.es
* Correspondence: iciariru@psi.ucm.es

Abstract: Eating disorders are vulnerability factors that increase the likelihood of intimate partner violence. However, the mechanisms underlying this relationship are unclear. Although eating disorders have been associated with increased perception and fear of loneliness, they have also been associated with increased social withdrawal resulting from decreased enjoyment of social situations and poorer social functioning. The purpose of the present study was to examine the mediating role of fear of loneliness in the relationship between the behavioural characteristics of eating disorders and intimate partner violence, as well as to explore the moderating role of social withdrawal in the relationship between fear of loneliness and intimate partner violence. The sample comprised 683 participants (78% female and 22% male) with a mean age of 21.14 years (SD = 2.72). The psychometric scales used were Eating Disorders Inventory (EDI 2), Emotional Dependency Questionnaire (EDQ), Coping Strategies Inventory (CSI) and the Violence Received, Exercised and Perceived in Youth and Adolescent Dating Relationships Scale (VREPS). The hypothesised model was tested by path analysis using maximum likelihood. The path analysis of the hypothesised model showed that inefficacy, fear of maturity, and impulsivity were the behavioural characteristics of eating disorders predominantly related to fear of loneliness. Fear of loneliness had no direct significant effect on any of the received violence variables. However, interaction effects indicated that there was a moderately significant effect of fear of loneliness on physical, psychological, and social violence received as a function of levels of social withdrawal. These findings show the need to take into account and work on fear of loneliness and social withdrawal among individuals with an eating disorder to decrease the likelihood of establishing violent intimate partner relationships. Improving interpersonal functioning and social support is key to recovery from eating disorders.

Keywords: eating disorders; intimate partner violence; violence received; social withdrawal; fear of loneliness; vulnerability factors; path analysis

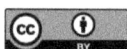

1. Introduction

Eating Disorders (EDs) are serious psychiatric disorders [1] that significantly impair the physical and psychological health of sufferers. Moreover, the mortality rate is one of the highest compared to other psychiatric conditions (5–10%) [2,3]. Currently, the main types of EDs that individuals suffer from worldwide are anorexia nervosa, bulimia nervosa, and binge eating disorder [4], characterised by persistent disturbance of eating behaviour [5]. It has been estimated that EDs affect 15% of the world population and their incidence continues to increase. Moreover, they begin to manifest themselves between early and late adolescence. It is at this stage of the life cycle that important physical, psychological and neuronal changes occur [6]. Its aetiology is multifactorial, and psychological, developmental, biological and/or sociocultural factors may influence it. However, the aetiology is not yet fully elucidated. In recent years, the need for further research has been noted [2,7].

In addition to the deterioration produced in physical and psychological health, EDs can also negatively impacts social functioning [8–11]. The perception of loneliness has been found to be present in individuals with this problem, and it is considered a negative emotion that contributes to and increases their symptomatology. Moreover, EDs also exacerbate feelings of loneliness [12]. Perceived loneliness is defined as emotional distress stemming from a feeling of rejection or isolation by others or the lack of a social partner to lean on and engage in activities with. Moreover, it has been shown to severely influence individuals' quality of life [13,14].

Recent research has highlighted the feeling of loneliness as one of the most commonly present issues among young adults [15]. However, very few studies have examined the feeling of loneliness in emerging adulthood [16] and even fewer in Spain (where the present study was carried out) in relation to EDs. Understanding the relationship between EDs and fear of loneliness is vital to address these intense emotions within prevention and treatment programs. Therefore, it is important to analyse the impact exerted by the fear of loneliness among individuals with this problem [12,17].

In addition, previous studies have noted the use of dysfunctional coping strategies by individuals with an ED [18,19] that contribute to the aetiology and maintenance of this problem [6,20]. Therefore, the behaviours characteristic of EDs can be employed as dysfunctional coping mechanisms to regain control over stressful circumstances [21]. More specifically, findings suggest that individuals with an ED predominantly employ coping strategies based on self-criticism and social isolation. Furthermore, the importance of further research has been pointed out because coping strategies play an important role in the prognosis and treatment of EDs [22], especially social isolation. Empirical studies suggest that social isolation and low sense of social support increase ED symptomatology and have a detrimental impact on recovery [23–26]. This may be because social isolation promotes increased maladaptive eating habits and body dissatisfaction [27]. Therefore, it has been noted that social support and adaptive social functioning are key to a more effective and complete recovery [28,29].

Likewise, the empirical literature has noted that EDs increase the probability of suffering intimate partner violence (IPV) throughout life [30]. Therefore, the prevalence of IPV among individuals with EDs is high [31]. It should be noted that previous literature has also posited a bidirectional relationship between IPV and EDs because the direction of causality can be in both directions [32]. However, the mechanisms underlying this relationship are unclear. Previous studies have found that social isolation and fear of loneliness are vulnerability factors for staying in violent relationships [33]. Despite this, the role they play in the relationship between EDs and IPV has not been established. Consequently, their study is of utmost importance in designing early and effective prevention and intervention programs [34].

In recent years, this line of research examining the relationship between EDs and IPV has gained relevance due to its clinical and prognostic implications. Therefore, the present study's main objectives were to: (i) analyse the relationships between core symptoms traversing Eds; (ii) explore the mediating role of fear of loneliness in the relationship between the behavioural characteristics of EDs and IPV; and (iii) explore the moderating role of social isolation in the relationship between fear of loneliness and IPV. Based on the aforementioned literature, the hypotheses of the present study were that: (i) the core symptoms traversing EDs will have a significant direct effect on received partner violence; and (ii) the core symptoms traversing EDs will have a significant indirect effect on received partner violence through the mediating role of fear of loneliness and the moderating role of social isolation.

2. Method

2.1. Participants

The sample comprised 683 emerging Spanish adults who participated in a cross-sectional survey study. The average age of the participants was 21.14 years old (SD = 2.72; 78% female and 22% male). The participants were mostly students (80.1%) and workers (19.3%). The remaining participants were unemployed (0.6%).

2.2. Procedure

Participants were recruited through two channels: online and face-to-face. For the online recruitment, surveys were made available through an online platform (*surveymonkey.com* accessed on 1 January 2020). Participation was promoted through different social networks and advertisements on research websites. For the face-to-face recruitment, participants were recruited at the Complutense University of Madrid and at gyms in the Madrid community. The only exclusion criterion was being under 18 years of age. All participants gave their informed consent by confirming or clicking on a button indicating that they had read the study information and agreed to participate voluntarily. The study followed the ethical principles of the 2013 Helsinki Declaration and was approved by the research team's university ethics committee.

2.3. Instruments

Eating disorder characteristics. The Eating Disorders Inventory-2 (EDI-2) [35] was used to assess clinically relevant behaviours and psychological traits that accompany EDs. The EDI-2 consists of 91 items divided into 11 scales (obsession with thinness, bulimia, body dissatisfaction, inefficacy, perfectionism, interpersonal distrust, interoceptive awareness, fear of maturity, asceticism, impulsivity and social insecurity). All items (e.g., *"I tend to eat when I am upset"*; *"I find it difficult to express my emotions to others"*; *"I think my stomach is too big"*) are rated on a six-point scale from 0 (*"Never"*) to 5 (*"Always"*). The higher the scores obtained on each scale, the greater the manifestations of the trait evaluated. The internal consistency (Cronbach's α) of the subscales in the present study ranged from 0.73 to 0.90.

Fear of loneliness. The fear of loneliness subscale from the Emotional Dependency Questionnaire (EDQ) [36] was used to assess fear of loneliness. All items (e.g., *"I feel helpless when I am alone"*; *"I feel a strong sense of emptiness when I am alone"*; *"I cannot tolerate loneliness"*) are rated on a six-point scale from 1 (*"Completely untrue of me"*) to 6 (*"Describes me perfectly"*). The higher the score obtained, the greater the fear of loneliness. The internal consistency in the present study was $\alpha = 0.82$.

Social avoidance. The Coping Strategies Inventory (CSI) [37] was used to assess social avoidance. The scale assesses eight styles of coping with stressful situations by means of 41 items (problem solving, cognitive restructuring, social support, emotional expression, problem avoidance, desiderative thinking, social withdrawal, self-criticism). All items (e.g., *"I avoided being with people"*; *"I didn't let anyone know how I felt"*) are rated on a five-point scale from 0 (*"Not at all"*) to 4 (*"Completely"*). The higher the score obtained, the greater the social avoidance. The internal consistency in the present study was $\alpha = 0.74$.

Received violence. The Violence Received, Exercised and Perceived in Youth and Adolescent Dating Relationships Scale (VREPS) [38] was used to assess received violence. The scale comprises 28 items including five violence subscales (physical violence, sexual violence, social psychological violence, psychological violence humiliation–coercion, and psychological violence control-jealousy) and encompassing three aspects of violence: received, exerted, and perceived. For violence received and exercised, items (e.g., *"My boyfriend/girlfriend tells me to change the way I dress, do my hair . . . and criticizes it"*; *"My boyfriend/girlfriend wants to know where I am at all times and who I am with"*; *"My boyfriend/girlfriend has run out of friends because I didn't like them and told him/her not to be with them"*) are rated on a six-point scale (0 *"Never"*, 1 *"Once"*, 2 *"From 2 to 5 times"*, 3 *"From 6 to 10 times"*, 4 *"From 11 to 15 times"* and 5 *"More than 15 times"*) and for perceived violence items (e.g., *"My boyfriend/girlfriend has forced me to have sex (any kind of oral or penetration) when I did not want to. Is this violence?"*) are rated on a five-point scale (1 *"No violence"*, 2 *"Little violence"*, 3 *"Somewhat violent"*, 4 *"Quite violent"* and 5 *"Very violent"*). In addition, participants indicate whether they consider the situations mentioned to be violence. The higher the score obtained, the greater the received violence. In the present study, the violence received was of particular interest in the analysis. The internal consistency of the five subscales of received violence in the present study ranged from α = 0.82 to 0.89.

2.4. Statistical Analysis

Data analyses were carried out using Mplus 7.0 [39]. The hypothesised model was tested by path analysis using maximum likelihood. Following the model described in Figure 1, the model included the eating disorder characteristics (i.e., obsession for thinness, bulimia, body dissatisfaction, ineffectiveness, perfectionism, interpersonal distrust, interoceptive awareness, fear of maturity, asceticism, impulsiveness and social insecurity) as independent variables, received violence as the dependent variable (i.e., physical, sexual, psychological humiliation–coercion, psychological control-jealousy and social), the fear of loneliness as the mediator, and social withdrawal as the moderator in the relationship between the mediator and the dependent variables. Gender and age were included as controls in the model.

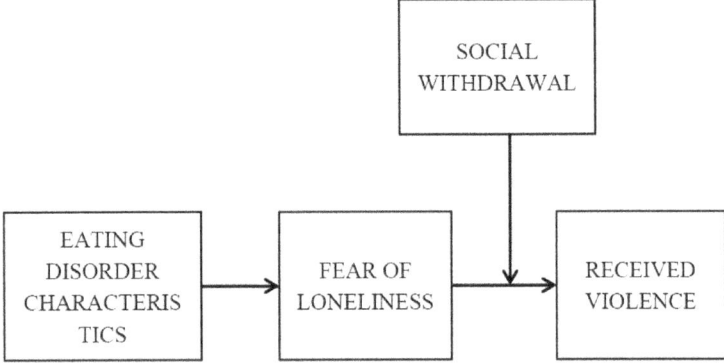

Figure 1. Hypothesised model.

The adequacy of the proposed model was analysed according to the following model fit indicators: ratio of chi-square (χ^2) and the degrees of freedom, the comparative fit index (CFI), the Tucker–Lewis index (TLI), the root mean squared error of approximation (RMSEA), and the standardised root mean square residual (SRMR). Values of χ^2/df of <3.0, CFI and TLI ≥ 0.90, and RMSEA and SRMR < 0.08 were considered indicators of good fit [40].

In order to test the moderated mediation, the direct effect of EDCs (eating disorder characteristics) on the dependent variables was included, and the variables of the products were standardised. Additionally, the analysis adapted the code provided by Stride et al. (2015) [41] in Model 1 and Model 14 to test the simple slopes of the direct and indirect effects. For the computation of the indirect effects, bootstrap was applied with 5000 samples. All significant moderations and moderated-mediations were tested at low (−1.5 SD), average (at the mean) and high levels (+1.5 SD) of the moderator to examine simple slopes.

3. Results

First, the descriptive statistics of the sample and the correlations between the study variables were calculated (see Tables 1 and 2). Some of the EDCs were not significantly correlated with any of the received violence indicators (i.e., bulimia, body dissatisfaction and fear of maturity). Fear of loneliness and social withdrawal were significantly correlated with all variables.

Table 1. Descriptive statistics and reliability of the study variables (n = 683).

Variables	Means and Standard Deviations				Reliability		
	M	SD	Min	Max	α	CR	AVE
Eating disorder characteristics							
Obsession for thinness	13.68	9.30	0	35	0.90	0.93	0.64
Bulimia	9.10	6.08	0	32	0.80	0.85	0.46
Body dissatisfaction	20.39	7.18	2	41	0.89	0.91	0.54
Ineffectiveness	15.14	8.78	0	48	0.88	0.90	0.48
Perfectionism	11.60	5.67	0	30	0.73	0.82	0.43
Interpersonal distrust	11.92	5.97	0	32	0.73	0.82	0.41
Interoceptive awareness	17.74	8.76	0	45	0.84	0.88	0.43
Fear of maturity	19.18	6.43	2	40	0.73	0.81	0.35
Asceticism	12.31	6.20	0	40	0.73	0.81	0.36
Impulsiveness	14.44	8.44	0	55	0.82	0.86	0.36
Social insecurity	13.84	6.51	0	40	0.79	0.84	0.41
Fear of loneliness	5.53	2.99	2	18	0.82	0.90	0.74
Social withdrawal	5.80	4.11	0	20	0.74	0.83	0.50
Received violence							
Physical	0.21	0.55	0	5	0.82	0.89	0.61
Sexual	0.33	0.73	0	5	0.88	0.91	0.64
Psychological humiliation–coercion	0.41	0.82	0	5	0.88	0.91	0.63
Psychological control-jealousy	0.60	0.96	0	5	0.89	0.92	0.65
Social	0.28	0.67	0	4.6	0.85	0.90	0.65

Note. Min = Minimum; Max = Maximum; α = Cronbach's alpha; CR = Composite reliability; AVE = Average variance extracted.

Second, the path analysis of the hypothesised model was performed. All model fit indicators showed a good fit of the model, $\chi^2/df = 2.26$, CFI = 0.99, TLI = 0.95, RMSEA = 0.04, SRMR < 0.01. Therefore, the model adequately explained the study data. As displayed in Table 3, the direct effects showed that ineffectiveness, fear of maturity, and impulsiveness were the EDCs related to fear of loneliness. Fear of loneliness had no direct significant effect on any of the variables of received violence. However, the interaction effects indicated that there was a significant moderated effect of fear of loneliness on physical, psychological humiliation–coercion, and social received violence depending on the levels of social withdrawal.

Based on the exposed variables, the simple slopes were examined to understand the moderation effects. Simple slopes showed that higher fear of loneliness was significantly related to more physical violence ($\beta = 0.16$, SE = 0.03, $p < 0.001$) and psychological humiliation–coercion received violence ($\beta = 0.11$, SE = 0.05, $p = 0.028$) when the social withdrawal was high, but there was no significant relationship when the social withdrawal was low (physical: $\beta = -0.07$, SE = 0.03, $p = 0.063$; psychological humiliation—coercion: $\beta = -0.06$, SE = 0.05, $p = 0.281$) or medium (physical: $\beta = 0.16$, SE = 0.03, $p = 0.053$; psychological humiliation—coercion: $\beta = 0.02$, SE = 0.03, $p = 0.444$).

Regarding social received violence, the simple slopes indicated that greater fear of loneliness was significantly related to lower social received violence when the social withdrawal was low ($\beta = -0.19$, SE = 0.04, $p = 0.043$), but was related to greater social violence when the social withdrawal was high ($\beta = 0.13$, SE = 0.04, $p = 0.002$). The relationship at medium levels of social withdrawal was not significant ($\beta = 0.01$, SE = 0.02, $p = 0.499$).

As a final step, the moderated mediation of the EDCs was tested on the variables of received violence (see Table 4). The indirect effects of ineffectiveness, fear of maturity and impulsiveness on physical violence, and social received violence, through fear of loneliness, were significant only at high social withdrawal levels. However, none of the indirect effects on psychological humiliation–coercion received violence was significant, although a tendency was observed towards high social withdrawal levels.

Table 2. Bivariate correlations between the study variables.

Variables	1	2	3	4	5	6	7	8	9	10	11	12	13	14	15	16	17	18
Eating disorder characteristics																		
1. Obsession for thinness	(0.90)																	
2. Bulimia	0.41 **	(0.80)																
3. Body dissatisfaction	0.58 **	0.32 **	(0.89)															
4. Ineffectiveness	0.45 **	0.39 **	0.35 **	(0.88)														
5. Perfectionism	0.27 **	0.39 **	0.15 **	0.26 **	(0.73)													
6. Interpersonal distrust	0.15 **	0.14 **	0.17 **	0.53 **	0.10 **	(0.73)												
7. Interoceptive awareness	0.49 **	0.56 **	0.38 **	0.65 **	0.39 **	0.46 **	(0.84)											
8. Fear of maturity	0.23 **	0.17 **	0.19 **	0.35 **	0.20 **	0.26 **	0.40 **	(0.73)										
9. Asceticism	0.44 **	0.57 **	0.34 **	0.49 **	0.48 **	0.17 **	0.60 **	0.25 **	(0.73)									
10. Impulsiveness	0.35 *	0.52 **	0.29 **	0.52 **	0.39 **	0.24 **	0.67 **	0.28 **	0.67 **	(0.82)								
11. Social insecurity	0.21 **	0.20 **	0.20 **	0.66 **	0.13 **	0.67 **	0.43 **	0.26 **	0.27 **	0.38 **	(0.79)							
12. Fear of loneliness	0.22 **	0.26 **	0.20 **	0.37 **	0.23 **	0.16 **	0.34 **	0.25 **	0.35 **	0.38 **	0.24 **	(0.82)						
13. Social withdrawal	0.19 **	0.23 **	0.17 **	0.39 *	0.22 **	0.42 **	0.38 **	0.21 **	0.31 **	0.30 **	0.43 **	0.19 **	(0.74)					
Received violence																		
14. Physical	0.05	0.04	−0.03	0.04	0.06	0.01	0.10 **	0.07	0.09 *	0.11 **	0.05	0.12 **	0.10 **	(0.82)				
15. Sexual	0.13 **	0.04	0.02	0.11 **	0.09 *	0.04	0.11 **	0.01	0.12 **	0.15 **	0.09 *	0.09 *	0.11 **	0.53 **	(0.88)			
16. Psychological humiliation-coercion	0.07 *	0.03	0.01	0.09 **	0.10 **	0.03	0.07 *	0.02	0.12 **	0.14 **	0.10 **	0.09 *	0.08 *	0.64 **	0.67 **	(0.88)		
17. Psychological control-jealousy	0.10 **	0.06	0.03	0.08 *	0.11 **	0.04	0.11 **	0.03	0.14 **	0.19 **	0.09 *	0.11 **	0.12 **	0.57 **	0.64 **	0.81 **	(0.89)	
18. Social	0.08 *	0.03	0.03	0.12 **	0.07	0.08 *	0.10 **	0.02	0.11 **	0.13 **	0.15 **	0.09 **	0.11 **	0.60 **	0.65 **	0.86 **	0.81 **	(0.85)

Note. * $p < 0.05$, ** $p < 0.01$.

Table 3. Standardised direct and interaction effects of the model based on path analysis.

Independent Variables	Dependent Variables											
	Received Violence											
	Fear of Loneliness		Physical		Sexual		Psychological Humiliation–Coercion		Psychological Control–Jealousy		Social	
	β	SE	β	SE	β	SE	β	SE	β	SE	β	SE
Eating disorder characteristics												
Obsession for thinness	−0.03	0.04	0.08	0.05	0.14 **	0.05	0.06	0.05	0.10 *	0.05	0.06	0.05
Bulimia	0.02	0.04	−0.06	0.04	−0.08	0.05	−0.08	0.05	−0.09 *	0.04	−0.08	0.05
Body dissatisfaction	0.05	0.04	−0.12 *	0.04	−0.09 *	0.04	−0.05	0.04	−0.04	0.04	0.04	0.04
Ineffectiveness	0.20 ***	0.05	−0.12	0.06	0.01	0.06	<−0.01	0.06	−0.08	0.06	<0.01	0.06
Perfectionism	0.05	0.04	<0.01	0.04	0.04	0.04	0.06	0.04	0.04	0.04	0.03	0.04
Interpersonal distrust	−0.03	0.04	−0.08	0.05	−0.03	0.05	−0.04	0.05	−0.02	0.05	−0.03	0.05
Interoceptive awareness	−0.04	0.06	0.14 *	0.06	<0.01	0.06	−0.03	0.06	0.01	0.06	<0.01	0.06
Fear of maturity	0.12 **	0.03	0.03	0.04	−0.06	0.04	−0.03	0.04	−0.03	0.04	−0.05	0.04
Asceticism	0.09	0.05	<0.01	0.05	<0.01	0.05	0.05	0.05	<0.01	0.05	0.05	0.05
Impulsiveness	0.17 **	0.05	0.03	0.05	0.13 *	0.05	0.11	0.05	0.18 **	0.05	0.06	0.05
Social insecurity	<0.01	0.05	0.07	0.05	0.02	0.06	0.08	0.06	0.05	0.05	0.12 *	0.05
Fear of loneliness			0.08	0.04	0.03	0.04	0.03	0.04	0.04	0.04	0.02	0.04
Social withdrawal			0.06	0.04	0.07	0.04	0.03	0.04	0.07	0.04	0.04	0.04
Fear of loneliness X Social withdrawal			0.15 ***	0.03	0.03	0.03	0.07 *	0.03	0.06	0.03	0.12 **	0.03
r^2	0.21 ***		0.07 ***		0.05 **		0.04 **		0.06 ***		0.05 **	

Note. * $p < 0.05$, ** $p < 0.01$, *** $p < 0.001$.

Table 4. Moderated indirect effects of ineffectiveness, fear of maturity and impulsiveness on physical, psychological humiliation–coercion and social received violence through fear of loneliness.

Independent variables	Level of the moderator	Dependent Variables (Received Violence)					
		Physical		Psychological Humiliation–Coercion		Social	
		z	p	z	p	z	p
Ineffectiveness	Low social withdrawal	−1.65	0.099	−1.03	0.302	−1.76	0.078
	Average social withdrawal	1.70	0.089	0.74	0.454	0.66	0.507
	High social withdrawal	2.81 *	0.005	1.86	0.062	2.34 *	0.019
Fear of maturity	Low social withdrawal	−1.60	0.109	−1.02	0.308	−1.71	0.088
	Average social withdrawal	1.65	0.099	0.74	0.456	0.66	0.509
	High social withdrawal	2.61 **	0.009	1.80	0.071	2.22 *	0.026
Impulsiveness	Low social withdrawal	−1.61	0.106	−1.02	0.306	−1.72	0.085
	Average social withdrawal	1.66	0.096	0.74	0.456	0.66	0.508
	High social withdrawal	2.66 **	0.008	1.82	0.068	2.25 *	0.024

Note. * $p < 0.05$, ** $p < 0.01$.

4. Discussion

The main objective of the present study was to analyse the association between core symptoms traversing eating disorders (EDs) and to explore the role of fear of loneliness and social isolation in relation to behavioural eating disorder characteristics (EDCs) and intimate partner violence (IPV) received. First, it was hypothesised that core symptoms traversing EDs would have a significant direct effect on received partner violence. Results showed that some of the EDCs were not significantly associated with any of the received violence indicators (e.g., bulimia, body dissatisfaction, and fear of maturity). However, other indicators such as obsession for thinness, ineffectiveness, perfectionism, interoceptive awareness, asceticism, impulsiveness, and social insecurity were all significantly and positively related to received violence.

These results are in accordance with previous scientific literature that EDs increase the likelihood of IPV among both females and males [30,31]. Although EDs have traditionally been considered female disorders, recent evidence suggests that it is not uncommon among males, and that males can present similar severe ED symptoms. In fact, there are specific risk factors for developing EDs among young and adolescent males, such as body image concerns related to muscularity and sexual orientation [1]. As mentioned, EDs can emerge as maladaptive coping mechanisms that enable individuals to regain control over adverse situations, as can be receiving violence [21,42].

Another factor associated with EDs and violence exposure among both sexes is social isolation, which has been associated with adoption of unhealthy weight control practices [26]. With the aim of exploring more deeply the role of social aspects, the second hypothesis was that core symptoms traversing EDs would have a significant indirect effect on received partner violence through the mediating role of fear of loneliness and the moderating role of social isolation.

On the one hand, results showed that ineffectiveness, fear of maturity, and impulsivity were the behavioural EDCs predominantly related to fear of loneliness. Fear of loneliness had no direct significant effect on any of the received violence variables. Nevertheless, interaction effects indicated a moderately significant influence of fear of loneliness on physical violence, psychological humiliation—coercion, and social received violence as a function of levels of social withdrawal.

It was also found that the indirect effects of ineffectiveness, fear of maturity, and impulsiveness on physical and social received violence, through fear of loneliness, were significant only at high social withdrawal levels. Results refine the understanding of the relationship between social withdrawal and the development of EDs in individuals exposed to partner violence. Individuals suffering loneliness appear to be more susceptible to developing disordered eating patterns [43].

Participants in the present study are characterised as being young. Moreover, it should be noted that emerging adulthood can be a critical period for developing mental health problems [15,16]. In particular, EDs are frequently initiated in this period, especially, considering the great relevance that acquire social interactions at this developmental stage [18]. Fear of loneliness and social isolation are among the most common concerns for young people, and results have evidenced their impact on the relation between EDs and IPV [15].

For instance, the pandemic and subsequent social restrictions have limited and deprived individuals of social interaction resulting in decreased social support and similar coping strategies in facing this unprecedented situation [44]. Therefore, eliminating social protection factors when coping with adverse events could increase risk and symptoms of ED [45]. In this sense, loneliness has been conceived as a mediator between emotional dysregulation and eating disorders-related psychopathology [46].

This lack of perceived social support associated with the exposure to partner violence could culminate in many psychological health consequences, such as depression, post-traumatic stress, anxiety, and EDs, among other mental health illnesses [47]. Low levels of social support have been related to increased risk of ED among women exposed to IPV. Social support has shown protective effects against ED by decreasing levels of anxiety and promoting mechanisms related to functional coping strategies [48]. However, IPV-exposure and trauma history can precede the development of ED symptoms. The extant literature highlights the presence of childhood abuse among individuals suffering IPV and EDs. Children who have experienced exposure to violent situations appear to be more susceptible to developing EDs [30,49]. Other studies have identified specific aspects related to altered-eating behaviours and IPV exposure including somatization, avoiding abuse, coping, self-harm, and challenging abusive partners [42].

Overall, results in the present study confirm the bidirectional relationship between ED and IPV, influenced by aspects such as fear of loneliness and social withdrawal. On the one hand, it was observed that childhood abuse is highly related to both EDs and IPV, so it could be considered a possible explanatory factor [32,49–51]. On the other hand, it should be noted that the association between EDs and IPV also depends on the type of ED, due to the fact that different EDs have diverse aetiology [52]. Nevertheless, the present study highlights social-related aspects in explaining some of the mechanisms underlying this bidirectional relationship between EDs and IPV. Individuals who suffer from EDs usually show fear of loneliness and social isolation patterns, which are also consequences of IPV, and could likewise derive in developing ED-related symptoms.

All of these aspects support the notion that ED-related behaviours are used as ways to cope with adverse and stressful situations such as received violence. This could be important information for therapists who work with those experiencing IPV and who develop interventions for patients with clinical symptoms of an ED. Results emphasise the importance of understanding the vulnerability and absence of coping resources among individuals who suffer IPV and develop EDs, with the aim of designing interventions focused on the promotion of coping through seeking social support and avoiding isolation.

5. Limitations

The present study has some limitations that should be noted. First, the cross-sectional design employed in the present study does not allow determining conclusions in terms of causality. Therefore, longitudinal studies are needed to determine any casual inferences among different variables examined in the present study. Secondly, the sample in the present study was limited to emerging adults, with an average age of 21 years old, therefore results cannot necessarily be generalised to other age groups.

In future research, it would be interesting to extend the study to other age populations, with the aim of exploring differences in ED-behaviour patterns and IPV related to social isolation aspects in other developmental phases. In addition, the present study did not explore differences by sex in the variables of interest. Efforts to increase the number of male participants would be of utility with the objective of homogenising the sample and analysing differences in ED patterns and different symptoms related to received violence in relationships.

6. Conclusions

Eating disorders are vulnerability factors that increase the likelihood of intimate partner violence. Nevertheless, the mechanisms underlying this relationship are unclear. The present study has explored the influence of withdrawal as a result of decreased enjoyment of social situations and poorer social functioning. Overall, the results of the present study demonstrate the role of social-related aspects in the relationship between EDs and IPV.

It is suggested that individuals exposed to violent situations in relationships may develop ED-related symptoms as a way of coping with adverse situations. However, this relationship is not direct, and it appears that underlying mechanisms related to fear to loneliness and social withdrawal prevent the developing of coping resources for facing received violence. These findings highlight the significance of working on fear of loneliness and social withdrawal among individuals with an ED to decrease the likelihood of establishing violent intimate partner relationships.

Future research should focus on finding ways of empowering victims through increasing social support and promoting resilience and adaptive coping resources as ways to reduce exposure to violent situations. Improving interpersonal functioning and social support is key to recovery from eating disorders.

Author Contributions: Writing, J.M. and P.M.; supervision, A.E., M.D.G. and I.I; methodology, L.O. and I.I.; formal analysis, M.H. All authors have read and agreed to the published version of the manuscript.

Funding: This research was funded by the Basque Government grant number [POS_2021_1_0031].

Institutional Review Board Statement: The study was conducted in accordance with the Declaration of Helsinki, and approved by the Deontological Commission of the Faculty of Psychology of the Complutense University of Madrid (with reference Ref. 2020/21-035) for studies involving humans.

Informed Consent Statement: Informed consent was obtained from all subjects involved in the study.

Data Availability Statement: The datasets generated during and/or analysed during the current study are available from the corresponding author on reasonable request.

Conflicts of Interest: The authors declare no conflict of interest.

References

1. Gorrell, S.; Murray, S.B. Eating disorders in males. *Child Adolesc. Psychiatr. Clin. N. Am.* **2019**, *28*, 641–651. [CrossRef] [PubMed]
2. Bhattacharya, A.; DeFilipp, L.; Timko, C.A. Feeding and eating disorders. In *Handbook of Clinical Neurology*; Elsevier: Amsterdam, The Netherlands, 2020; Volume 175, pp. 387–403. [CrossRef]
3. Jagielska, G.; Kacperska, I. Outcome, comorbidity and prognosisin anorexia nervosa. *Psychiatr. Pol.* **2017**, *51*, 205–218. [CrossRef]
4. Hay, P. Current approach to eating disorders: A clinical update. *Intern. Med. J.* **2020**, *50*, 24–29. [CrossRef]
5. Maon, I.; Horesh, D.; Gvion, Y. Siblings of individuals with eating disorders: A review of the literature. *Front. Psychol.* **2020**, *11*, 604. [CrossRef] [PubMed]
6. Aouad, P.; Hay, P.; Foroughi, N.; Cosh, S.M.; Mannan, H. Associations between defence-style, eating disorder symptoms, and quality of life in community sample of women: A longitudinal exploratory study. *Front. Psychol.* **2021**, *12*, 671652. [CrossRef] [PubMed]
7. Treasure, J.; Duarte, T.A.; Schmidt, U. Eating disorders. *Lancet* **2020**, *395*, 899–911. [CrossRef]
8. Brown, S.M.; Opitz, M.C.; Peebles, A.I.; Sharpe, H.; Duffy, F.; Newman, E. A qualitative exploration of the impact of COVID-19 on individuals with eating disorders in the UK. *Appetite* **2021**, *156*, 104977. [CrossRef]
9. Mason, T.B.; Heron, K.E.; Braitman, A.L.; Lewis, R.J. A daily diary study of perceived social isolation, dietary restraint, and negative affect in binge eating. *Appetite* **2016**, *97*, 94–100. [CrossRef]
10. Mason, T.B.; Heron, K.E. Do depressive symptoms explain associations between binge eating symptoms and later psychosocial adjustment in young adulthood? *Eat. Behav.* **2016**, *23*, 126–130. [CrossRef]
11. Mehl, A.; Rohde, P.; Gau, J.M.; Stice, E. Disaggregating the predictive effects of impaired psychosocial functioning on future DSM-5 eating disorder onset in high-risk female adolescents. *Int. J. Eat. Disord.* **2019**, *52*, 817–824. [CrossRef]
12. Wiedemann, A.A.; Ivezaj, V.; Barnes, R.D. Characterizing emotional overeating among patients with and without binge-eating disorder in primary care. *Gen. Hosp. Psychiatry* **2018**, *55*, 38–43. [CrossRef] [PubMed]
13. Cacioppo, J.T.; Cacioppo, S. The growing problem of loneliness. *Lancet* **2018**, *3*, 426. [CrossRef]
14. Johnson, D.; Dupuis, G.; Piche, J.; Clayborne, Z.; Colman, I. Adult mental health outcomes of adolescent depression: A systematic review. *Depress. Anxiety* **2018**, *35*, 700–716. [CrossRef]
15. Pitman, A.; Mann, F.; Johnson, S. Advancing our understanding of loneliness and mental health problems in young people. *Lancet Psychiatry* **2018**, *5*, 955–956. [CrossRef]
16. Arnett, J.J.; Žukauskienė, R.; Sugimura, K. The new life stage of emerging adulthood at ages 18–29 years: Implications for mental health. *Lancet Psychiatry* **2014**, *1*, 569–576. [CrossRef]
17. Kim, S.; Wang, W.L.; Mason, T. Eating disorders and trajectory of mental health across the COVID-19 pandemic: Results from the understanding America study. *J. Affect. Disord. Rep.* **2021**, *5*, 100187. [CrossRef] [PubMed]
18. Han, W.; Zheng, Z.; Zhang, N. Three mediating pathways of anxiety and security in the relationship between coping style and disordered eating behaviors among Chinese female college students. *Neural Plast.* **2021**, *2021*, 7506754. [CrossRef]
19. Hernando, A.; Pallás, R.; Cebolla, A.; García-Campayo, J.; Hoogendoorn, C.J.; Roy, J.F. Mindfulness, rumination, and coping skills in young women with eating disorders: A comparative study with healthy controls. *PLoS ONE* **2019**, *14*, e0213985. [CrossRef]
20. Brown, J.M.; Selth, S.; Stretton, A.; Simpson, S. Do dysfunctional coping modes mediate the relationship between perceived parenting style and disordered eating behaviours? *J. Eat. Disord.* **2016**, *4*, 21. [CrossRef]
21. Schlegl, S.; Maier, J.; Meule, A.; Voderholzer, U. Eating disorders in times of the COVID-19 pandemic-Results from an online survey of patients with anorexia nervosa. *Int. J. Eat. Disord.* **2020**, *53*, 1791–1800. [CrossRef]
22. Richardson, C.E.; Magson, N.R.; Fardouly, J.; Oar, E.L.; Forbes, M.K.; Johnco, C.J.; Rapee, R.M. Longitudinal associations between coping strategies and psychopathology in pre-adolescence. *J. Youth Adolesc.* **2021**, *50*, 1189–1204. [CrossRef] [PubMed]

23. Branley-Bell, D.; Talbot, C.V. Exploring the impact of the COVID-19 pandemic and UK lockdown on individuals with experience of eating disorders. *J. Eat. Disord.* **2020**, *8*, 44. [CrossRef] [PubMed]
24. Cooper, M.; Reilly, E.E.; Siegel, J.A.; Coniglio, K.; Sadeh-Sharvit, S.; Pisetsky, E.M.; Anderson, L.M. Eating disorders during the COVID-19 pandemic and quarantine: An overview of risks and recommendations for treatment and early intervention. *Eat. Disord.* **2022**, *30*, 54–76. [CrossRef] [PubMed]
25. Hajek, A.; König, H.H. Do lonely and socially isolated individuals think they die earlier? The link between loneliness, social isolation and expectations of longevity based on a nationally representative sample. *Psychogeriatrics* **2021**, *21*, 571–576. [CrossRef]
26. Martins, L.; Ramos, R.; Gravas, G.; Bertazzi, R.; Machado, C. Association between exposure to interpersonal violence and social isolation, and the adoption of unhealthy weight control practices. *Appetite* **2019**, *142*, 104384. [CrossRef]
27. Robertson, M.; Duffy, F.; Newman, E.; Prieto, C.; Husevin, H.; Sharpe, H. Exploring changes in body image, eating and exercise during the COVID-19 lockdown: A UK survey. *Appetite* **2021**, *159*, 105062. [CrossRef]
28. Barkus, E.; Badcock, J.C. A transdiagnostic perspective on social anhedonia. *Front. Psychiatry* **2019**, *10*, 216. [CrossRef]
29. Harney, M.B.; Fitzsimmons-Craft, E.E.; Maldonado, C.R.; Bardone-Cone, A.M. Negative affective experiences in relation to stages of eating disorder recovery. *Eat. Behav.* **2014**, *15*, 24–30. [CrossRef]
30. Claydon, E.A.; Davidov, D.M.; DeFazio, C.; Zullig, K.J.; Ward, R.M.; Smith, K.Z. The relationship between sexual assault, intimate partner violence, and eating disorder symptomatology among college students. *Violence Vict.* **2022**, *37*, 63–76. [CrossRef]
31. Huston, J.C.; Grillo, A.R.; Iverson, K.M.; Mitchell, K.S.; Boston Healthcare System. Associations between disordered eating and intimate partner violence mediated by depression and posttraumatic stress disorder symptoms in a female veteran sample. *Gen. Hosp. Psychiatry* **2019**, *58*, 77–82. [CrossRef]
32. Bundock, L.; Howard, L.M.; Trevillion, K.; Malcolm, E.; Feder, G.; Oram, S. Prevalence and risk of experiences of intimate partner violence among people with eating disorders: A systematic review. *J. Psychiatr. Res.* **2013**, *47*, 1134–1142. [CrossRef]
33. Lausi, G.; Pizzo, A.; Cricenti, C.; Baldi, M.; Desiderio, R.; Giannini, A.M.; Mari, E. Intimate partner violence during the COVID-19 pandemic: A review of the phenomenon from victims' and help professionals' perspectives. *Int. J. Environ. Res. Public Health* **2021**, *18*, 6204. [CrossRef] [PubMed]
34. Bauer, S.; Kindermann, S.S.; Moessner, M. Prevention of eating disorder: A review. *Z. fur Kinder Jugendosychiatrie Psychoter.* **2017**, *45*, 403–413. [CrossRef] [PubMed]
35. Garner, D.M. *Eating Disorder Inventory EDI 2*; TEA Ediciones: Madrid, Spain, 1998.
36. Lemos, M.; Londoño, N.H. Construcción y validación del cuestionario de dependencia emocional en población Colombiana. *Acta Colomb. Psicol.* **2006**, *9*, 127–140.
37. Tobin, D.L.; Holroyd, K.A.; Reynolds, R.V.; Wigal, J.K. The hierarchical factor structure of the Coping Strategies Inventory. *Cogn. Ther. Res.* **1989**, *13*, 343–361. [CrossRef]
38. Urbiola, I.; Estévez, A.; Momeñe, J. Desarrollo y validación del cuestionario VREP (Violencia Recibida, Ejercida y Percibida) en las relaciones de pareja en adolescentes. *Apunt. Psicol.* **2020**, *38*, 103–114.
39. Muthén, L.K.; Muthén, B.O. *Mplus User's Guide: Statistical Analysis with Latent Variables*, 7th ed.; Muthén & Muthén: Los Angeles, CA, USA, 2012.
40. Hu, L.T.; Bentler, P.M. Cutoff criteria for fit indexes in covariance structure analysis: Conventional criteria versus new alternatives. *Struct. Equ. Model.* **1999**, *6*, 1–55. [CrossRef]
41. Stride, C.B.; Gardner, S.E.; Catley, N.; Thomas, F. Mplus Code for Mediation, Moderation and Moderated Mediation Models (1 to 80). 2015. Available online: http://www.figureitout.org.uk (accessed on 16 June 2022).
42. Wong, S.P.; Chang, J.C. Altered eating behaviors in female victims of intimate partner violence. *J. Interpers. Violence* **2016**, *31*, 3490–3505. [CrossRef]
43. Wright, A.; Pritchard, M.E. An examination of the relation of gender, mass media influence, and loneliness to disordered eating among college students. *Eat. Weight Disord.* **2009**, *14*, e144–e147. [CrossRef]
44. Monteleone, A.M.; Cascino, G.; Marciello, F.; Abbate-Daga, G.; Baiano, M.; Balestrieri, M.; Barone, E.; Bertelli, S.; Carpiniello, B.; Castellini, G.; et al. Risk and resilience factors for specific and general psychopathology worsening in people with eating disorders during COVID-19 pandemic: A retrospective Italian multicentre study. *Eat. Weight Disord.* **2021**, *26*, 2443–2452. [CrossRef]
45. Rodgers, R.F.; Lombardo, C.; Cerolini, S.; Franko, D.L.; Omori, M.; Fuller-Tyszkiewicz, M.; Linardon, J.; Courtet, P.; Guillaume, S. The impact of the COVID-19 pandemic on eating disorder risk and symptoms. *Int. J. Eat. Disord.* **2020**, *53*, 1166–1170. [CrossRef] [PubMed]
46. Southward, M.W.; Christensen, K.A.; Fettich, K.C.; Weissman, J.; Berona, J.; Chen, E.Y. Loneliness mediates the relationship between emotion dysregulation and bulimia nervosa/binge eating disorder psychopathology in a clinical sample. *Eat. Weight Disord.* **2014**, *19*, 509–513. [CrossRef] [PubMed]
47. Mazza, M.; Marano, G.; Del Castillo, A.G.; Chieffo, D.; Monti, L.; Janiri, D.; Moccia, L.; Sani, G. Intimate partner violence: A loop of abuse, depression and victimization. *World J. Psychiatry* **2021**, *11*, 215–221. [CrossRef] [PubMed]
48. Schirk, D.K.; Lehman, E.B.; Perry, A.N.; Ornstein, R.M.; McCall-Hosenfeld, J.S. The impact of social support on the risk of eating disorders in women exposed to intimate partner violence. *Int. J. Women's Health* **2015**, *7*, 919–931. [CrossRef]
49. Kimber, M.; McTavish, J.R.; Couturier, J.; Boven, A.; Gill, S.; Dimitropoulos, G.; MacMillan, H.L. Consequences of child emotional abuse, emotional neglect and exposure to intimate partner violence for eating disorders: A systematic critical review. *BMC Psychol.* **2017**, *5*, 33. [CrossRef]

50. Rayworth, B.B.; Wise, L.A.; Harlow, B.L. Childhood abuse and risk of eating disorders in women. *Epidemiology* **2004**, *15*, 271–278. [CrossRef]
51. Emery, R.L.; Yoon, C.; Mason, S.M.; Neumark-Sztainer, D. Childhood maltreatment and disordered eating attitudes and behaviors in adult men and women: Findings from project EAT. *Appetite* **2021**, *163*, 105224. [CrossRef]
52. Collier, D.A.; Treasure, J.L. The aetiology of eating disorders. *Br. J. Psychiatry* **2004**, *185*, 363–365. [CrossRef]

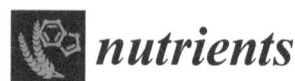

Article

The Association of Perceived Vulnerability to Disease with Cognitive Restraint and Compensatory Behaviors

Lindzey V. Hoover *, Joshua M. Ackerman, Jenna R. Cummings † and Ashley N. Gearhardt

Department of Psychology, University of Michigan, Ann Arbor, MI 48109, USA
* Correspondence: lindzeyh@umich.edu
† Current address: Social and Behavioral Sciences Branch, Division of Intramural Population Health Research, the *Eunice Kennedy Shriver* National Institute of Child Health and Human Development, Bethesda, MD 20892, USA.

Abstract: Individual differences exist in perceived vulnerability to disease (PVD). PVD is associated with negative responses (e.g., disgust) towards individuals with obesity and heightened sensitivity regarding personal appearance. Through increasing fear of fat (FOF), PVD may be associated with cognitive restraint and compensatory behaviors. We utilized an adult sample (n = 247; 53.3% male sex assigned at birth) recruited through Amazon's MTurk prior to the COVID-19 pandemic to investigate associations between PVD, cognitive restraint and compensatory behaviors. Participants completed the Perceived Vulnerability to Disease Scale, Eating Disorder Diagnostic Scale, Dutch Eating Behaviors Questionnaire, and Goldfarb's Fear of Fat Scale. Mediation analyses were used to test our hypotheses. Perceived infectability (PVD-Infection) was associated with cognitive restraint and compensatory behaviors through increased FOF. Perceived germ aversion (PVD–Germ) was associated with cognitive restraint, but FOF did not mediate this association. Sex-stratified analyses revealed no significant sex differences. PVD may be an overlooked factor associated with cognitive restraint and compensatory behaviors in males and females. FOF was an important mediating factor in these associations. Increased engagement in cognitive restraint and compensatory behaviors may reflect attempts to reduce FOF. Future longitudinal research should explore whether PVD is a risk factor for cognitive restraint and compensatory behaviors.

Keywords: cognitive restraint; compensatory behaviors; perceived vulnerability to disease; fear of fat

Citation: Hoover, L.V.; Ackerman, J.M.; Cummings, J.R.; Gearhardt, A.N. The Association of Perceived Vulnerability to Disease with Cognitive Restraint and Compensatory Behaviors. *Nutrients* 2023, 15, 8. https://doi.org/10.3390/nu15010008

Academic Editor: Sébastien Guillaume

Received: 13 November 2022
Revised: 15 December 2022
Accepted: 16 December 2022
Published: 20 December 2022

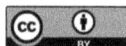

Copyright: © 2022 by the authors. Licensee MDPI, Basel, Switzerland. This article is an open access article distributed under the terms and conditions of the Creative Commons Attribution (CC BY) license (https://creativecommons.org/licenses/by/4.0/).

1. Introduction

The coronavirus pandemic has brought the dangers of infectious disease to the forefront, but the dangers of pathogen transmission are not new. The near-constant threat of disease has fostered the development of defense mechanisms to protect our bodies from new and potentially deadly disease threats. The most well-known of these defenses is the immune system, which destroys pathogens detected within the body. However, humans also seem to have a second immune system known as the "behavioral immune system" [1–3] which, in contrast to the role of the reactive physiological immune system in combating internal pathogens, proactively prevents infection by facilitating detection of sensory cues (e.g., physical characteristics) in the environment that may indicate risk of disease exposure [1–3].

Perceived vulnerability to disease (PVD) is a trait-level indicator of behavioral immune activity that reflects both perceived infectability (PVD-Infection), a personal belief about susceptibility to infectious disease (e.g., if a disease is going around you will get it [4]) and germ aversion (PVD-Germ), the level of emotional discomfort experienced in situations where risk of disease transmission is high (e.g., someone sneezing without covering their mouth [4]). From an evolutionary perspective, PVD is highly beneficial to survival. Heightened sensitivity to environmental cues and higher perception of personal risk both encourage early detection and avoidance of potentially deadly pathogens before they can enter the body [3]. However, detection processes within the behavioral immune system are not perfect—because we cannot directly observe pathogens, these processes are sensitive to cues associated with disease but also can activate in response to cues that merely resemble or are heuristically associated with disease threat [3]. For example, physical characteristics (e.g., accident-related limb amputations), which are logically irrelevant to disease transmission, may activate this system and can result in negative responses toward the person associated with the cue [3,5].

1.1. Obesity as a Disease Cue

Obesity is a physical characteristic and chronic disease associated with disease-related perceptions [2,6,7]. Individuals with higher PVD are more likely to label individuals who appear heavier as obese [8] and are more prone to stigmatize individuals with higher body weight [6,8–11]. PVD has been directly associated with negative behavioral (e.g., avoidance) and cognitive (e.g., disgust) responses towards individuals with obesity [3]. PVD has also been associated with heightened sensitivity regarding one's own appearance, including weight-related features [12]. Heightened attention to one's own appearance combined with increased weight stigma may lead individuals with higher PVD to develop a fear of fat (FOF, i.e., avoidance of or aversion to fatness [13,14]) regarding their own body. Thus, heightened perceptions of vulnerability to disease could contribute to disordered eating behavior due to heightened FOF.

1.2. Fear of Fat and Disordered Eating

FOF is associated with cognitive restraint and compensatory behaviors [15–17]. Cognitive restraint refers to the desire to control or restrict food consumption (regardless of success [18,19]). Cognitive restraint is associated with FOF in clinical [20,21] and community samples [16,22–25]. FOF is also associated with restrictive eating disorders marked by compensatory behaviors (i.e., anorexia nervosa, bulimia nervosa [18,26–28]. Compensatory behaviors (e.g., fasting, abuse of laxatives/diuretics, vomiting, excessive exercising) are intended to counteract caloric intake to achieve a desired shape/weight or avoid fatness [18]. If PVD is also associated with FOF, then PVD may be a factor contributing to both cognitive restraint and compensatory behaviors.

1.3. The Current Study

We investigated the hypothesis that greater PVD is associated with cognitive restraint and compensatory behaviors through FOF in a community sample of 247 adults (age 21–70). This is (to our knowledge) the first study to investigate whether two dimensions of PVD (perceived germ aversion and perceived infectability) are associated with FOF, cognitive restraint and compensatory behaviors.

Female participants have been found to have higher PVD [4] and to be more prone to cognitive restraint and eating disorders than male participants [29]. Thus, we decided a priori to conduct exploratory sex-stratified analyses to investigate potential sex differences in the associations between PVD and FOF with cognitive restraint and compensatory behaviors.

2. Materials and Methods

2.1. Participants

We conducted secondary analyses using data from participants recruited on Amazon's Mechanical Turk platform (MTurk) in 2019 prior to the COVID-19 pandemic. Participants completed questionnaires on their beliefs, behaviors, thoughts, and feelings related to eating and drinking (Qualifications: U.S. Location, HIT Approval Rate > 95%, Age > 18). Additional information (e.g., quality assurance steps) can be found in previously published work [30]. Original data have been shared on the Open Science Framework at https://osf.io/8kspw/, accessed on 10 August 2019.

All available data (n = 247, 53.3% male sex at birth) were included in the current study. The average age of participants was 36.8 years old (SD = 11.3, min–max = 21–70).

The racial/ethnic distribution of the study was: 74.5% White, 15.4% Black, 6.9% Hispanic/Latinx, 4.5% Asian, 2.4% American Indian or Alaskan Native, and 0.8% other (percentages exceed 100% because participants could select one or multiple race/ethnicity). The sample overall was well-educated (12.1% high-school graduates, 18.2% some college, 9.7% associates degree, 47.4% bachelor's degree, and 12.6% advanced degree (masters, Ph.D., M.D., J.D., etc.) Average participant body mass index (BMI) was "overweight" (M = 26.3, SD = 5.9, min–max = 17.7–55.8) with 3.1% of participants "underweight", 42.3% "normal" weight, 36.6%, "overweight", and 18.1% "obese". Additional information about sample characteristics is presented in Table 1.

Table 1. Demographic characteristics.

	n (%)
Age (M = 36.8, SD = 11.3, min–max = 21–70)	
21–29	73 (29.6%)
30–39	101 (40.8%)
40–49	33 (13.4%)
50–59	23 (9.3%)
60–69	16 (6.5%)
70	1 (0.4%)
Sex at Birth	
Male	131 (53.3%)
Female	115 (46.7%)
Racial Identity ±	
American Indian/Alaskan Native	6 (2.4%)
Hispanic/Latino	17 (6.9%)
Asian	11 (4.5%)
Black/African American	38 (15.4%)
White	184 (74.5%)
Other	2 (0.8%)
Education	
High school graduate	30 (12.1%)
Some college	45 (18.2%)
Associates degree	24 (9.7%)
Bachelor's degree	117 (47.4%)
Advanced degree	31 (12.6%)
Income	
Less than USD 10,000	15 (6.1%)
USD 10,000–USD 19,999	18 (7.3%)
USD 20,000–USD 29,999	31 (12.7%)
USD 30,000–USD 39,999	45 (18.4%)
USD 40,000–USD 49,999	31 (12.7%)
USD 50,000–USD 59,999	25 (10.2%)
USD 60,000–USD 69,999	19 (7.8%)
USD 70,000–USD 79,999	20 (8.2%)
USD 80,000–USD 89,999	8 (3.3%)
USD 90,000–USD 99,999	10 (4.1%)
USD 100,000–USD 149,999	16 (6.5%)
More than USD 150,000	7 (2.9%)

Table 1. Cont.

	n (%)
Subjective Socioeconomic Status [¥]	
1	3 (1.2%)
2	19 (7.7%)
3	32 (13.0%)
4	32 (13.0%)
5	60 (24.3%)
6	32 (13.0%)
7	35 (14.2%)
8	23 (9.3%)
9	9 (3.6%)
10	2 (0.8%)
BMI (M = 26.3, SD = 5.9, min–max = 17.7–55.8)	
Underweight (BMI < 18.5)	7 (3.1%)
Normal Weight (BMI 18.5–24.9)	96 (42.3%)
Overweight (BMI 25.0–29.9)	84 (36.6%)
Obese (BMI > 30)	41 (18.1%)

Notes: Differences in n are due to "prefer not to answer" responses. [±] Percentages for Race/Ethnicity exceed 100% because of the option to select multiple response options. [¥] Subjective Socioeconomic Status indicates participants self-ranking on a ladder representing people in the US with 10 = people who are best off (most money, most education, most respected jobs) and 1 = worst off (least money, least education, least respected jobs).

2.2. Procedures

Research procedures were approved by the University of Michigan Institution Review Board in accordance with provisions of the World Medical Association Declaration of Helsinki. Participants consented and completed questionnaires in randomized order through the MTurk platform. Participants were compensated USD 1.00 for their time (~25 min).

2.3. Measures

2.3.1. Perceived Vulnerability to Disease Scale (PVD)

The Perceived Vulnerability to Disease Scale (PVD) [4] is a 15-item questionnaire that measures trait-level concerns about the transmission of infectious diseases. Participants rated each item on a 7-point Likert scale (1 = strongly disagree to 7 = strongly agree). The PVD questionnaire measures two factors: perceived germ aversion (PVD-Germ) and perceived infectability (PVD-Infection). Subscales were scored by averaging the items. The PVD-Germ subscale measures affective response to situations where pathogen transmission is likely (e.g., It really bothers me when people sneeze without covering their mouth, M = 4.4, SD = 1.1, min–max = 1.1–7.0, α = 0.76). The PVD-Infection Subscale assesses subjective beliefs about one's own susceptibility to infectious disease as well as one's personal beliefs about their immune functioning (e.g., In general, I am very susceptible to colds, flu and other infectious diseases, M = 3.4, SD = 1.2, min–max = 1.0–7.0, α = 0.82).

2.3.2. Goldfarb Fear of Fat Scale (FOF)

The Goldfarb Fear of Fat Scale (FOF) [26] is a 10-item measure developed to differentiate normal versus abnormal FOF for early identification of patients at risk for bulimia nervosa. Participants rate how representative each statement is on a 4-point scale (1 = very untrue to 4 = very true). Questions include, "I am afraid to gain even a little weight", and, "If I eat even a little, I may lose control and not stop eating". The scale is scored by averaging all items (M = 2.4, SD = 0.9, min–max = 1.0–4.0, α = 0.92).

2.3.3. Dutch Eating Behaviors Scale (DEBQ)

The Dutch Eating Behaviors Scale [19] is a 33-item self-report scale assessing restraint, emotional, and external eating behaviors. Participants answer questions about their eating behaviors on a 5-point scale (1 = Never to 5 = Always). Only the restraint subscale was included in analyses. Questions included on the restraint scale ask about frequency of engagement in cognitive restraint, such as "Do you try to eat less at mealtimes than you would like to eat?" The restraint subscale was calculated by averaging the 10 restraint items (M = 3.0, SD = 1.0, min–max = 1.0–5.0, α = 0.94).

2.3.4. Eating Disorder Diagnostic Scale (EDDS)

The Eating Disorder Diagnostic Scale [31] is a brief, self-report measure of eating disorder diagnostic criteria (DSM–IV). Questions asked about the average number of occurrences of eating disorder symptoms per week over the past 3 months, for example, "How many times per week on average over the past 3 months have you made yourself vomit to prevent weight gain or counteract the effects of eating?" This scale assesses 4 types of compensatory behaviors (vomiting, laxatives/diuretics, excessive exercising, fasting) and possible scores range from 0 to 14 for each behavior. Endorsement was highest for fasting (M = 3.5, SD = 4.1, min–max = 0–14) followed by exercise (M = 2.9, SD = 4.1, min–max = 0–14), vomiting, (M = 2.3, SD = 4.2, min–max = 0–14) and laxative/diuretics (M = 2.2, SD = 3.9, min–max = 0–14). A compensatory eating behavior subscale was created by summing the total number of compensatory behaviors endorsed on these 4 questions (M = 10.8, SD = 15.6, min–max = 0.0–54.0, α = 0.95).

2.4. Data Analytic Plan

Analyses were conducted in IBM SPSS Statistics version 27, IBM Corp, Armonk, NY, USA [32]. Data were reviewed for normality, outliers (± 3 SD), and missing values. Distributions met normality assumptions. Missing data were highest for BMI ($n = 19$). All other missing data ranged from $n = 0$ to $n = 4$. Missing data were removed using pairwise deletion. Thus, differences in n are a result of missing data.

Zero-order correlational analyses were conducted between demographic variables (age, sex, race/ethnicity, education, and BMI), cognitive restraint and compensatory behaviors to identify potential covariates (see Table A1). We created dummy codes for biological sex at birth (0 = male, 1 = female), race/ethnicity (0 = non-White, 1 = White), and education level (0 = associates or lower, 1 = bachelors or higher). Education was positively correlated with cognitive restraint (r = 0.20, p = 0.001) and compensatory behaviors (r = 0.29, p < 0.001). Including education in regression models for the relations of PVD subscales with cognitive restraint and compensatory behaviors did not alter significance (see Table A2). Thus, we report the unadjusted models.

Correlational analyses were conducted to investigate the hypothesized associations between PVD subscales, FOF, cognitive restraint and compensatory behaviors. Separate mediational analyses were conducted using the SPSS PROCESS Model 4 macro [33] to investigate whether FOF mediated the associations between PVD subscales, cognitive restraint, and compensatory behaviors. Both PVD subscales were included in the same model to account for shared variance between the subscales [4]. We used 10,000 bootstrap samples to create 95% bias-corrected confidence intervals to test the significance of indirect effects. Significance at p < 0.05 was indicated if the 95% confidence interval did not include zero. Sex-stratified mediation analyses were also conducted to investigate potential sex differences.

3. Results

3.1. Associations between PVD Subscales, Cognitive Restraint and Compensatory Behaviors

Table 2 presents zero-order correlations between PVD subscales, FOF, cognitive restraint and compensatory behaviors. PVD-Germ was positively associated with FOF (r = 0.15, p = 0.02) and cognitive restraint (r = 0.18, p = 0.005), but was not significantly associated with compensatory behaviors (r = 0.03, p = 0.66). PVD-Infection was positively associated with FOF (r = 0.45, p < 0.001), cognitive restraint (r = 0.21, p = 0.001) and compensatory behaviors (r = 0.35, p < 0.001).

Table 2. Zero-Order Correlation Matrix PVD, FOF, Cognitive Restraint, and Compensatory Behaviors.

		PVD-Germ	PVD-Infection	FOF	Cognitive Restraint	Comp Behaviors
PVD–Germ	r		0.25 ***	0.15 *	0.18 **	0.03
	n		245	245	245	245
PVD–Infection	r			0.45 ***	0.21 **	0.35 ***
	n			245	245	245
FOF	r				0.65 ***	0.60 ***
	n				246	246
Cognitive Restraint	r					0.48 ***
	n					247
Comp Behaviors	r					
	n					

Notes: * indicates significance at $p < 0.05$. ** indicates significance at $p < 0.01$. *** indicates significance at $p < 0.001$. "FOF" indicates Goldberg's Fear of Fat Scale. "PVD–Germ" indicates the Perceived Vulnerability to Disease Germ Subscale. "PVD–Infection" indicates the Perceived Vulnerability to Disease Infectability Subscale. "Cognitive Restraint" indicates the Dutch Eating Behavior Questionnaire Restraint Scale. "Comp Behaviors" indicates Eating Disorder Diagnostic Scale—Compensatory Behaviors Subscale.

3.2. Indirect Effects of PVD Subscales on Cognitive Restraint through FOF

Figure 1 presents results of mediational analyses for FOF as a potential mediator of the association between the PVD Subscales and cognitive restraint. The indirect effect of PVD-Infection on cognitive restraint through FOF was positive and significant, B (SE) = 0.26 (0.04), 95% CI [0.18, 0.34]. The direct effect of PVD-Infection on cognitive restraint was also significant. However, the indirect effect of PVD-Germ on cognitive restraint through FOF was not significant, B (SE) = 0.02 (0.04), 95% CI [−0.05, 0.09]. The direct effect of PVD-Germ on cognitive restraint was significant. Standardized coefficient betas suggest small-to-medium effect sizes of the associations between PVD subscales, FOF, and cognitive restraint.

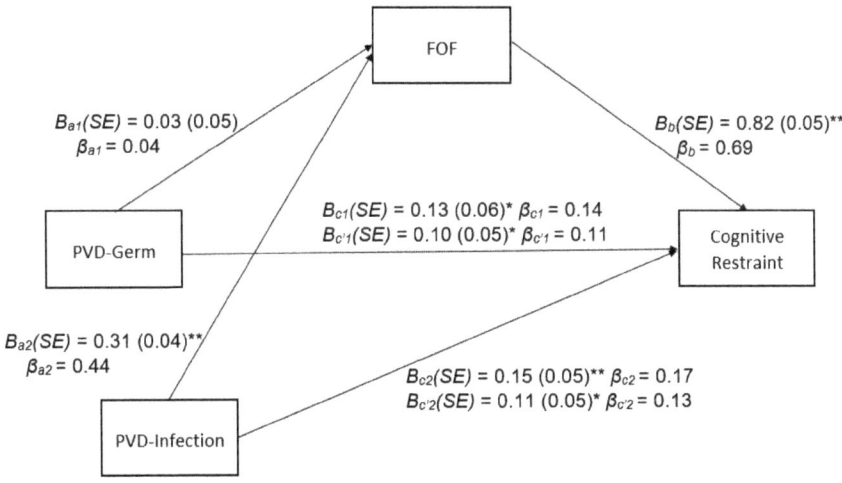

Figure 1. PVD Subscales and Cognitive Restraint Mediated by FOF. Process Model—4 path estimates from testing the indirect effect of perceived germ aversion (PVD-Germ) and perceived infectability (PVD-Infection) on cognitive restraint through fear of fat (FOF). Standardized coefficients (β), unstandardized coefficients (B), and standard errors (SE) are presented (* $p < 0.05$, ** $p < 0.01$).

3.3. Indirect Effects of PVD Subscales on Compensatory Behaviors through FOF

Figure 2 presents results of mediational analyses for FOF as a potential mediator of the association between the PVD subscales and compensatory behaviors. The indirect effect of PVD-Infection on compensatory behaviors through FOF was significant, B (SE) = 3.16 (0.61), 95% CI [2.08, 4.47]. The direct effect of PVD-Infection on compensatory behaviors was also significant. In contrast, the indirect effect of PVD-Germ on compensatory behaviors through FOF was not significant, B (SE) = 0.30 (0.43), 95% CI [−0.55, 1.15]. The direct effect of PVD-Germ on compensatory behaviors was also not significant. Standardized coefficient betas suggest small-to-medium effect sizes of the associations between PVD subscales, FOF, and compensatory behaviors.

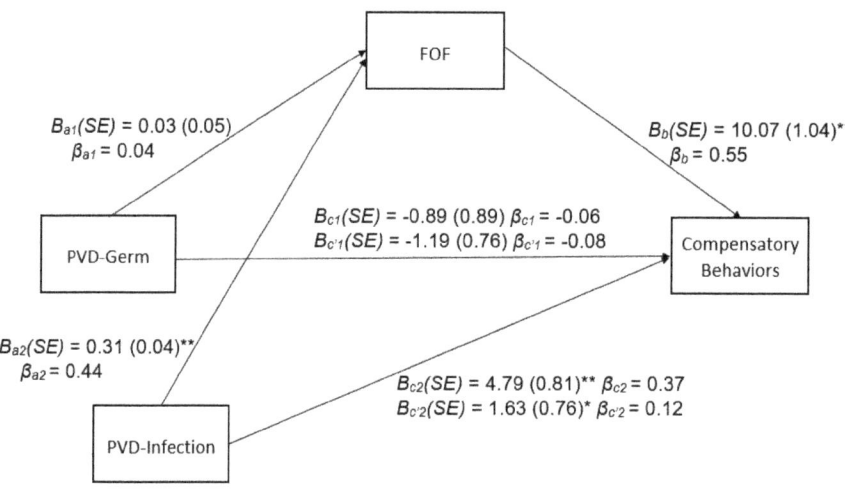

Figure 2. PVD Subscales and Compensatory Behaviors Mediated by FOF. Process Model—4 path estimates from testing the indirect effect of perceived germ aversion (PVD-Germ) and perceived infectability (PVD-Infection) on compensatory behaviors through fear of fat (FOF). Standardized coefficients (β), unstandardized coefficients (B) and standard errors (SE) are presented (* $p < 0.05$, ** $p < 0.01$).

3.4. Sex-Stratified Analyses

Exploratory sex-stratified mediation analyses were conducted to investigate potential sex differences. Results indicated no significant sex differences between male and female participants. FOF did not significantly mediate associations between PVD-Germ and cognitive restraint or PVD-Germ and compensatory behaviors for male or female participants. FOF also remained a significant mediator of the associations between PVD-Infection and cognitive restraint and PVD-Infection and compensatory behaviors for both male and female participants (see Figures A1 and A2).

4. Discussion

This is, to our knowledge, the first study to investigate the association between PVD, cognitive restraint, and compensatory behaviors. In a community sample of 247 adult participants, we found that perceived infectability was associated with cognitive restraint and compensatory behaviors and that FOF partially mediated these associations. Perceived germ aversion was significantly associated with cognitive restraint (but not compensatory behaviors). However, FOF did not significantly mediate the association between perceived germ aversion and cognitive restraint. Sex-stratified analyses revealed no significant sex differences between male and female participants. Perceived infectability may be an overlooked factor associated with cognitive restraint and compensatory behaviors in males and females through FOF. Implications of these findings are discussed below.

4.1. PVD, FOF, Cognitive Restraint, and Compensatory Behaviors

Perceived infectability refers to personal beliefs about susceptibility to infectious disease that stem, in large part, from one's history of infections [4]. Results indicated that those with a heightened concern about their own susceptibility to disease endorsed both higher cognitive restraint and compensatory behaviors, which was partially explained by higher FOF. One possible explanation for these findings is that those higher in perceived infectability may perceive themselves as being more susceptible to obesity. This hypothesis aligns with past research indicating obesity is a physical condition that can be erroneously identified as an indicator of disease transmission by the behavioral immune system [2,6,7]. The misidentification of obesity as a disease cue in those high in perceived infectability could lead to an increased fear of the "disease" of fatness.

FOF mediation findings suggest possible future directions for reducing cognitive restraint and compensatory behaviors. Reducing FOF in individuals with high perceived infectability may be important for reducing disordered eating. For example, delivering interventions designed to reduce internalized weight stigma (e.g., cognitive-behavioral treatment to cope with internalized weight stigma [34]) to individuals with high perceived infectability may be useful in reducing cognitive restraint and compensatory behaviors. Illness during childhood is an important predictor of heightened perceived infectability in adults [35], so reducing FOF in children and adolescents who have experienced significant illness may also be useful in preventing the development of cognitive restraint and compensatory behaviors.

FOF partially mediated the associations between perceived infectability, cognitive restraint, and compensatory behaviors, leaving the possibility of other mediators. For instance, the associations between perceived infectability, cognitive restraint, and compensatory behaviors could reflect broader concerns about negative health outcomes associated with obesity. Perceived infectability is strongly associated with health anxiety [4], and it is plausible that those high in perceived infectability may engage in cognitive restraint and compensatory behaviors to minimize the risk of negative health outcomes associated with obesity.

Contrary to our hypothesis, perceived germ aversion was not related to compensatory behaviors. Although perceived germ aversion demonstrated a small, but significant association with cognitive restraint, FOF did not significantly mediate this association. Perceived germ aversion is thought to reflect emotional discomfort with situations, indicating an increased risk of disease transmission [4] and has been found to significantly overlap with pathogen disgust [9]. A growing body of research suggests that disgust-based avoidance is an important factor contributing to the development and maintenance of cognitive restraint and compensatory behaviors [36]. Future research should explore the role of disgust in the association between perceived germ aversion and cognitive restraint.

4.2. Sex-Stratified Analyses

Results of sex-stratified analyses reflected results in the full sample. FOF remained a significant mediator for associations between perceived infectability (but not perceived germ aversion), cognitive restraint, and compensatory behaviors in male and female participants. Males have historically been under researched in the context of disordered eating behaviors [37]. Our results suggest that evolutionary processes associated with disease threat could be one factor contributing to disordered eating for males and females, warranting further investigation.

4.3. Strengths and Limitations

The current study had several notable strengths. We had a relatively large sample size ($n = 247$) with a balanced sex distribution (53.3% male). The sample included a wide range of ages (M = 36.8, min–max = 21–70) and BMI (M = 26.28, min–max = 17.7–55.8). Study data included assessments of both cognitive restraint and compensatory behaviors and, to our knowledge, was the first to investigate their association with perceived disease vulnerability.

There are limitations of this study that should also be considered. Cognitive restraint and compensatory behaviors were assessed using self-report measures. Although these are validated scales [19,31], self-reported measures tend to over-represent disordered eating behavior [38–40]. Future research should utilize clinical interviews to assess cognitive restraint and compensatory behaviors. Data were collected using Amazon's MTurk, which has historically raised some concerns about data quality. Recommended approaches (95% approval, 5000 HITS, attention check questions [41]) were implemented to minimize these concerns. Another important next step is to utilize clinical samples with disordered eating to explore associations between PVD, cognitive restraint, and compensatory behaviors. Although there was some diversity in this sample, it consisted predominantly of White participants (74.5%) and was underpowered to investigate differences in race/ethnicity. Future research should recruit a more diverse sample to allow for investigation of racial/ethnic differences in PVD, cognitive restraint, and compensatory behaviors. Factors other than FOF likely contribute to an association between PVD and disordered eating. Both PVD and disordered eating are associated with anxiety more broadly [42,43], disgust sensitivity [44–46], and obsessive-compulsive tendencies [43,44,46–48]. This dataset did not include measures on these constructs, but future research that investigates anxiety, disgust sensitivity, and OCD as potential mediators is an important future direction. While eating disorders and obesity are distinct constructs, they are not mutually exclusive of each other. Rates of eating disorders are elevated in individuals with obesity [49] and binge eating often occurs when restrictive eating fails [50,51]. While we did assess BMI as a potential covariate in this study, the study was not well suited to disentangle the complex associations between eating disorders and obesity. Future research should aim to investigate these complex associations. The study utilized a cross-sectional design, which does not allow for us to make causal inferences. Future research should utilize experimental or longitudinal designs that are better positioned to investigate causal inferences. For example, it may be possible to experimentally prime pathogen threat cues [52,53] to investigate whether being primed for PVD increases fear of fat, stigmatizing attitudes, or desire to engage in disordered eating behaviors. Assessing PVD in childhood would allow for follow-up during adolescence (a high-risk period for onset of eating disorders [54]) to see if childhood PVD is predictive of adolescent disordered eating behaviors. If PVD was predictive of future onset of disordered eating behaviors, it may be a useful screening tool for early intervention. Understanding the causal effect of disease salient environmental cues in increasing FOF and engagement in cognitive restraint and compensatory behaviors may be particularly important considering heightened media coverage surrounding disease transmission during the pandemic.

5. Conclusions

The role that evolved psychological mechanisms play in cognitive restraint and compensatory behaviors is an important and understudied area of psychological research. Our results indicate that people who perceive themselves to be more susceptible to infection (i.e., perceived infectability) are more likely to engage in cognitive restraint and compensatory behaviors. No differences were found between male and female participants, suggesting that perceived infectability might be a novel factor that can contribute to existing gaps in the understanding of disordered eating in males. Increased engagement in cognitive restraint and compensatory behaviors due to perceptions of obesity as a disease-relevant cue may be an attempt to reduce risk or fear of becoming fat. Future longitudinal research is needed to explore whether individual differences in perceived infectability is a risk factor for the development of cognitive restraint and compensatory behaviors.

Although data were collected before the coronavirus pandemic, consideration of how the pandemic might relate to these findings is particularly relevant. Increased salience of vulnerability to coronavirus combined with the specific identification of obesity as a risk factor for severe disease trajectory could have concerning implications for engagement in cognitive restraint and compensatory behaviors. Early research during the pandemic found that participants with a current or history of an eating disorder endorsed increased cognitive restraint and compensatory behaviors [55]. Such findings might be particularly likely in individuals with high PVD. Future research should explore the potential impact of the coronavirus pandemic on cognitive restraint and compensatory behaviors.

Author Contributions: L.V.H., J.M.A., J.R.C. and A.N.G. developed the study concept and contributed to the study design. J.R.C. collected data. L.V.H. performed the data analysis and interpretation under the supervision of A.N.G. and L.V.H. drafted the paper with assistance from L.V.H., J.M.A., J.R.C. and A.N.G., L.V.H., J.M.A., J.R.C. and A.N.G. approved the final version of the paper for submission. All authors have read and agreed to the published version of the manuscript.

Funding: J.R.C. was supported by *Eunice Kennedy Shriver* National Institute of Child Health and Human Development (NICHD) Award T32-HD079350 and the NICHD Intramural Research Program. The content of the article is solely the responsibility of the authors and does not necessarily represent the official views of the NICHD.

Institutional Review Board Statement: Research procedures were approved by the University of Michigan Institution Review Board (HUM00158499) in accordance with provisions of the World Medical Association Declaration of Helsinki.

Informed Consent Statement: Informed consent was obtained from all subjects involved in the study.

Data Availability Statement: Original data have been shared on the Open Science Framework at https://osf.io/8kspw/, accessed on 10 August 2019. No new data were collected for this study.

Conflicts of Interest: The authors declare no conflict of interest.

Appendix A

Table A1. Correlation matrix with potential covariates.

		PVD-Germ	PVD—Inf	FOF	Cog Restraint	Comp Behaviors	BMI	Age	Sex	Education	Race/Ethnicity
PVD—Germ	r		0.25 ***	0.15 *	0.18 *	0.03	−0.13	0.02	−0.22 **	−0.06	0.11
	n		245	245	245	245	226	245	244	245	245
PVD—Inf	r			0.45 ***	0.21 **	0.35 ***	0.06	0.09	−0.10	0.14 *	0.13 *
	n			245	245	245	226	245	244	245	245
FOF	r				0.65 ***	0.60 ***	0.07	<0.01	−0.03	0.19 **	≤0.01
	n				246	246	227	246	245	246	246
Cog Restraint	r					0.48 ***	0.01	0.02	−0.02	0.21 **	−0.04
	n					247	228	247	246	247	247
Comp Behaviors	r						−0.12	≤0.01	−0.07	0.29 ***	≤0.01
	n						228	247	246	247	247
BMI	r							−0.03	−0.05	−0.16 *	−0.03
	n							228	227	228	228
Age	r								0.18 **	0.09	0.19 **
	n								246	247	247
Sex	r									−0.10	0.16 *
	n									246	246
Education	r										−0.16 *
	n										247
Race/Ethnicity	r										
	n										

Notes: * indicates significance at $p < 0.05$. ** indicates significance at $p < 0.01$. *** indicates significance at $p < 0.001$. "FOF" indicates Goldberg's Fear of Fat Scale. "PVD—Germ" indicates the Perceived Vulnerability to Disease Germ Subscale. "PVD—Inf" indicates the Perceived Vulnerability to Disease Infectability Subscale. "Cog Restraint" indicates the Dutch Eating Behavior Questionnaire Restraint Scale. "Comp Behaviors" indicates Eating Disorder Diagnostic Scale—Compensatory Behaviors Subscale. "BMI" indicates body mass index.

Appendix B

Table A2. Regression analyses for potential covariates.

	t	p	b (SE)	β	f	p	Adj. R^2
Cog Restraint							
Overall model					9.51	<0.001	0.07
Constant	7.40	<0.001	2.03 (0.28)				
Education	3.29	0.001	0.42 (0.13)	0.20			
PVD—Germ	3.04	0.003	0.18 (0.06)	0.19			
Cog Restraint							
Overall model					8.86	<0.001	0.06
Constant	11.67	<0.001	2.31 (0.20)				
Education	2.68	0.01	0.35 (0.13)	0.17			
PVD—Infection	2.93	0.004	0.16 (0.05)	0.18			
Comp Behaviors							
Overall model					11.16	<0.001	0.08
Constant	0.62	0.54	2.58 (4.19)				
Education	4.70	<0.001	9.22 (1.96)	0.29			
PVD-Germ	0.71	0.48	0.63 (0.88)	0.04			
Comp Behaviors							
Overall model					26.72	<0.001	0.17
Constant	−2.77	0.01	−7.91 (2.85)				
Education	4.13	<0.001	7.72 (1.87)	0.24			
PVD-Infection	5.39	<0.001	4.15 (0.77)	0.32			

Notes: "PVD—Germ" indicates the Perceived Vulnerability to Disease Germ Subscale. "PVD—Infection" indicates the Perceived Vulnerability to Disease Infectability Subscale. "Cog Restraint" indicates the Dutch Eating Behavior Questionnaire Restraint Scale. "Comp Behaviors" indicates Eating Disorder Diagnostic Scale–Compensatory Behaviors Subscale.

Appendix C

Male Participants

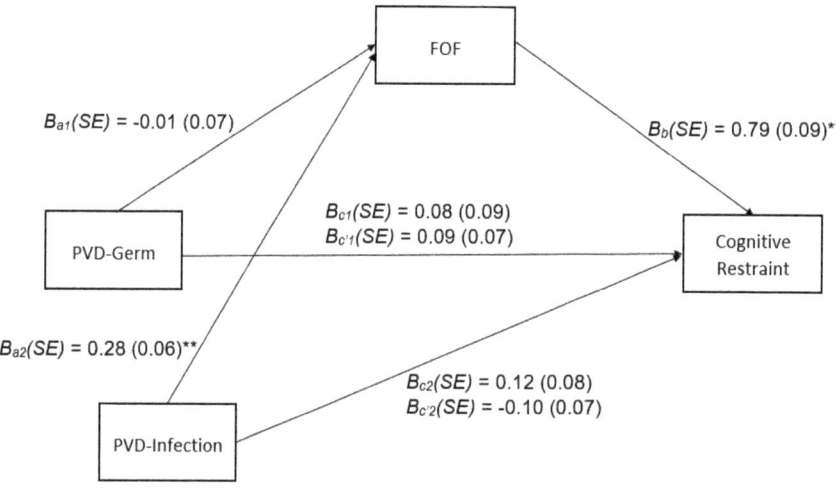

Figure A1. Cont.

Female Participants

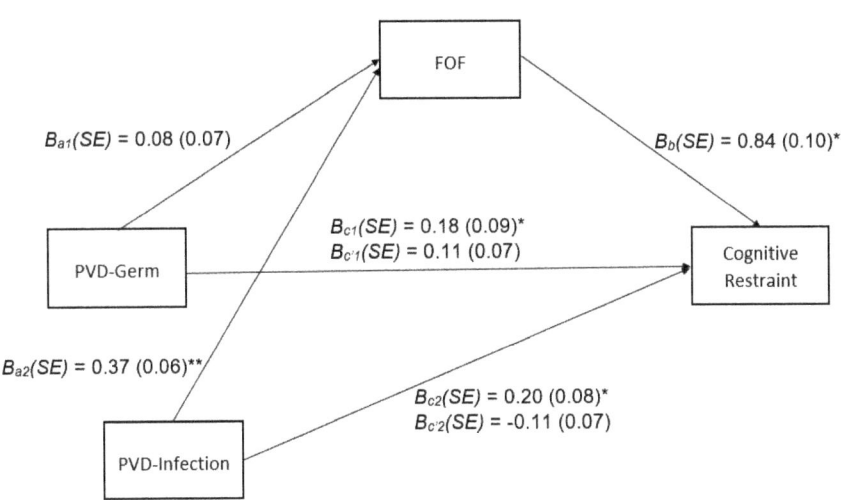

Figure A1. *Sex—Stratified Analyses for PVD Subscales, FOF, and Cognitive Restraint.* Process Model—4 path estimates from sex-stratified analyses testing the indirect effect of perceived germ aversion and perceived infectability on cognitive restraint through fear of fat. Unstandardized coefficients and standard errors are presented (* $p < 0.05$, ** $p < 0.01$). Indirect effect of PVD-Germ path for male, B (SE) = −0.02 (0.05), 95% CI [−0.11, 0.75], and female, B (SE) = 0.07 (0.06), 95% CI [−0.03, 0.19], participants. Indirect effect of PVD-Infection path for male, B (SE) = 0.22 (0.05), 95% CI [0.12, 0.34], and female, B (SE) = 0.31 (0.06), 95% CI [0.21, 0.45], participants.

Appendix D

Male Participants

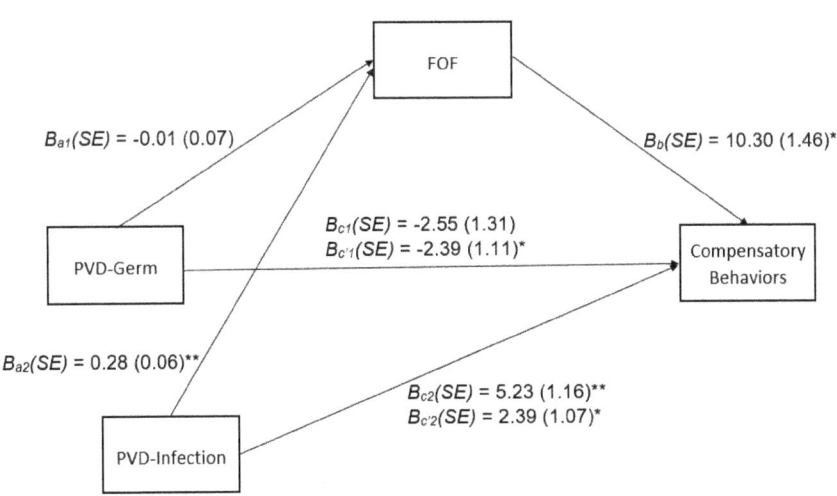

Female Participants

Figure A2. *Cont.*

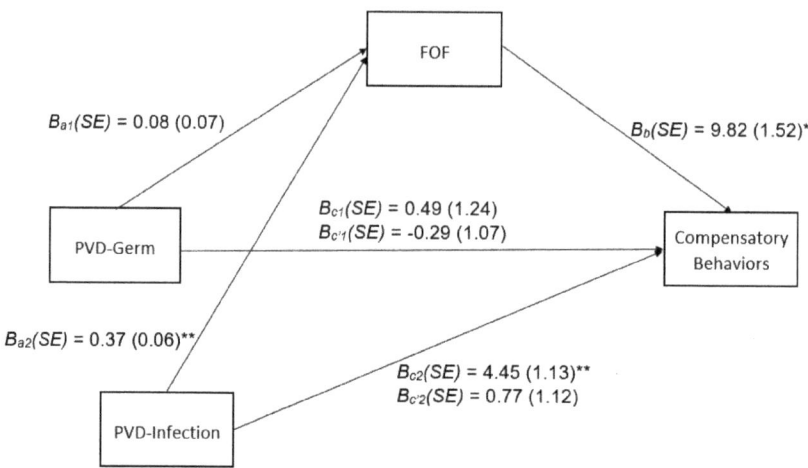

Figure A2. *Sex—Stratified Analyses for PVD-Infection, FOF, and Compensatory Behaviors.* Process Model—4 path estimates from sex-stratified analyses testing the indirect effect of perceived germ aversion and perceived infectability on compensatory behaviors through fear of fat. Unstandardized coefficients and standard errors are presented (* $p < 0.05$, ** $p < 0.01$). Indirect effect of PVD-Germ path for male, B (SE) = −0.15 (0.63), 95% CI [−1.53, 1.00] and female, B (SE) = 0.77 (0.68), 95% CI [−0.36, 2.35], participants. Indirect effect of PVD-Infection path for male, B (SE) = 2.84 (0.83), 95% CI [1.47, 4.73] and female, B (SE) = 3.68 (0.96), 95% CI [2.09, 5.88], participants.

References

1. Ackerman, J.M.; Hill, S.E.; Murray, D.R. The behavioral immune system: Current concerns and future directions. *Soc. Personal. Psychol. Compass* **2018**, *12*, e12371. [CrossRef]
2. Park, J.H.; Van Leeuwen, F.; Chochorelou, Y. Disease-Avoidance Processes and Stigmatization: Cues of Substandard Health Arouse Heightened Discomfort with Physical Contact. *J. Soc. Psychol.* **2013**, *153*, 212–228. [CrossRef] [PubMed]
3. Schaller, M.; Park, J.H. The behavioral immune system (and why it matters). *Curr. Psychol.* **2011**, *20*, 99–103. [CrossRef]
4. Duncan, L.A.; Schaller, M.; Park, J.H. Perceived vulnerability to disease: Development and validation of a 15-item self-report instrument. *Personal. Individ. Differ.* **2009**, *47*, 541–546. [CrossRef]
5. Park, J.H.; Faulkner, J.; Schaller, M. Evolved Disease-Avoidance Processes and Contemporary Anti-Social Behavior: Prejudicial Attitudes and Avoidance of People with Physical Disabilities. *J. Nonverbal Behav.* **2003**, *27*, 65–87. [CrossRef]
6. Park, J.H.; Schaller, M.; Crandall, C.S. Pathogen-avoidance mechanisms and the stigmatization of obese people. *Evol. Hum. Behav.* **2007**, *28*, 410–414. [CrossRef]
7. Tapp, C.; Oaten, M.; Stevenson, R.; Occhipinti, S.; Thandi, R. Is obesity treated like a contagious disease? *J. Appl. Soc. Psychol.* **2019**, *50*, 205–212. [CrossRef]
8. Miller, S.L.; Maner, J.K. Overperceiving disease cues: The basic cognition of the behavioral immune system. *J. Personal. Soc. Psychol.* **2012**, *102*, 1198–1213. [CrossRef]
9. Lieberman, D.L.; Tybur, J.M.; Latner, J.D. Disgust Sensitivity, Obesity Stigma, and Gender: Contamination Psychology Predicts Weight Bias for Women, Not Men. *Obesity* **2012**, *20*, 1803–1814. [CrossRef]
10. Lund, E.M.; Miller, S.L. Is obesity un-American? Disease concerns bias implicit perceptions of national identity. *Evol. Hum. Behav.* **2014**, *35*, 336–340. [CrossRef]
11. Magallares, A.; Jáuregui-Lobera, I.; Carbonero-Carreño, R.; Ruiz-Prieto, I.; Bolaños-Ríos, P.; Cano-Escoriaza, A. Perceived vulnerability to disease and antifat attitudes in a sample of children and teenagers. *Eat. Weight Disord.* **2015**, *20*, 483–489. [CrossRef] [PubMed]
12. Ackerman, J.M.; Tybur, J.M.; Mortensen, C.R. Infectious Disease and Imperfections of Self-Image. *Psychol. Sci.* **2018**, *29*, 228–241. [CrossRef] [PubMed]
13. Burmeister, J.M.; Hinman, N.; Koball, A.; Hoffmann, D.A.; Carels, R.A. Food addiction in adults seeking weight loss treatment. Implications for psychosocial health and weight loss. *Appetite* **2013**, *60*, 103–110. [CrossRef] [PubMed]
14. Durso, L.E.; Latner, J.D.; White, M.A.; Masheb, R.M.; Blomquist, K.K.; Morgan, P.T.; Grilo, C.M. Internalized weight bias in obese patients with binge eating disorder: Associations with eating disturbances and psychological functioning. *Int. J. Eat. Disord.* **2012**, *45*, 423–427. [CrossRef]

15. American Psychiatric Association. Feeding and Eating Disorders. In *Diagnostic and Statistical Manual of Mental Disorders*, 5th ed.; American Psychiatric Association: Arlington, VA, USA, 2013. [CrossRef]
16. Dalley, S.E.; Buunk, A.P. "Thinspiration" vs. "fear of fat". Using prototypes to predict frequent weight-loss dieting in females. *Appetite* **2009**, *52*, 217–221. [CrossRef]
17. Levitt, D.H. Drive for Thinness and Fear of Fat: Separate Yet Related Constructs? *Eat. Disord.* **2003**, *11*, 221–234. [CrossRef]
18. Fairburn, C.G.; Cooper, Z.; Shafran, R. Cognitive behaviour therapy for eating disorders: A "transdiagnostic" theory and treatment. *Behav. Res. Ther.* **2003**, *41*, 509–528. [CrossRef]
19. van Strien, T.; Frijters, J.E.; Bergers, G.; Defares, P.B. The Dutch Eating Behavior Questionnaire (DEBQ) for assessment of restrained, emotional, and external eating behavior. *Int. J. Eat. Disord.* **1986**, *5*, 295–315. [CrossRef]
20. Calugi, S.; Grave, R.D. Body image concern and treatment outcomes in adolescents with anorexia nervosa. *Int. J. Eat. Disord.* **2019**, *52*, 582–585. [CrossRef] [PubMed]
21. Calugi, S.; El Ghoch, M.; Conti, M.; Grave, R.D. Preoccupation with shape or weight, fear of weight gain, feeling fat and treatment outcomes in patients with anorexia nervosa: A longitudinal study. *Behav. Res. Ther.* **2018**, *105*, 63–68. [CrossRef]
22. Chow, C.M.; Ruhl, H.; Tan, C.C.; Ellis, L. Fear of fat and restrained eating: Negative body talk between female friends as a moderator. *Eat. Weight Disord.* **2019**, *24*, 1181–1188. [CrossRef] [PubMed]
23. Dalley, S.E.; Toffanin, P.; Pollet, T.V. Dietary restraint in college women: Fear of an imperfect fat self is stronger than hope of a perfect thin self. *Body Image* **2012**, *9*, 441–447. [CrossRef] [PubMed]
24. MacLeod, J.S.; MacLeod, C.; Dondzilo, L.; Bell, J. The Role of Fear of Fatness and Avoidance of Fatness in Predicting Eating Restraint. *Cogn. Ther. Res.* **2020**, *44*, 196–207. [CrossRef]
25. Wellman, J.D.; Araiza, A.M.; Newell, E.E.; McCoy, S.K. Weight stigma facilitates unhealthy eating and weight gain via fear of fat. *Stigma Health* **2018**, *3*, 186–194. [CrossRef]
26. Goldfarb, L.A.; Dykens, E.M.; Gerrard, M. The Goldfarb Fear of Fat Scale. *J. Personal. Assess.* **1985**, *49*, 329–332. [CrossRef]
27. Goldschmidt, A.B.; Crosby, R.D.; Cao, L.; Moessner, M.; Forbush, K.T.; Accurso, E.C.; Le Grange, D. Network analysis of pediatric eating disorder symptoms in a treatment-seeking, transdiagnostic sample. *J. Abnorm. Psychol.* **2018**, *127*, 251–264. [CrossRef] [PubMed]
28. Levinson, C.A.; Zerwas, S.; Calebs, B.; Forbush, K.; Kordy, H.; Watson, H.; Hofmeier, S.; Levine, M.; Crosby, R.D.; Peat, C.; et al. The core symptoms of bulimia nervosa, anxiety, and depression: A network analysis. *J. Abnorm. Psychol.* **2017**, *126*, 340–354. [CrossRef]
29. De Coninck, D.; D'Haenens, L.; Matthijs, K. Perceived vulnerability to disease and attitudes towards public health measures: COVID-19 in Flanders, Belgium. *Personal. Individ. Differ.* **2020**, *166*, 110220. [CrossRef]
30. Cummings, J.R.; Joyner, M.A.; Gearhardt, A.N. Development and preliminary validation of the Anticipated Effects of Food Scale. *Psychol. Addict. Behav.* **2020**, *34*, 403–413. [CrossRef]
31. Stice, E.; Telch, C.F.; Rizvi, S.L. Development and validation of the Eating Disorder Diagnostic Scale: A brief self-report measure of anorexia, bulimia, and binge-eating disorder. *Psychol. Assess.* **2000**, *12*, 123–131. [CrossRef]
32. IBM Corporation. *Released 2020. IBM SPSS Statistics for Windows*; Version 27; IBM Corp.: Armonk, NY, USA.
33. Hayes, A.F. *Introduction to Mediation, Moderation, and Conditional Process Analysis: A Regression-Based Approach*; The Guilford Press: New York, NY, USA, 2013.
34. Pearl, R.L.; Hopkins, C.H.; Berkowitz, R.I.; Wadden, T.A. Group cognitive-behavioral treatment for internalized weight stigma: A pilot study. *Eat. Weight Disord.* **2018**, *23*, 357–362. [CrossRef] [PubMed]
35. Makhanova, A.; Shepherd, M.A.; Plant, E.A.; Gerend, M.A.; Maner, J.K. Childhood illness as an antecedent of perceived vulnerability to disease. *Evol. Behav. Sci.* **2020**, *16*, 53–66. [CrossRef]
36. Anderson, L.M.; Berg, H.; Brown, T.A.; Menzel, J.; Reilly, E.E. The Role of Disgust in Eating Disorders. *Curr. Psychiatry Rep.* **2021**, *23*, 4. [CrossRef]
37. Mitchison, D.; Mond, J.M. Epidemiology of eating disorders, eating disordered behaviour, and body image disturbance in males: A narrative review. *J. Eat. Disord.* **2015**, *3*, 20. [CrossRef] [PubMed]
38. Berg, K.C.; Peterson, C.B.; Frazier, P.; Crow, S.J. Psychometric evaluation of the eating disorder examination and eating disorder examination-questionnaire: A systematic review of the literature. *Int. J. Eat. Disord.* **2011**, *45*, 428–438. [CrossRef] [PubMed]
39. Fairburn, C.G.; Beglin, S.J. Assessment of eating disorders: Interview or self-report questionnaire? *Int. J. Eat. Disord.* **1994**, *16*, 363–370. [CrossRef]
40. Keel, P.K.; Crow, S.; Davis, T.L.; Mitchell, J.E. Assessment of eating disorders comparison of interview and questionnaire data from a long-term follow-up study of bulimia nervosa. *J. Psychosom. Res.* **2002**, *53*, 1043–1047. [CrossRef] [PubMed]
41. Buhrmester, M.D.; Talaifar, S.; Gosling, S.D. An Evaluation of Amazon's Mechanical Turk, Its Rapid Rise, and Its Effective Use. *Perspect. Psychol. Sci.* **2018**, *13*, 149–154. [CrossRef]
42. De Pasquale, C.; Pistorio, M.L.; Sciacca, F.; Hichy, Z. Relationships Between Anxiety, Perceived Vulnerability to Disease, and Smartphone Use during Coronavirus Disease 2019 Pandemic in a Sample of Italian College Students. *Front. Psychol.* **2021**, *12*, 692503. [CrossRef]
43. Swinbourne, J.M.; Touyz, S. The co-morbidity of eating disorders and anxiety disorders: A review. *Eur. Eat. Disord. Rev.* **2007**, *15*, 253–274. [CrossRef]

44. Brady, R.E.; Badour, C.L.; Arega, E.A.; Levy, J.J.; Adams, T.G. Evaluating the mediating effects of perceived vulnerability to disease in the relation between disgust and contamination-based OCD. *J. Anxiety Disord.* **2021**, *79*, 102384. [CrossRef] [PubMed]
45. Bektas, S.; Keeler, J.L.; Anderson, L.M.; Mutwalli, H.; Himmerich, H.; Treasure, J. Disgust and Self-Disgust in Eating Disorders: A Systematic Review and Meta-Analysis. *Nutrients* **2022**, *14*, 1728. [CrossRef] [PubMed]
46. Eyal, T.; Dar, R.; Liberman, N. Is disgust in obsessive-compulsive disorder mediated by fear of pathogens? *J. Anxiety Disord.* **2021**, *77*, 102340. [CrossRef] [PubMed]
47. Altman, S.E.; Shankman, S.A. What is the association between obsessive–compulsive disorder and eating disorders? *Clin. Psychol. Rev.* **2009**, *29*, 638–646. [CrossRef] [PubMed]
48. Liu, T.; Ackerman, J.M.; Preston, S.D. Dissociating compulsive washing and hoarding tendencies through differences in comorbidities and the content of concerns. *J. Behav. Cogn. Ther.* **2021**, *31*, 291–308. [CrossRef]
49. Da Luz, F.Q.; Hay, P.; Touyz, S.; Sainsbury, A. Obesity with Comorbid Eating Disorders: Associated Health Risks and Treatment Approaches. *Nutrients* **2018**, *10*, 829. [CrossRef]
50. Burton, A.L.; Abbott, M.J. Processes and pathways to binge eating: Development of an integrated cognitive and behavioural model of binge eating. *J. Eat. Disord.* **2019**, *7*, 18. [CrossRef]
51. Mathes, W.F.; Brownley, K.A.; Mo, X.; Bulik, C.M. The biology of binge eating. *Appetite* **2009**, *52*, 545–553. [CrossRef]
52. Mortensen, C.R.; Becker, D.V.; Ackerman, J.M.; Neuberg, S.L.; Kenrick, D.T. Infection Breeds Reticencer: The Effects of Disease Salience on Self-Perceptions of Personality and Behavioral Avoidance Tendencies. *Psychol. Sci.* **2010**, *21*, 440–447. [CrossRef]
53. Wang, I.M.; Ackerman, J.M. The Infectiousness of Crowds: Crowding Experiences Are Amplified by Pathogen Threats. *Personal. Soc. Psychol. Bull.* **2019**, *45*, 120–132. [CrossRef]
54. Allen, K.L.; Crosby, R.D.; Oddy, W.H.; Byrne, S.M. Eating disorder symptom trajectories in adolescence: Effects of time, participant sex, and early adolescent depressive symptoms. *J. Eat. Disord.* **2013**, *1*, 32. [CrossRef] [PubMed]
55. Termorshuizen J., D.; Watson, H.J.; Thornton, L.M.; Borg, S.; Flatt, R.E.; MacDermod, C.M.; Harper, L.E.; van Furth, E.F.; Peat, C.M.; Bulik, C.M. Early impact of COVID-19 on individuals with self-reported eating disorders: A survey of ~1000 individuals in the United States and the Netherlands. *Int. J. Eat. Disord.* **2020**, *53*, 1780–1790. [CrossRef] [PubMed]

Disclaimer/Publisher's Note: The statements, opinions and data contained in all publications are solely those of the individual author(s) and contributor(s) and not of MDPI and/or the editor(s). MDPI and/or the editor(s) disclaim responsibility for any injury to people or property resulting from any ideas, methods, instructions or products referred to in the content.

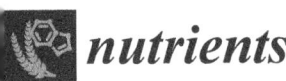

Article

The Role of Food Addiction and Lifetime Substance Use on Eating Disorder Treatment Outcomes

Romina Miranda-Olivos [1,2,3,†], Zaida Agüera [1,3,4,5,*,†], Roser Granero [1,3,6], Susana Jiménez-Murcia [1,2,3,7], Montserrat Puig-Llobet [4,5], Maria Teresa Lluch-Canut [4,5], Ashley N. Gearhardt [8] and Fernando Fernández-Aranda [1,2,3,7,*]

1. CIBER Fisiopatología Obesidad y Nutrición (CIBERobn), Instituto de Salud Carlos III, 28029 Madrid, Spain; rmiranda@idibell.cat (R.M.-O.)
2. Clinical Psychology Unit, L'Hospitalet de Llobregat, Hospital Universitari de Bellvitge, 08907 Barcelona, Spain
3. Psychoneurobiology of Eating and Addictive Behaviors Group, Neurosciences Programme, Bellvitge Biomedical Research Institute (IDIBELL), L'Hospitalet de Llobregat, 08908 Barcelona, Spain
4. Departament d'Infermeria de Salut Pública, Salut Mental i Materno-Infantil, Escola d'Infermeria, Facultat de Medicina i Ciències de la Salut, L'Hospitalet de Llobregat, Universitat de Barcelona (UB), 08007 Barcelona, Spain; monpuigllob@ub.edu (M.P.-L.); tlluch@ub.edu (M.T.L.-C.)
5. Research Group in Mental Health, Psychosocial and Complex Nursing Care (NURSEARCH), Facultat de Medicina i Ciències de la Salut, L'Hospitalet de Llobregat, Universitat de Barcelona (UB), 08007 Barcelona, Spain
6. Departament de Psicobiologia i Metodologia de les Ciències de la Salut, Universitat Autònoma de Barcelona, 08193 Barcelona, Spain
7. Department of Clinical Sciences, School of Medicine and Health Sciences, University of Barcelona, 08007 Barcelona, Spain
8. Department of Psychology, University of Michigan, Ann Arbor, MI 48109, USA; agearhar@umich.edu
* Correspondence: zaguera@ub.edu (Z.A.); ffernandez@bellvitgehospital.cat (F.F.-A.); Tel.: +34-93-260-72-27 (Z.A. & F.F.-A.)
† These authors contributed equally to this work.

Abstract: Food addiction (FA) and substance use (SU) in eating disorders (ED) have been associated with a more dysfunctional clinical and psychopathological profile. However, their impact on treatment outcomes has been poorly explored. Therefore, this transdiagnostic study is aimed at examining whether the presence of FA and/or SU is associated with treatment outcomes in patients with different ED types. The results were not able to reveal significant differences in treatment outcomes between patients with and without FA and/or SU; however, the effect sizes suggest higher dropout rates in the group with both FA and SU. The predictive models of treatment outcomes showed different features associated with each group. High persistence (i.e., tendency to perseverance and inflexibility) was the personality trait most associated with poor treatment outcomes in patients without addictions. High harm avoidance and younger age at ED onset were the variables most related to poor outcomes in patients with FA or SU. Finally, in the group with both addictive behaviors (FA and SU), the younger patients presented the poorest outcomes. In conclusion, our results suggest that, regardless of presenting addictive behaviors, patients with ED may similarly benefit from treatment. However, it may be important to consider the differential predictors of each group that might guide certain treatment targets.

Keywords: food addiction; substance use; treatment outcomes; eating disorders

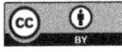

1. Introduction

The comorbidity between eating disorders (ED) and some addictive-related patterns, such as food addiction (FA), behavioral addictions, and substance use (SU), has been widely described in the literature. The construct of FA combines the concepts of substance-based and behavioral addictions. Thus, there is no consensus on whether FA should be integrated within substance use disorders (SUDs) [1] or, on the contrary, within behavioral addictions [2]. However, many studies increasingly point out that the mere application of criteria based on the addictive chemical properties of food (as in SU) does not seem sufficient to fully capture the phenomenological aspects of an FA, hence the need to study FA and SU as distinct addictive behaviors [3]. A high prevalence rate of FA has been widely reported in individuals with obesity and/or ED, mainly in those with bulimia nervosa (BN) and binge eating disorder (BED) (70–90%) [4,5]. Intriguingly, the presence of FA has also been described in patients with anorexia nervosa (AN), especially in those of the bulimic-purging subtype (AN-BP), compared to the restricting subtype (AN-R) (75.0% and 54.2%, respectively) [6–8]. The presence of FA in patients with ED has been associated with greater severity of ED-related symptomatology (e.g., a higher frequency of binge-eating episodes, emotional eating, and compulsive eating) [5,7–9], as well as more dysfunctional personality traits (i.e., high impulsivity), and greater general psychopathology (mainly more depressive symptoms) [5,8]. The impact of FA on the prognosis of EDs has not yet been fully investigated. Hilker et al. [10] reported that the severity of both FA and binge/purge episodes decreased after a psychoeducational program in patients with BN. Likewise, Romero et al. [4] found that the association between FA and treatment outcomes appeared to be mediated by the severity of the ED. Additionally, this study found that FA was indirectly associated with poorer treatment outcomes in BED, but not in BN [4]. There are currently no studies exploring the impact of FA on the prognosis of AN. However, a recent study suggested that FA in AN-R could increase the likelihood of a crossover diagnosis to AN-BP [6].

In terms of SU in ED, numerous studies over the last years have addressed this topic of interest, reporting SU prevalence rates in EDs ranging from 21% to 50%, with tobacco being the most prevalent addictive substance, but also caffeine, alcohol, and illicit drugs [11]. The comorbidity of lifetime SU varies among the ED diagnoses, being more prevalent in BN (34%), followed by BED (18%), AN (13%), and other specified feeding or eating disorders (OSFED) (12%) [8] The coexistence of EDs and SU has been associated with high levels of impulsivity and sensation-seeking that may promote addictive-like behaviors towards a stimulus perceived as rewarding [12,13]. Additionally, SU in BN has been linked to increased emotional dysregulation, suggesting that certain substances might be used as a maladaptive strategy to cope with negative emotions [14,15] The purpose of substance misuse in patients with ED is a relevant aspect to consider [16]. It is important to identify whether SU is part of the ED symptomatology as a strategy aimed at weight control (e.g., caffeine, tobacco, psychostimulant substances), or whether it acts as a maladaptive coping mechanism to deal with negative emotions (e.g., alcohol, psychoactive substances) [16,17]. In both cases, the functional role of SU may guide different targeted intervention strategies [11]. In addition, the co-occurrence of ED with SU has been associated with a poorer prognosis, contributing to a longer duration of the disorder, greater psychopathology and presence of other psychiatric disorders, and an increased risk of mortality [18,19]. This co-occurrence may accentuate the symptomatology of ED, hampering its recovery [11]. However, research directly testing the role of SU on ED treatment outcomes is limited.

The comorbidity of FA and SU in ED have usually been addressed separately. Nevertheless, some studies have indicated the presence of a potential common brain substrate in FA and SU, suggesting shared neurobiological vulnerabilities and genetic predispositions [20]. For instance, certain polymorphisms of the dopamine (DA) receptor D2 have been linked to an increased risk for both FA and SU [21,22]. Considering that the DA system plays a role in appetite regulation and reward pathways, it is plausible that this neurotransmitter system underlies maladaptive eating behaviors in EDs. Based on this premise, it is plausible to hypothesize that the concurrent occurrence of multiple addictive behaviors could have epidemiological implications on treatment outcomes in EDs. However, to date, there have been no studies that have explored the potential effects that the simultaneous presence of both addictive-related patterns could have on treatment outcomes in individuals with EDs. One recent study by our research group explored the joint involvement of FA and/or lifetime problematic alcohol and illicit drug use in EDs [23]. Patients with at least one addictive-like behavior (either current FA or lifetime SU) exhibited more general psychopathology and ED-related symptomatology than those without FA and/or SU. However, the cross-sectional design of this study was not able to address whether this dysfunctional clinical and personality profile has implications for treatment outcomes. Therefore, the main goals of this study were threefold: (a) to examine the sociodemographic and clinical characteristics of patients with different types of ED (including AN, BN, BED, and OSFED) who reported FA and/or lifetime problematic alcohol and illicit drug use (i.e., between those with both addictive behaviors (FA+ and SU+), those with only one addictive behavior (FA+ or SU+), and those with no addictive behaviors (FA− and SU−)); (b) to analyze whether there are differences in treatment outcomes, including dropout rates, between patients with and without current FA and/or lifetime problematic SU; and (c) to describe predictors of treatment outcomes in patients with or without addictive-like behaviors.

2. Materials and Methods

2.1. Participants

A total of 303 patients with ED composed the sample of this study (32 AN, 132 BN, 67 BED, and 72 OSFED). All patients were attended to at the ED Unit of the Hospital Universitario de Bellvitge (Barcelona, Spain) for assessment and treatment.

2.2. Instruments

In the assessment process, sociodemographic and clinical data were collected through a semi-structured face-to-face interview using the SCID-5 [24]. Clinical data covered lifetime alcohol or illegal drug misuse by utilizing module E of the SCID-5 [24]. For the present study, problematic lifetime SU was defined as a problematic pattern of continued use of alcohol and/or illicit drugs at some time throughout the patient's life, and with negative consequences. These consequences may comprise, for example, higher consumption than intended; craving to, or unsuccessful efforts to control, consumption; consumption despite physical or psychological problems; interpersonal problems; being in dangerous situations; etc. Furthermore, the usually applied questionnaires in the field of EDs were administered, namely:

- The Yale Food Addiction Scale 2.0 (YFAS 2.0), Spanish validation [25]. This is a 35-item, self-report questionnaire to assess FA, based on 11 substance-dependence-related symptoms and adapted to the context of food consumption. This scale allows the classifying of FA into binary categories, namely present (at least 2 symptoms and self-reported clinically significant impairment or distress) and absent. The internal consistency of our sample was excellent ($\alpha = 0.97$).
- The Eating Disorder Inventory-2 (EDI-2), Spanish validation [26]. It is a 91-item, self-reported questionnaire that assesses 11 ED-related cognitive and behavioral domains. A total score is also provided to report overall ED severity. For this sample, the internal consistency was excellent ($\alpha = 0.94$).
- The Symptom Checklist-90 Revised (SCL-90-R), Spanish validation [27]. The questionnaire is composed of 90 items that assess 9 dimensions of psychopathology: somatization, obsession–compulsion, interpersonal sensitivity, depression, anxiety, hostility, phobic anxiety, paranoid ideation, and psychoticism. Additionally, it includes three global indices related to overall psychological distress (i.e., the global severity index, GSI), the intensity of symptoms (i.e., the positive symptom distress index, PSDI), and self-reported symptoms (i.e., a total of positive symptoms). The questionnaire demonstrated excellent internal consistency, with a Cronbach's alpha coefficient of 0.97.
- The Temperament and Character Inventory Revised (TCI-R), Spanish validation [28]. It is a self-reported assessment, consisting of 240 items, that evaluates 4 temperament dimensions (harm avoidance, novelty seeking, reward dependence, and persistence) and

3 character dimensions (self-directedness, cooperativeness, and self-transcendence). Our internal consistency ranged from $\alpha = 0.81$ to $\alpha = 0.89$.
- The Impulsive Behavior Scale (UPPS-P), Spanish validation [29]. This self-report questionnaire consists of 59 items that assess 5 distinct facets of impulsivity: positive and negative urgency (a tendency to act rashly in response to positive mood or distress), lack of perseverance (an inability to sustain focus on a task), lack of premeditation (acting without considering the consequences of an action), and sensation seeking (a tendency to seek novel and exciting experiences). The internal consistency for the sample ranged from very good (negative urgency $\alpha = 0.83$) to excellent (positive urgency $\alpha = 0.92$).

2.3. Treatment

Treatment for BN, BED, and OSFED was provided by experienced psychologists through 16 weekly outpatient group therapy sessions of 90 min each. Separate therapeutic groups were conducted for patients with different diagnoses, but all were on the same cognitive–behavioral therapy (CBT) program. Patients diagnosed with AN (not requiring inpatient treatment for underweight) underwent a day hospital treatment program, which included ten weekly CBT group sessions for about 3 months.

Upon discharge, patients were assessed and assigned into one of three previously defined categories: full remission, partial remission, and non-remission. Criteria for full remission were based on the DSM-5, indicating a complete absence of ED symptoms for at least four weeks of treatment. Partial remission referred to substantial symptomatic improvement with residual symptoms, while non-remission was used to describe poor outcomes. These categories have been employed to evaluate the efficacy of ED treatments in previous studies [4,30–32]. Treatment discontinuation was classified as dropout, defined as being absent for at least three consecutive therapy sessions. In addition, patients were also subsequently recategorized into a dichotomous variable (i.e., good versus poor outcomes), which has been previously used to examine ED treatments [33], in order to facilitate the interpretation of the results, especially in the predictive models, namely good outcomes (i.e., full and partial remission) and poor outcomes (i.e., non-remission and dropout).

2.4. Statistical Analyses

Stata 17 for Windows was used for the statistical analysis. The comparison between the groups was performed using chi-square tests (χ^2) for categorical variables, and analysis of variance (ANOVA) for quantitative variables. Bonferroni's correction was applied for post hoc comparisons in chi-square tests, while post hoc pairwise comparisons for ANOVA were performed using the Bonferroni method. Effect size was considered in the range of mild-moderate to large-high when $|CV| > 0.15$, mild-moderate if $OR > 1.86$, and large-high when $OR > 3.00$. The comparisons of the treatment outcomes (0 = good versus 1 = poor) between the groups were performed by odds ratio coefficients (OR), obtained in logistic regression, and adjusted by the ED type. Stepwise logistic regressions were also used to identify the significant predictors of the treatment outcomes (0 = good versus 1 = poor) for the list of measures at the baseline. Given the exploratory approach of this analysis, we tried to include the maximum number of predictors, while minimizing adjustment problems due to high collinearity. For this reason, in addition to the sociodemographic profile and the personality profile, the global measures associated with the severity of the ED (EDI-2 total), the psychopathological state (SCL-90R GSI), and impulsivity (UPPS-P total) were included. The goodness-of-fit was assessed with the Hosmer–Lemeshow test, and the global predictive capacity with the pseudo-Nagelkerke R^2 coefficient.

3. Results

3.1. Descriptive of the Sample

Most participants in the study were women ($n = 277$, 91.4%), single ($n = 201$, 66.3%), or married ($n = 65$, 21.5%), with primary ($n = 114$, 37.6%) or secondary ($n = 140$, 46.2%)

education levels, and employed ($n = 170$, 56.1%). The mean age was 32.3 years (SD = 12.3), the mean age of onset of the ED was 20.7 years (SD = 9.9), and the mean duration of the ED was 12.1 years (SD = 9.6).

Table S1 (see Supplementary Materials) includes the comparison of the sociodemographic data, the onset of the ED, the duration, and the BMI between the groups defined by the ED types. Table S1 also contains the distribution of FA, SU, and both FA + SU for each diagnostic type.

Table 1 shows the comparisons between the groups defined by the presence of FA and/or SU. These analyses were performed with bivariate analyses, separately assessing the associations of each variable (defined in the rows) with the created groups (displayed in the columns). Results of these analyses contribute to the first objective of the study. No differences between the groups were found for gender, civil status, education, onset of the ED, and BMI. Differences between the groups were found for the employment status, age, and duration of the ED. The distribution of the ED subtypes was also different for the FA and SU groups being the OSFED condition most associated with FA− and SU−, and BN in the presence of FA+ and/or SU+.

Table 1. Descriptive statistics of the sample based on the presence of FA and SU.

		FA− and SU− $n = 56$		FA+ or SU+ $n = 159$		FA+ and SU+ $n = 88$			
		n	%	n	%	n	%	p	Groups with Significant Differences
Gender	Women	49	87.5%	148	93.1%	80	90.9%	0.430	
	Men	7	12.5%	11	6.9%	8	9.1%		
Civil status	Single	42	75.0%	99	62.3%	60	68.2%	0.413	
	Married/partner	9	16.1%	40	25.2%	16	18.2%		
	Divorced/separated	5	8.9%	20	12.6%	12	13.6%		
Education	Primary	23	41.1%	55	34.6%	36	40.9%	0.539	
	Secondary	26	46.4%	73	45.9%	41	46.6%		
	University	7	12.5%	31	19.5%	11	12.5%		
Employment	Unemployed	13	23.2%	30	18.9%	17	19.3%	0.001 *	All pairwise comparisons with $p < 0.05$
	Student	23	41.1%	41	25.8%	9	10.2%		
	Employed	20	35.7%	88	55.3%	62	70.5%		
		Mean	SD	Mean	SD	Mean	SD	p	
Age (years old)		29.04	12.90	32.56	12.56	34.19	10.93	0.046 *	(FA− and SU−) ≠ (FA+ and SU+)
Onset ED (years old)		21.68	9.95	20.84	9.80	19.89	9.96	0.556	
Duration ED (years)		7.98	8.34	11.94	10.00	15.05	9.74	0.001 *	All pairwise comparisons with $p < 0.05$
BMI (kg/m^2)		25.34	10.59	28.05	9.42	28.09	9.22	0.160	
		n	%	n	%	n	%	p	Groups with significant differences
ED subtypes	AN	11	19.6%	17	10.7%	4	4.5%	0.001 *	All pairwise comparisons with $p < 0.05$
	BN	7	12.5%	71	44.7%	54	61.4%		
	BED	12	21.4%	38	23.9%	17	19.3%		
	OSFED	26	46.4%	33	20.8%	13	14.8%		

Note. AN: anorexia nervosa. BN: bulimia nervosa. BED: binge eating disorder. ED: eating disorder. OSFED: other specified feeding or eating disorder. FA−: food addiction negative screening score. FA+: food addiction positive screening score. SU−: lifetime substances use absent. SU+: lifetime substances use present. SD: standard deviation. * Bold: significant parameter.

3.2. Association of the Treatment Outcomes with the Presence of FA and SU

Table 2 shows the distribution of the treatment outcomes classified into four categories, namely dropout, non-remission, partial remission, and full remission for each group, defined by the presence of FA and/or lifetime SU. Results of these analyses contribute to the second objective of the study. The results of the chi-square test comparing the treatment outcomes between the clinical conditions showed no statistical differences, but an effect size in the moderate range was found comparing the treatment outcomes between FA+ and SU+, and FA− and SU−. The comorbid condition of FA+ and SU+ was associated with a higher risk of dropout. The other comparisons in Table 2 obtained non-significant results and poor effect sizes.

Table 2. Distribution of the treatment outcomes.

	Total		FA− and SU−		FA+ or SU+		FA+ and SU+		FA+ or SU+ vs. FA− and SU−		FA+ and SU+ vs. FA− and SU−		FA+ and SU+ vs. FA+ or SU+	
	n = 303		n = 56		n = 159		n = 88							
	n	%	n	%	n	%	n	%	p	|CV|	p	|CV|	p	|CV|
Dropout	125	41.3%	21	37.5%	61	38.4%	43	48.9%	0.233	0.141	0.108	0.205 †	0.421	0.107
Non-remission	24	7.9%	9	16.1%	11	6.9%	4	4.5%						
Partial remission	72	23.8%	12	21.4%	40	25.2%	20	22.7%						
Full remission	82	27.1%	14	25.0%	47	29.6%	21	23.9%						

Note. FA−: food addiction negative screening score. FA+: food addiction positive screening score. SU−: lifetime substances use absent. SU+: lifetime substances use present. † Bold: effect size into the range mild-moderate to large-high (|CV| > 0.15).

Table 3 displays the distribution of treatment outcomes categorized into two levels, namely poor outcome and good outcome. A logistic regression model was employed, with the group serving as the independent variable, the treatment outcome as the criterion (i.e., dependent variable), and the ED type as a covariate. These analyses contribute to addressing the second objective of the study. Adjusted for the ED type, no statistically significant differences were observed in the pairwise comparisons (effect size was also in the low range).

Table 3. Comparisons of the treatment outcomes in the study: results adjusted by the ED type.

	Total		FA− and SU−		FA+ or SU+		FA+ and SU+		FA+ or SU+ vs. FA− and SU−		FA+ & SU+ vs. FA− and SU−		FA+ and SU+ vs. FA+ or SU+	
	n = 303		n = 56		n = 159		n = 88							
	n	%	n	%	n	%	n	%	p	OR	p	OR	p	OR
Poor outcome	149	49.2%	30	53.6%	72	45.3%	47	53.4%	0.238	0.68	0.762	0.89	0.238	1.48
Good outcome	154	50.8%	26	46.4%	87	54.7%	41	46.6%		*1.47*		*1.12*		

Note. FA−: food addiction negative screening score. FA+: food addiction positive screening score. SU−: lifetime substances use absent. SU+: lifetime substances use present. Poor outcome: dropout or non-remission. Good outcome: partial remission or full remission. Italics font: inverse of the OR (1/OR).

3.3. Predictors of the Treatment Outcomes in the Study

Table 4 presents the results of the stepwise logistic regression analyses conducted to identify the significant predictors of treatment outcomes for each group. The list of potential predictors (independent variables) were the ED types, sociodemographic data (i.e., gender, civil status, education, employment status, and age), onset, duration of the ED, and clinical profile considering the ED symptomatology (EDI-2 total), general psychopathology (SCL-90R), impulsivity levels (UPPS-P total), and personality traits (TCI-R scales). The criterion in the model (dependent variable) was represented by 1 = poor outcome (dropout and non-remission) and 0 = good outcome (partial and full remission). Then, three separate models were tested for each group: the FA− and SU− group (n = 56), the FA+ or SU+ group (n = 159), and the FA+ and SU+ group (n = 88). The results of these analyses contributed to addressing the third objective of the study.

Table 4. Predictors of poor treatment outcomes in the study.

Subsample	Predictors	B	SE	p	OR	95%CI (OR)		H–L	NR²
FA− and SU− (n = 56)	TCI-R Persistence	0.043	0.018	0.017	1.44	1.01	1.08	0.158	0.167
FA+ or SU+ (n = 159)	Onset at the ED (years)	−0.048	0.019	0.010	0.953	0.919	0.989	0.181	0.109
	TCI-R harm avoidance	0.021	0.009	0.018	1.021	1.004	1.039		
FA+ and SU+ (n = 88)	Age (years)	−0.049	0.021	0.021	0.952	0.914	0.993	0.338	0.084

Note. List of predictors: ED type, sociodemographic variables (gender, civil status, education, employment status, age), age at onset of ED, duration of ED, ED symptom severity level (EDI-2 total), psychopathology distress (SCL-90R GSI), impulsivity (UPPS-P total), and personality (TCI-R scales). H–L: Hosmer–Lemeshow test (p-value). NR^2: Nagelkerke's pseudo-R^2.

Significant predictors that referred to a higher likelihood for a poor outcome in each group were: (a) high persistence levels (TCI-R) in the FA− and SU− group; (b) an earlier onset of the ED and higher harm avoidance level (TCI-R) in the FA+ or SU+ group; and (c) being younger in the FA+ and SU+ group. These three logistic models in Table 4 achieved an adequate fit ($p > 0.05$ in the Hosmer–Lemeshow tests) and global predictive capacity, considering a Nagelkerke R^2 coefficient of between 0.08 and 0.17.

Table S2 (see Supplementary Materials) includes comparisons of good and poor outcomes in groups defined for the presence or absence of current FA and lifetime SU. For the FA− and SU− group, a poor treatment outcome was associated with lower levels of body dissatisfaction (EDI-2), lack of perseverance (UPPS-P), harm avoidance (TCI-R), and higher levels of persistence (TCI-R). For the FA+ or SU+ group, a poor treatment outcome was related to higher scores in the EDI-2 ineffectiveness, TCI-R impulse regulation, a poor psychopathological state in the SCL-90-R (interpersonal sensitivity, depression, psychotic, GSI, and PSDI), and a higher TCI-R harm avoidance. For the group with FA+ and SU+, no differences between patients with good and poor treatment outcomes were found.

Table S3 (see Supplementary Material) presents the results for the subsample of patients who had a poor treatment outcome (n = 149). The pairwise comparisons between the FA+ or SU+ group versus the FA+ and SU+ group revealed few statistical differences. Notably, statistical differences were observed in the UPPS-P impulsivity measures and TCI-R novelty seeking, with higher scores in the FA+ and SU+ group compared to the FA+ or SU+ group. In contrast, the FA− and SU− group, when compared to the other conditions, exhibited lower scores in the EDI-2, SCL-90-R, and UPPS-P scales. Additionally, their personality profile was characterized by lower novelty seeking and harm avoidance, as well as higher persistence and self-directedness.

Table S4 (see Supplementary Materials) includes a comparison of the treatment outcomes of the three groups stratified by the ED type. No statistical differences were found, but a moderate effect size was found in the AN group, suggesting that the comorbid condition of FA+ and SU+ in AN was associated with an increased risk of a poor treatment outcome.

4. Discussion

In recent years, there has been increasing interest in understanding the role of FA and other comorbid addictions on the clinical status and prognosis of patients with ED. However, to the best of our knowledge, this is the first study that aims to address whether the presence of one (i.e., FA or SU) or multiple lifetime addictive behaviors (i.e., FA and SU) might have an impact on the treatment outcomes of these patients. Because most patients with an ED have a co-occurrence with some addictive behavior, it is essential to study them to understand and consider how the addiction perspective can be included in the care of these patients. Intriguingly, the results suggest that there are no differences related to the presence of addictive-like behaviors, in terms of treatment outcomes of patients with ED. However, despite not reaching statistical significance, a moderate effect size was observed in the group with both FA and SU, in terms of higher dropout rates than the non-addiction group.

Similarly to previous findings [23], when comparing patients with a poor treatment outcome, we found that those with at least one addiction-related behavior were characterized by greater overall psychopathology, more severity of ED, and more dysfunctional personality traits, compared to the non-addiction group. However, in contrast with our hypothesis, our findings did not show significant differences in treatment outcomes between individuals without addictive behaviors and those with FA and/or SU. These results are in line with a previous study reporting that FA mediates the severity of ED but is not, per se, directly associated with the treatment response [4]. However, despite the absence of significant results, when considering diagnostic types separately, the effect size of the comparisons suggests that the FA+ and SU+ condition was associated with an increased risk of poor treatment outcomes in patients with AN. Further studies with higher sampling power are needed to corroborate this hypothesis.

We also hypothesized that patients with one or more addictive behaviors would have higher dropout rates; however, no statistically significant differences were found between the three groups. This finding is in line with another study that found no differences in treatment outcomes between patients with ED who were either with or without SU disorder [16]. However, it is not consistent with other studies that found greater treatment dropout rates in patients with addictions [34,35]. In this vein, it should be noted that these previous studies were conducted with current SU disorders, and not with lifetime problematic SU, as in this current study, which could explain the lack of differences. Nonetheless, we observed a moderate effect size, suggesting the comorbid condition of FA+ and SU+ was associated with a higher risk of dropout. It might represent a very relevant point for clinical practice that deserves further investigation. For instance, it would be interesting to identify in which treatment session they are most likely to drop out in order to identify strategies to reduce dropout, as well as to include relevant treatment goals from the early stages of care, and to discuss addiction.

Regarding predictive models of treatment outcome, our results showed different features associated with a poor outcome in each group. Firstly, for the group with no addictive-related behavior (i.e., FA− and SU−), a higher persistence (i.e., higher perfectionism and tendency to perseverance and inflexibility) was associated with a poor outcome. Although some studies have reported that a higher persistence is related to more adherence to treatment and less risk of dropout [36], other studies have related a high persistence to the risk of non-remission of the symptomatology, and even relapse, due to the perpetuation of ED-related maladaptive behaviors [37–41]. In this regard, persistence might be linked to the motivational processes of these patients. That is, if they are motivated to initiate treatment, persistence could act as a positive factor related to treatment adherence, despite the considerable effort involved. However, if patients are maladaptively motivated to perpetuate ED-related behaviors, persistence may be associated with a poorer treatment outcome.

Secondly, higher harm avoidance, and an earlier onset of the disorder, were predictors of poor treatment outcomes in patients who reported FA+ or SU+. Overall, a higher harm avoidance has been previously associated with a positive FA score [25], and with other comorbid addictions [42–44]. Some authors have proposed that the link between harm avoidance and outcomes is based on a lack of functional coping strategies, increasing the risk of engaging in dysfunctional patterns in food or drug consumption [45,46]. Therefore, the decrease of harm avoidance through interventions, based on the promotion of adaptive coping strategies in response to distressing events, could be a good therapeutic target to reduce the risk of engaging in addictive patterns as well. The relationship between the age of the onset of ED and a poor treatment outcome is consistent with previous studies postulating that a younger age of onset of ED may increase its severity and even the risk of presenting comorbidities such as SU [47,48]. In addition, it has also been associated with greater difficulties in adapting to the treatment recommendations [49]. Finally, poor treatment outcomes in patients with both addictive-related behaviors were associated with younger age at the time of treatment. This may be related to the postulation that younger people are more prone to impulsivity [50] and, therefore, could be more prone to engage in addictive behaviors [51,52].

Limitations and Strengths

The current study has some limitations that should be considered. First, one has to be cautious in interpreting these results related to lifetime SU, as our results refer to patients with a history of substance misuse having a non-full diagnosis of SU disorder. Second, all participants were recruited from a hospital setting and, therefore, the results may not be representative of the entire population with EDs. Finally, the sample size did not allow for meaningful comparisons between groups to assess the severity of SU, or compare between alcohol and other illicit drug users. In addition, it would be interesting to consider how many different substances the participants had consumed in their lifetime, data that were not available in this study. Further research with larger sample sizes should analyze these shortcomings, as well as analyze whether there are differences between the FA+ and SU− and the FA− and SU+ groups, which were not possible to analyze in this study, due to the low proportion of patients with ED and lifetime SU but without FA ($n = 6$). Despite these limitations, the current study also presents several strengths that should be considered. In terms of treatment outcomes, identifying predictors of each group (FA+ and SU+, FA+ or SU+, and FA− and SU−) would improve our ability to better understand the differences related to these patients' profiles and, thus, provide better treatment options. Further research is needed to investigate this further.

5. Conclusions

In conclusion, it is noteworthy that most patients with EDs suffered from FA and/or lifetime SU, and only the minority did not represent an addictive-related phenotype. Our results did not show significant differences between the three groups in terms of treatment outcomes. However, the effect sizes, when comparing the FA+ and SU+ group with those who did not present any addictive behaviors, suggest higher dropout rates in the former. Additionally, when comparing those patients with poor outcomes, we found that those with at least one addiction-related behavior also present greater symptomatological and psychopathological severity, as well as more dysfunctional personality traits, ratifying the clinical importance of screening for the presence of addictive behavioral patterns in EDs. Furthermore, distinctive predictors were found in each group, highlighting the need to select specific therapeutic strategies to improve the efficacy and adherence to treatments in these patients with different addictive profiles. Further studies are also needed to analyze the possible genetic predisposition to FA and SU in these patients, with special attention to dopamine receptor genes.

Supplementary Materials: The following are available online at https://www.mdpi.com/article/10.3390/nu15132919/s1; Table S1: Descriptive statistics of the sample based on the ED types; Table S2: Distribution of the measures in the study; Table S3: Comparison between groups with a poor outcome; and Table S4: Comparison of the treatment outcomes in the study, stratified by the ED subtype.

Author Contributions: Conceptualization, R.M.-O., Z.A., S.J.-M. and F.F.-A.; methodology, R.M.-O., Z.A. and R.G.; formal analysis, R.G.; investigation, R.M.-O. and Z.A.; data curation, R.M.-O., Z.A. and R.G.; resources, F.F.-A.; writing—original draft preparation, R.M.-O., Z.A. and R.G.; writing—review and editing, R.M.-O., Z.A., R.G., S.J.-M., M.P.-L., M.T.L.-C., A.N.G. and F.F.-A.; supervision, Z.A. and F.F.-A.; funding acquisition, S.J.-M. and F.F.-A. All authors have read and agreed to the published version of the manuscript.

Funding: This manuscript and research were supported by grants from the Delegación del Gobierno para el Plan Nacional sobre Drogas (2021I031), Ministerio de Ciencia e Innovación (PDI2021-124887OB-I00), Instituto de Salud Carlos III (ISCIII) (FIS PI20/00132), and co-funded by FEDER funds/European Regional Development Fund (ERDF), a way to build Europe. Additional funding was received by

AGAUR-Generalitat de Catalunya (2021-SGR-00824). CIBERObn is an initiative of ISCIII. RG is supported by the Catalan Institution for Research and Advanced Studies (ICREA-Academia, 2021-Programme). The funders had no role in the study design, data collection, analysis, decision to publish, or preparation of the manuscript.

Institutional Review Board Statement: The study was conducted according to the guidelines of the Declaration of Helsinki and approved by the Ethics Committee of the University Hospital of Bellvitge (PR205/17).

Informed Consent Statement: Written informed consent was obtained from all participants involved in the study.

Data Availability Statement: Data is not available in any repository. Contact with corresponding authors.

Acknowledgments: We thank CERCA Programme/Generalitat de Catalunya for institutional support. We also thank Ministerio de Ciencia, Innovación y Universidades, Delegación del Gobierno para el Plan Nacional sobre Drogas, Instituto de Salud Carlos III (ISCIII), CIBERobn (an initiative of ISCIII), FEDER funds/European Regional Development Fund (ERDF), a way to build Europe, and European Social Fund (ESF, investing in your future). RG is supported by The Catalan Institution for Research and Advanced Studies (ICREA-2021 Academia Program).

Conflicts of Interest: Fernando Fernández-Aranda and Susana Jiménez-Murcia received consultancy honoraria from Novo Nordisk and Fernando Fernández-Aranda editorial honoraria as EIC from Wiley. The other authors declared no conflicts of interest. The funders had no role in the design of the study; in the collection, analyses, or interpretation of data; in the writing of the manuscript; or in the decision to publish the results.

References

1. Gordon, E.; Ariel-Donges, A.; Bauman, V.; Merlo, L. What Is the Evidence for "Food Addiction?" A Systematic Review. *Nutrients* **2018**, *10*, 477. [CrossRef]
2. Albayrak, Ö.; Wölfle, S.M.; Hebebrand, J. Does Food Addiction Exist? A Phenomenological Discussion Based on the Psychiatric Classification of Substance-Related Disorders and Addiction. *Obes. Facts* **2012**, *5*, 165–179. [CrossRef]
3. Hebebranda, J.; Albayrak, Ö.; Adanb, R.; Antel, J.; Dieguezc, C.; De Jongb, J.; Lenge, G.; Menziese, J.; Mercer, J.G.; Murphy, M.; et al. "Eating Addiction", Rather than "Food Addiction", Better Captures Addictive-like Eating Behavior. *Neurosci. Biobehav. Rev.* **2014**, *47*, 295–306. [CrossRef]
4. Romero, X.; Agüera, Z.; Granero, R.; Sánchez, I.; Riesco, N.; Jiménez-Murcia, S.; Gisbert-Rodriguez, M.; Sánchez-González, J.; Casalé, G.; Baenas, I.; et al. Is Food Addiction a Predictor of Treatment Outcome among Patients with Eating Disorder? *Eur. Eat. Disord. Rev.* **2019**, *27*, 700–711. [CrossRef] [PubMed]
5. Jiménez-Murcia, S.; Agüera, Z.; Paslakis, G.; Munguia, L.; Granero, R.; Sánchez-González, J.; Sánchez, I.; Riesco, N.; Gearhardt, A.N.; Dieguez, C.; et al. Food Addiction in Eating Disorders and Obesity: Analysis of Clusters and Implications for Treatment. *Nutrients* **2019**, *11*, 2633. [CrossRef]
6. Sanchez, I.; Lucas, I.; Munguía, L.; Camacho-Barcia, L.; Giménez, M.; Sánchez-González, J.; Granero, R.; Solé-Morata, N.; Gearhardt, A.N.; Diéguez, C.; et al. Food Addiction in Anorexia Nervosa: Implications for the Understanding of Crossover Diagnosis. *Eur. Eat. Disord. Rev.* **2022**, *30*, 278–288. [CrossRef]
7. Gearhardt, A.N.; Boswell, R.G.; White, M.A. The Association of "Food Addiction" with Disordered Eating and Body Mass Index. *Eat. Behav.* **2014**, *15*, 427–433. [CrossRef] [PubMed]
8. Tran, H.; Poinsot, P.; Guillaume, S.; Delaunay, D.; Bernetiere, M.; Bégin, C.; Fourneret, P.; Peretti, N.; Iceta, S. Food Addiction as a Proxy for Anorexia Nervosa Severity: New Data Based on the Yale Food Addiction Scale 2.0. *Psychiatry Res.* **2020**, *293*, 113472. [CrossRef] [PubMed]
9. Fauconnier, M.; Rousselet, M.; Brunault, P.; Thiabaud, E.; Lambert, S.; Rocher, B.; Challet-Bouju, G.; Grall-Bronnec, M. Food Addiction among Female Patients Seeking Treatment for an Eating Disorder: Prevalence and Associated Factors. *Nutrients* **2020**, *12*, 1897. [CrossRef]
10. Hilker, I.; Sánchez, I.; Steward, T.; Jiménez-Murcia, S.; Granero, R.; Gearhardt, A.N.; Rodríguez-Muñoz, R.C.; Dieguez, C.; Crujeiras, A.B.; Tolosa-Sola, I.; et al. Food Addiction in Bulimia Nervosa: Clinical Correlates and Association with Response to a Brief Psychoeducational Intervention. *Eur. Eat. Disord. Rev.* **2016**, *24*, 482–488. [CrossRef]
11. Bahji, A.; Mazhar, M.N.; Hudson, C.C.; Nadkarni, P.; MacNeil, B.A.; Hawken, E. Prevalence of Substance Use Disorder Comorbidity among Individuals with Eating Disorders: A Systematic Review and Meta-Analysis. *Psychiatry Res.* **2019**, *273*, 58–66. [CrossRef]
12. Dawe, S.; Loxton, N.J. The Role of Impulsivity in the Development of Substance Use and Eating Disorders. *Neurosci. Biobehav. Rev.* **2004**, *28*, 343–351. [CrossRef]

13. Zorrilla, E.P.; Koob, G.F. The Dark Side of Compulsive Eating and Food Addiction: Affective Dysregulation, Negative Reinforcement, and Negative Urgency. In *Compulsive Eating Behavior and Food Addiction: Emerging Pathological Constructs*; Academic Press: Cambridge, MA, USA, 2019; pp. 115–192. [CrossRef]
14. Spindler, A.; Milos, G. Links between Eating Disorder Symptom Severity and Psychiatric Comorbidity. *Eat. Behav.* **2007**, *8*, 364–373. [CrossRef] [PubMed]
15. Calero-Elvira, A.; Krug, I.; Davis, K.; López, C.; Fernández-Aranda, F.; Treasure, J. Meta-Analysis on Drugs in People with Eating Disorders. *Eur. Eat. Disord. Rev.* **2009**, *17*, 243–259. [CrossRef]
16. Michael, M.L.; Juarascio, A. Differences in Eating Disorder Symptoms and Affect Regulation for Residential Eating Disorder Patients with Problematic Substance Use. *Eat. Weight. Disord.* **2020**, *25*, 1805–1811. [CrossRef]
17. Gregorowski, C.; Seedat, S.; Jordaan, G.P. A Clinical Approach to the Assessment and Management of Co-Morbid Eating Disorders and Substance Use Disorders. *BMC Psychiatry* **2013**, *13*, 289. [CrossRef] [PubMed]
18. Keel, P.K.; Dorer, D.J.; Eddy, K.T.; Franko, D.; Charatan, D.L.; Herzog, D.B. Predictors of Mortality in Eating Disorders. *Arch. Gen. Psychiatry* **2003**, *60*, 179–183. [CrossRef]
19. Mellentin, A.I.; Mejldal, A.; Guala, M.M.; Støving, R.K.; Eriksen, L.S.; Stenager, E.; Skøt, L. The Impact of Alcohol and Other Substance Use Disorders on Mortality in Patients with Eating Disorders: A Nationwide Register-Based Retrospective Cohort Study. *Am. J. Psychiatry* **2022**, *179*, 46–57. [CrossRef] [PubMed]
20. Davis, C.; Loxton, N.J. A Psycho-Genetic Study of Hedonic Responsiveness in Relation to "Food Addiction". *Nutrients* **2014**, *6*, 4338–4353. [CrossRef] [PubMed]
21. Mattioni, J.; Vansteene, C.; Poupon, D.; Gorwood, P.; Ramoz, N. Associated and Intermediate Factors between Genetic Variants of the Dopaminergic D2 Receptor Gene and Harmful Alcohol Use in Young Adults. *Addict. Biol.* **2023**, *28*, e13269. [CrossRef] [PubMed]
22. Küçükkasap Cömert, T.; Muşlu, Ö.; Ağagündüz, D. Associations among SNPs in Two Addictive Genes, Food Addiction, and Antioxidant Markers in Recreationally Active Young Women. *Nutr. Hosp.* **2023**, *40*, 332–339. [CrossRef]
23. Miranda-Olivos, R.; Agüera, Z.; Granero, R.; Vergeer, R.R.; Dieguez, C.; Jiménez-Murcia, S.; Gearhardt, A.N.; Fernández-Aranda, F. Food Addiction and Lifetime Alcohol and Illicit Drugs Use in Specific Eating Disorders. *J. Behav. Addict.* **2022**, *11*, 102–115. [CrossRef] [PubMed]
24. First, M.; Williams, J.; Karg, R.; Spitzer, R. *Structured Clinical Interview for DSM-5—Research Version (SCID-5 for DSM-5, Research Version; SCID-5-RV)*; American Psychiatric Association: Arlington, VA, USA, 2015.
25. Granero, R.; Jiménez-Murcia, S.; Gerhardt, A.N.; Agüera, Z.; Aymamí, N.; Gómez-Peña, M.; Lozano-Madrid, M.; Mallorquí-Bagué, N.; Mestre-Bach, G.; Neto-Antao, M.I.; et al. Validation of the Spanish Version of the Yale Food Addiction Scale 2.0 (YFAS 2.0) and Clinical Correlates in a Sample of Eating Disorder, Gambling Disorder, and Healthy Control Participants. *Front. Psychiatry* **2018**, *9*, 208. [CrossRef] [PubMed]
26. Garner, D. *Inventario de Trastornos de La Conducta Alimentaria (EDI-2)*; TEA Ediciones: Madrid, Spain, 1998.
27. Derogatis, L.R. *SCL-90-R. Cuestionario de 90 Síntomas-Manual*; TEA Editorial: Madrid, Spain, 2002.
28. Gutiérrez-Zotes, J.A.; Bayón, C.; Montserrat, C.; Valero, J.; Labad, A.; Cloninger, C.R. Temperament and Character Inventory-Revised (TCI-R). Standardization and Normative Data in a General Population Sample. *Actas Esp. Psiquiatr.* **2004**, *32*, 8–15. [PubMed]
29. Verdejo-García, A.; Lozano, O.; Moya, M.; Alcázar, M.A.; Pérez-García, M. Psychometric Properties of a Spanish Version of the UPPS-P Impulsive Behavior Scale: Reliability, Validity and Association with Trait and Cognitive Impulsivity. *J. Pers. Assess.* **2010**, *92*, 70–77. [CrossRef] [PubMed]
30. Agüera, Z.; Sánchez, I.; Granero, R.; Riesco, N.; Steward, T.; Martín-Romera, V.; Jiménez-Murcia, S.; Romero, X.; Caroleo, M.; Segura-García, C.; et al. Short-Term Treatment Outcomes and Dropout Risk in Men and Women with Eating Disorders. *Eur. Eat. Disord. Rev.* **2017**, *25*, 293–301. [CrossRef]
31. Agüera, Z.; Vintró-Alcaraz, C.; Baenas, I.; Granero, R.; Sánchez, I.; Sánchez-González, J.; Menchón, J.M.; Jiménez-Murcia, S.; Treasure, J.; Fernández-Aranda, F. Lifetime Weight Course as a Phenotypic Marker of Severity and Therapeutic Response in Patients with Eating Disorders. *Nutrients* **2021**, *13*, 2034. [CrossRef]
32. Sauchelli, S.; Jiménez-Murcia, S.; Sánchez, I.; Riesco, N.; Custal, N.; Fernández-García, J.C.; Garrido-Sánchez, L.; Tinahones, F.J.; Steiger, H.; Israel, M.; et al. Orexin and Sleep Quality in Anorexia Nervosa: Clinical Relevance and Influence on Treatment Outcome. *Psychoneuroendocrinology* **2016**, *65*, 102–108. [CrossRef]
33. Lucas, I.; Miranda-Olivos, R.; Testa, G.; Granero, R.; Sánchez, I.; Sánchez-González, J.; Jiménez-Murcia, S.; Fernández-Aranda, F. Neuropsychological Learning Deficits as Predictors of Treatment Outcome in Patients with Eating Disorders. *Nutrients* **2021**, *13*, 2145. [CrossRef]
34. Bonfà, F.; Cabrini, S.; Avanzi, M.; Bettinardi, O.; Spotti, R.; Uber, E. Treatment Dropout in Drug-Addicted Women: Are Eating Disorders Implicated? *Eat. Weight. Disord.* **2008**, *13*, 81–86. [CrossRef]
35. Robinson, L.D.; Kelly, P.J.; Larance, B.K.; Griffiths, S.; Deane, F.P. Eating Disorder Behaviours and Substance Use in Women Attending Treatment for Substance Use Disorders: A Latent Class Analysis. *Int. J. Ment. Health Addict.* **2022**, *20*, 2006–2023. [CrossRef]
36. Dalle Grave, R.; Calugi, S.; Brambilla, F.; Marchesini, G. Personality Dimensions and Treatment Drop-Outs among Eating Disorder Patients Treated with Cognitive Behavior Therapy. *Psychiatry Res.* **2008**, *158*, 381–388. [CrossRef] [PubMed]

37. Waller, G.; Shaw, T.; Meyer, C.; Haslam, M.; Lawson, R.; Serpell, L. Persistence, Perseveration and Perfectionism in the Eating Disorders. *Behav. Cogn. Psychother.* **2012**, *40*, 462–473. [CrossRef] [PubMed]
38. Tchanturia, K.; Davies, H.; Roberts, M.; Harrison, A.; Nakazato, M.; Schmidt, U.; Treasure, J.; Morris, R. Poor Cognitive Flexibility in Eating Disorders: Examining the Evidence Using the Wisconsin Card Sorting Task. *PLoS ONE* **2012**, *7*, e28331. [CrossRef]
39. Rohde, P.; Stice, E.; Gau, J.M. Predicting Persistence of Eating Disorder Compensatory Weight Control Behaviors. *Int. J. Eat. Disord.* **2017**, *50*, 561–568. [CrossRef]
40. Abbate-Daga, G.; Amianto, F.; Rogna, L.; Fassino, S. Do Anorectic Men Share Personality Traits with Opiate Dependent Men? A Case-Control Study. *Addict. Behav.* **2007**, *32*, 170–174. [CrossRef]
41. King, J.A.; Frank, G.K.W.; Thompson, P.M.; Ehrlich, S. Structural Neuroimaging of Anorexia Nervosa: Future Directions in the Quest for Mechanisms Underlying Dynamic Alterations. *Biol. Psychiatry* **2018**, *83*, 224–234. [CrossRef]
42. del Pino-Gutiérrez, A.; Fernández-Aranda, F.; Granero, R.; Tárrega, S.; Valdepérez, A.; Agüera, Z.; Håkansson, A.; Sauvaget, A.; Aymamí, N.; Gómez-Peña, M.; et al. Impact of Alcohol Consumption on Clinical Aspects of Gambling Disorder. *Int. J. Ment. Health Nurs.* **2017**, *26*, 121–128. [CrossRef]
43. Lara-Huallipe, M.L.; Granero, R.; Fernández-Aranda, F.; Gómez-Peña, M.; Moragas, L.; del Pino-Gutierrez, A.; Valenciano-Mendoza, E.; Mora-Maltas, B.; Baenas, I.; Etxandi, M.; et al. Clustering Treatment Outcomes in Women with Gambling Disorder. *J. Gambl. Stud.* **2021**, *38*, 1469–1491. [CrossRef]
44. Seyed Hashemi, S.G.; Merghati Khoei, E.; Hosseinnezhad, S.; Mousavi, M.; Dadashzadeh, S.; Mostafaloo, T.; Mahmoudi, S.; Yousefi, H. Personality Traits and Substance Use Disorders: Comparative Study with Drug User and Non-Drug User Population. *Pers. Individ. Dif.* **2019**, *148*, 50–56. [CrossRef]
45. Francesconi, M.; Flouri, E.; Harrison, A. Change in Decision-Making Skills and Risk for Eating Disorders in Adolescence: A Population-Based Study. *Eur. Psychiatry* **2020**, *63*, e93. [CrossRef]
46. Fernández-Aranda, F.; Jiménez-Murcia, S.; Álvarez-Moya, E.; Granero, R.; Vallejo, J.; Bulik, C.M. Impulse Control Disorders in Eating Disorders: Clinical and Therapeutic Implications. *Compr. Psychiatry* **2006**, *47*, 482–488. [CrossRef]
47. Wiseman, C.V.; Sunday, S.R.; Halligan, P.; Korn, S.; Brown, C.; Halmi, K.A. Substance Dependence and Eating Disorders: Impact of Sequence on Comorbidity. *Compr. Psychiatry* **1999**, *40*, 332–336. [CrossRef]
48. Ho, V.; Arbour, S.; Hambley, J.M. Eating Disorders and Addiction: Comparing Eating Disorder Treatment Outcomes among Clients with and without Comorbid Substance Use Disorder. *J. Addict. Nurs.* **2011**, *22*, 130–137. [CrossRef]
49. Jacobi, C.; Hayward, C.; de Zwaan, M.; Kraemer, H.C.; Agras, W.S. Coming to Terms with Risk Factors for Eating Disorders: Application of Risk Terminology and Suggestions for a General Taxonomy. *Psychol. Bull.* **2004**, *130*, 19–65. [CrossRef]
50. Casey, B.J.; Caudle, K. The Teenage Brain: Self Control. *Curr. Dir. Psychol. Sci.* **2013**, *22*, 82–87. [CrossRef]
51. Tang, K.T.Y.; Kim, H.S.; Hodgins, D.C.; McGrath, D.S.; Tavares, H. Gambling Disorder and Comorbid Behavioral Addictions: Demographic, Clinical, and Personality Correlates. *Psychiatry Res.* **2020**, *284*, 112763. [CrossRef]
52. Hauck, C.; Weiß, A.; Schulte, E.M.; Meule, A.; Ellrott, T. Prevalence of 'Food Addiction" as Measured with the Yale Food Addiction Scale 2.0 in a Representative German Sample and Its Association with Sex, Age and Weight Categories'. *Obes. Facts* **2017**, *10*, 12–24. [CrossRef]

Disclaimer/Publisher's Note: The statements, opinions and data contained in all publications are solely those of the individual author(s) and contributor(s) and not of MDPI and/or the editor(s). MDPI and/or the editor(s) disclaim responsibility for any injury to people or property resulting from any ideas, methods, instructions or products referred to in the content.

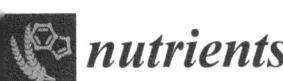

Article

Underlying Mechanisms Involved in Gambling Disorder Severity: A Pathway Analysis Considering Genetic, Psychosocial, and Clinical Variables

Neus Solé-Morata [1,†], Isabel Baenas [1,2,3,†], Mikel Etxandi [1,4], Roser Granero [2,3,5], Manel Gené [6], Carme Barrot [6], Mónica Gómez-Peña [1,3], Laura Moragas [1,3], Nicolas Ramoz [7], Philip Gorwood [7], Fernando Fernández-Aranda [1,2,3,8] and Susana Jiménez-Murcia [1,2,3,8,*]

1. Behavioral Addictions Unit, Department of Psychiatry, Bellvitge University Hospital, Feixa Llarga s/n, 08907 L'Hospitalet de Llobregat, 08907 Barcelona, Spain
2. CIBER Physiopathology of Obesity and Nutrition (CIBERObn), Instituto de Salud Carlos III, 28029 Madrid, Spain
3. Psychoneurobiology of Eating and Addictive Behaviors Group, Neurosciences Programme, Bellvitge Biomedical Research Institute (IDIBELL), 08908 Barcelona, Spain
4. Department of Psychiatry, Hospital Universitari Germans Trias i Pujol, IGTP Campus Can Ruti, 08916 Badalona, Spain
5. Department of Psychobiology and Methodology, Autonomous University of Barcelona, 08193 Barcelona, Spain
6. Genetics Laboratory, Legal Medicine and Toxicology Unit, Public Health Department, Faculty of Medicine, University of Barcelona, 08907 Barcelona, Spain
7. Institute of Psychiatry and Neuroscience of Paris (IPNP), INSERM U1266, Team Vulnerability of Psychiatric and Addictive Disorders, Université de Paris, 75014 Paris, France
8. Department of Clinical Sciences, School of Medicine and Health Sciences, University of Barcelona, 08907 Barcelona, Spain

* Correspondence: sjimenez@bellvitgehospital.cat; Tel.: +34-93-260-79-88; Fax: +34-93-260-76-58
† These authors contributed equally to this work.

Abstract: Gambling Disorder (GD) has a complex etiology that involves biological and environmental aspects. From a genetic perspective, neurotrophic factors (NTFs) polymorphisms have been associated with the risk of developing GD. The aim of this study was to assess the underlying mechanisms implicated in GD severity by considering the direct and mediational relationship between different variables including genetic, psychological, socio-demographic, and clinical factors. To do so, we used genetic variants that were significantly associated with an increased risk for GD and evaluated its relationship with GD severity through pathway analysis. We found that the interaction between these genetic variants and other different biopsychological features predicted a higher severity of GD. On the one hand, the presence of haplotype block 2, interrelated with haplotype block 3, was linked to a more dysfunctional personality profile and a worse psychopathological state, which, in turn, had a direct link with GD severity. On the other hand, having rs3763614 predicted higher general psychopathology and therefore, higher GD severity. The current study described the presence of complex interactions between biopsychosocial variables previously associated with the etiopathogenesis and severity of GD, while also supporting the involvement of genetic variants from the NTF family.

Keywords: gambling disorder; severity; neurotrophic genes; socio-demographics; personality traits; psychopathology

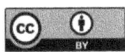

1. Introduction

Gambling is a ubiquitous and generally acceptable activity in our society [1]. Although most people gamble without suffering health issues, some individuals develop gambling disorder (GD) [2]. According to the *Diagnostic and Statistical Manual of Mental Disorders*

(DSM-5), GD is an addictive disorder characterized by recurrent gambling that leads to severe psychological, social, and economic consequences [3]. Moreover, recent changes in availability, promotion, and legislation of gambling activity have resulted in an unprecedented growth of the gambling industry, also accompanied by remarkable increases in the GD prevalence [4,5]. In Europe, GD prevalence is up to 3% while in North America and Asia it increases to 5% and 6%, respectively [6,7]; it is therefore defined as a major public health issue which needs to be properly addressed [8].

Even though GD is a relatively recently recognized mental disorder, several risk factors have already been identified that involve individual or biological variables and environmental factors [9]. For instance, cultural background and gambling availability, as well as socio-demographic characteristics (i.e., being single and having low socioeconomic and educational levels) of the individuals who gamble play an important role in the development of the disorder [1,10]. Similarly, being male [11,12] and young [10,13] have been classically considered individual risk factors for GD. Moreover, compared to women, men present an early GD onset [14,15], although the time between the onset of gambling activity and the development of gambling problems appears to be shorter in women (i.e., telescoping effect) [16,17]. Likewise, both males and younger people have preferences for strategic gambling where the gambler's skills play a role in the result of the gambling activity regardless of chance (e.g., casino, cards, sports betting) [9]. Noticeably, they usually bet higher amounts of money than their counterparts [18], which previous literature has linked to the severity of the disorder [19]. In contrast, women and older individuals are characterized by non-strategic gambling preferences (e.g., bingo, lotteries, slot machines) and higher frequency of comorbid general psychopathology (e.g., anxiety, depressive symptoms) [20]. In fact, a worse psychological state has been associated with the severity of gambling behavior among people with GD [21].

In this line, psychological variables have also been of interest and several studies have found that impulsivity is a nuclear characteristic of addictive-related disorders [22]. Indeed, higher scores on impulsivity measures and related constructs such as personality traits (i.e., sensation seeking) have been described in GD [22] that are, overall, linked to younger age, gambling preferences, and higher GD severity [23–25]. Individuals with high impulsivity are usually younger males with preferences for strategic gambling, whereas characteristic traits for individuals with a personality profile defined by high harm avoidance tend to be female sex, older age, higher emotional vulnerability, and non-strategic gambling preferences [20,26]. Taken together, these findings point to the fact that GD represents a phenotypically heterogeneous disorder [27,28].

From a genetic perspective, several studies have shown that inherited factors account for approximately 50% of the risk for GD [29,30]. Hence, genetic mechanisms underlying GD onset, maintenance, and severity are of particular interest. Before genome-wide association studies (GWAS) were made possible in GD, molecular genetic studies applied candidate gene approaches, mainly reporting an involvement of neurochemical systems, such as the dopaminergic and serotonergic systems [9]. Although GWAS have made considerable progress towards an understanding of many complex diseases [31], the single case–control GWAS study in GD did not identify significant regions associated with the disorder. However, an association between a polygenic risk score for alcoholism and severity of problem gambling was reported, which also supported the idea of a link between different psychiatric disorders, such as addictive-related disorders (e.g., substance use disorders and GD), based on shared biopsychosocial vulnerability features [32,33].

Searching for potential genetic targets, previous studies have associated neurotrophic factors (NTF) with the pathophysiology of neuropsychiatric disorders [34,35]. Precisely, a recent study by our group [36] analyzed the involvement of NTF genetic variants in the vulnerability of developing GD. As interesting results, some genetic polymorphisms related to neurotrophin 3 (NTF3) and the BDNF's tyrosine kinase receptor type 2 (NTRK2) genes were significantly related to a higher risk for GD.

The dysfunctions found in these genetic variants may have endocrine implications since the expression of the corresponding endogenous ligands would be altered and would therefore imply changes in normal brain signaling cross-talk. Specifically, NTF3 develops neurogenetic and neuroprotective functions in dopaminergic and noradrenergic neurons [37] that are involved in addiction and rewards pathways [38,39]. Meanwhile, NTRK2 binds the brain neurotrophic factor (BDNF), which has been the most studied NTF among addictive-related disorders to date [34,40,41]. In GD, an increase in its circulating concentrations has been described, as well as an association between BDNF concentrations and GD severity [42–45]. At the same time, NTRK2 seems to be binding not only BDNF but also NTF3 [46]. These findings support the involvement of the NTF family in the pathophysiology of GD at both genetic and endocrine levels.

Going one step further, clinical implications of these findings should be highlighted since genetic and endocrine dysfunctions in the complex NTF3 and its receptor (i.e., NTRK3), as well as in NTRK2 and their targets (i.e., BDNF and NTF3), have also been reported in affective disorders, attention deficit/hyperactivity disorder (ADHD), and eating disorders (EDs), among others [47–50], which are not infrequently comorbid conditions with GD [9,51]. With regard to the NTF family, these findings reinforced the idea of common vulnerability factors among different psychiatric disorders, which may be underlying transdiagnostic features, such as impulsivity [52,53].

At this stage, there has been a broad consensus that GD is a complex and heterogeneous disorder, and several phenotypic profiles of vulnerability have been identified, which also influence its severity [28,54]. Furthermore, it has also been proposed that GD probably relates to small genetic contributions in affected individuals' interaction with other biopsychosocial variables [9]. While the identification of risk factors associated with the disorder has been crucial so far, a more comprehensive approach to the multifactorial interplay (i.e., genotypic, and phenotypic factors) that underlies not only the development but also the severity of GD would be truly valuable for clinical application.

Characterizing GD severity phenotypes and endophenotypes could also allow clinicians to design more personalized preventive and therapeutic interventions aimed at modifying the course of the disorder since early clinical stages, with a special focus on those people with more vulnerable characteristics. Furthermore, since research based on the biological basis of GD is underexplored and no pharmacological treatment is officially approved in GD to date, a growing body of knowledge related to biological mechanisms involved in GD could help to elucidate new biological therapeutic targets, such as those related to the NTF family.

Regrettably, the complex relationship between genotypic and phenotypic features (e.g., genetic, psychological, clinical, and socio-demographic factors, etc.) means that the association between genotypes and phenotypes is not straightforward. To the best of our knowledge, this is the first clinical study that examined potential interactions between genotype and phenotype in GD with the aim of delineating profiles of vulnerability, which could also predict GD severity. Regarding genetics, NTF genetic variants significantly associated with an increased risk for GD were used [36]. Other biopsychosocial variables were also assessed, namely socio-demographic features (i.e., sex, chronological age, civil and employment status, educational level), personality profile, general psychopathology, and some characteristics of the gambling behavior (i.e., age of GD onset, GD duration, gambling preferences, gambling activity, debts, bets). For that purpose, whereas classical approaches only allow researchers to test for genotype-phenotype associations, structural equation models (SEM) are a powerful tool to model complex interactions between risk factors and consider the direct and indirect (mediational) links between a broad set of biopsychosocial variables.

Bearing all this in mind, we hypothesized the existence of interactions between genetic polymorphisms and GD severity. Therefore, the presence of certain genetic variants would not only predict the presence of the disorder [36] but also its severity. However, considering that GD is a complex multifactorial entity, we also envisaged a mediational role of other biopsychosocial factors in this interaction between genetics and GD severity.

2. Materials and Methods

2.1. Participants and Procedure

The sample was composed of 146 adult outpatients with GD linked to the Behavioral Addictions Unit in the Department of Psychiatry at the Bellvitge University Hospital (Catalonia, Spain). All patients in this study fulfilled the DSM-5 criteria for GD [3]. The recruitment took place between January 2005 and June 2006 [36]. They were evaluated at the Behavioral Addictions Unit in the Department of Psychiatry at the Bellvitge University Hospital (Catalonia, Spain). The assessment consisted of two pre-treatment sessions. In the first session, a semi-structured clinical interview [55] was conducted by experienced psychologists and psychiatrists with a large clinical and research trajectory in the field of behavioral addiction such as GD. In the second session, psychometric assessments and biological samples to analysis genetic variables were obtained. We received completed clinical assessments and biological samples analysis from all the participants included in this study.

2.2. Clinical Measurements

Diagnostic Questionnaire for Pathological Gambling According to DSM criteria [56]; Spanish validation [15]. This is a self-report questionnaire with 19 items, coded in a binary scale (yes–no), which is used for the GD diagnosis regarding DSM-IV-TR [57] and DSM-5 [3] criteria. In our sample, the internal consistency was adequate (Cronbach's alpha $\alpha = 0.81$).

South Oaks Gambling Screen (SOGS) [58]; Spanish validation [59]. This questionnaire assesses cognitive, emotional, and behavioral aspects related to problem gambling by measuring the severity of gambling activity (responses ranging from 0 to 20). With 20 items, it allows for the differentiation between non-problem gambling (from 0 to 2), light problem gambling (from 3 to 4), and problem gambling (from 5 to 20, with higher scores being indicative of higher gambling severity). In our study, the internal consistency was adequate ($\alpha = 0.79$).

Symptom Checklist-90 Items Revised (SCL-90-R) [60]; Spanish validation [61]. This is a self-report questionnaire with 90 items that explores psychological distress and psychopathology using 9 symptomatic dimensions: somatization, obsession-compulsion, interpersonal sensitivity, depression, anxiety, anger-hostility, phobic anxiety, paranoid ideation, and psychoticism. It also includes three global indices: Global Severity Index (GSI), Positive Symptom Total (PST), and Positive Symptom Distress Index (PSDI). In our sample, the internal consistency was excellent ($\alpha = 0.98$).

Temperament and Character Inventory-Revised (TCI-R) [62]; Spanish validation [63]. Personality traits are evaluated according to seven personality factors that are divided into four factors for temperament (sensation seeking, harm avoidance, reward dependence and persistence) and three for character (self-directedness, cooperation, and self-transcendence). This questionnaire consists of 240 items. The internal consistency in our study ranged between $\alpha = 0.71$ (novelty seeking) and $\alpha = 0.85$ (persistence).

2.3. Other Variables

Additional socio-demographic (i.e., sex, chronological age, civil status, educational level, and employment status) and clinical variables related to gambling (i.e., age of GD onset and GD duration, type of gambling which motivated seeking-treatment, and type of gambling modality regarding the preference for strategic gambling, non-strategic or mixed, the presence of debts, and maximum bets) were measured within the first pre-treatment evaluation session [64].

2.4. Genetic Information

Since this study is a continuation of a previous work by our group, genetic data analyzed in the present study came from the analysis performed by [36]. Briefly, single nucleotide polymorphisms (SNPs) of several NTF genes (nerve growth factor (NGF) gene and its receptor (NGFR), neurotrophic tyrosine kinase receptor type 1 (NTRK1), type 2 (NTRK2) and type 3 (NTRK3), BDNF and neurotrophins 3 and 4/5 (NTF3, NTF4), ciliary neurotrophic factor (CNTF), and its receptor (CNTFR) were selected and genotyped as previously described by Mercader, Saus et al. [50]. Overall, 183 SNPs were genotyped using the SNPlex Genotyping System (Applied Biosystems, Foster City, CA, USA) at the genotyping facilities of CeGen in the Barcelona Node (Centro Nacional de Genotipado, Genoma España). Of the whole available sample, genotyped SNPs which had a call rate lower than 80%, were outside the Hardy–Weinberg equilibrium (HWE), or were monomorphic, were not considered for further analyses ($n = 25$).

2.5. Statistical Analyses

Statistical analysis was conducted using Stata17 for Windows. The underlying mechanisms between the variables of the study were assessed using path analysis, a straightforward extension of multiple regressions used for modeling a set of hypothesized associations into a group of variables, including direct and indirect effects (mediational links) [65]. Path analysis is currently employed for both exploratory and confirmatory modeling, and therefore it allows theory testing and theory development [66]. In this work, path analysis was implemented through structural equation modeling (SEM), all parameters were free-estimated, and the maximum-likelihood method of parameter estimation was used. Because of the existence of multiple dimensions for the personality profile, a latent variable was defined by the observed indicators measured with the TCI-R scores, which allowed the data structure to be simplified and facilitated a more parsimonious fitting [67]. Additionally, with the aim to obtain a final parsimonious model and increase statistical power, an initial model that included all the potential associations between the variables was defined. Next, parameters without significant tests were deleted, and the model was respecified and readjusted. Adequate goodness-of-fit was evaluated for nonsignificant results in the chi-square test (χ^2), root mean square error of approximation RMSEA < 0.08, Bentler's Comparative Fit Index CFI > 0.90, Tucker–Lewis Index TLI > 0.90, and standardized root mean square residual SRMR < 0.10 [68].

3. Results

3.1. Description of the Participants and Distribution of the Genetic Measures

Table 1 summarizes the distribution of socio-demographic and clinical variables in the study. Most participants were men ($n = 134$, 91.8%), married ($n = 83$, 56.8%) or single ($n = 46$, 31.5%), with low education levels (primary, $n = 104$, 71.2%), and employed ($n = 100$, 68.5%). Mean age was 40.2 years (SD = 12.5), mean age of GD onset was 34.2 years (SD = 11.9), and mean duration of the gambling problems was 13.7 years (SD = 8.6). The gambling preference with the highest prevalence was non-strategic ($n = 125$, 85.6%), followed by mixed gambling (non-strategic and strategic, $n = 16$, 11.0%). Slot machines were the games with the highest prevalence ($n = 131$, 89.7%), followed by bingo ($n = 32$, 21.9%), casino ($n = 15$, 10.3%), lotteries ($n = 13$, 8.9%), and cards ($n = 10$, 6.8%).

Table 2 summarizes the distribution of the genetic variables in the study, all of which were identified in the study by Solé-Morata et al. [36]. We included four single SNPs significantly related to GD according to different genetic models: (a) rs796189, the presence of genotype "AG/GG" (dominant model) and "AG" (overdominant model); (b) rs3763614, the presence of genotype "CC" (codominant and dominant models) and genotype "CC/TT" (overdominant model); (c) rs11140783, the presence of genotype "CC" (codominant model); and, (d) rs3739570 the presence of genotype "CC" (dominant model) and "CC/TT" (overdominant model).

Table 1. Descriptive for the sample (*n* = 146).

Socio-Demographics		n	%
Sex	Women	12	8.2%
	Men	134	91.8%
Civil status	Single	46	31.5%
	Married—couple	83	56.8%
	Divorced—separated	17	11.6%
Education level	Primary	104	71.2%
	Secondary	36	24.7%
	University	6	4.1%
Employment status	Unemployed	46	31.5%
	Employed	100	68.5%
Age-onset-duration		Mean	SD
Chronological age (years-old)		40.2	12.52
Onset of gambling problems		34.24	11.89
Duration of gambling problems		13.72	8.60
Gambling activity (reason treatment)		n	%
Slot-machines		131	89.7%
Bingo		32	21.9%
Lotteries		13	8.9%
Casino		15	10.3%
Cards		10	6.8%
Preference (reason treatment)		n	%
Only non-strategic		125	85.6%
Only strategic		5	3.4%
Both (non-strategic and strategic)		16	11.0%
Bets		Median	IQR
Maximum euros per episode		400	300
Debts due to gambling activity		n	%
Yes		100	71.9%
No		46	28.1%

Note. SD: standard deviation. IQR: interquartile range. * Defined as the risk condition for the sample.

Table 2. Distribution of the genetic variables in the study (*n* = 146).

		n	%			n	%
Block 1 (SNPs: rs6489630, rs7956189)				SNP: rs7956189	AA		
Haplotype	A	85	58.2%		AA	98	67.1%
	TA	13	8.9%		AG *	45	30.8%
	TG *	48	32.9%		GG *	3	2.1%
Block 2 (SNPs: rs4412435, rs10868241, rs4361832)				SNP: rs3739570	CC *		
Haplotype	CAA	2	1.4%		CC *	130	89.0%
	CAG	4	2.7%		CT	15	10.3%
	CGG	9	6.2%		TT	1	0.7%
	TGG *	131	89.7%	SNP: rs3763614	CC *		
Block 3 (SNPs: rs11140783, rs3739570)					CC *	137	93.8%
Haplotype	CC *	119	81.5%		CT	9	6.2%
	CT	14	9.6%	SNP: rs11140783	CC *		
	TC	13	8.9%		CC *	133	91.1%
					CT	13	8.9%

Note. SNP: single nucleotide polymorphism. * Defined as the risk condition for the sample.

We also analyzed three haplotypes significantly related to GD. Haplotype block 1 included SNPs rs6489630 and rs7956189 in the NTF3 gene, and haplotype "TG" was significantly related to an increase in the risk of GD (p = 0.045); haplotype block 2 included the SNPs rs4412435, rs10868241, and rs4361832 in the NTRK2 gene, and haplotype CAG (p = 0.048) was related to a decreased risk of GD. Finally, haplotype block 3, defined by the SNPs rs11140783 and rs3739570 among the NTRK2 gene, showed a significant association of haplotype CC with an increased risk of GD (p = 0.012) [36].

3.2. Path Analysis

Table 3 shows the association between the genetic variables. Because of the strong association between haplotype 1 with rs7956189 (Cramer-V = 1.00) and haplotype 3 with rs3739570 (Cramer-V = 0.737), both SNPs were excluded from the path analysis.

Table 3. Association of the genetic variables in the study (n = 146).

Cramer-V Values		2	3	4	5	6	7
1	Haplotype-1	−0.003	−0.042	1.000	−0.035	−0.124	−0.088
2	Haplotype-2	—	0.187	−0.003	0.315	−0.087	−0.106
3	Haplotype-3		—	−0.042	0.737	−0.122	0.656
4	rs7956189			—	−0.035	−0.124	−0.088
5	rs3739570				—	−0.090	0.044
6	rs3763614					—	−0.080
7	rs11140783						—

Note. SNP: single nucleotide polymorphism. Haplotype 1: SNPs: rs6489630, rs7956189. Haplotype 2: SNPs: rs4412435, rs10868241, rs4361832. Haplotype 3: SNPs: rs11140783, rs3739570.

Figure 1 includes the path diagram with the standardized coefficients for the final model. Adequate goodness-of-fit was achieved: χ^2 = 95.99 (p = 0.239), RMSEA = 0.027 (95% confidence interval: 0.001 to 0.054), CFI = 0.970, TLI = 0.963 and SRMR = 0.059. The global predictive capacity valued with the coefficient of determination was CD = 0.490.

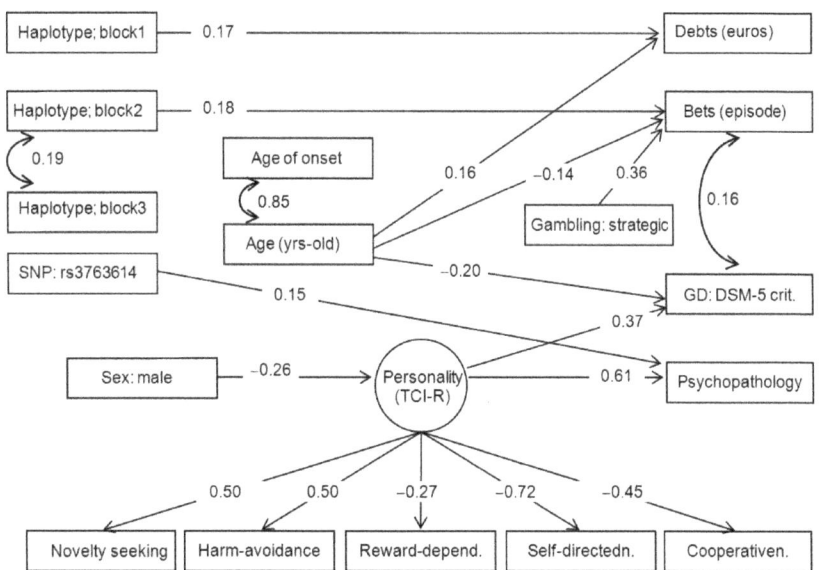

Figure 1. Path diagram: standardized coefficients (n = 146). Note: Only significant parameter estimates were retained in the final model. SNP: single nucleotide polymorphism. GD: Gambling Disorder.

The risk group for haplotype block 1 predicted higher debts due to gambling behavior, the group carrying the non-protective allele for haplotype block 2 predicted higher bets in the gambling episodes, and the risk group for SNP rs3763614 predicted worse psychopathological state. Within the SEM, no direct effect was observed for haplotype block 3 (this predictor only significantly correlated with haplotype 2), and SNP rs11140783 was excluded since there were no significant associations within the structural paths. No mediational links appeared between the genetic variables with socio-demographics (sex and age), personality and gambling-related measures.

The latent variable with the personality profile retained five TCI-R scales with significant coefficients (persistence and self-transcendence were excluded because of estimates with $p > 0.05$). Based on the coefficient's values, higher scores in the latent variable are characterized by higher scores in novelty seeking and harm avoidance, and lower scores in reward-dependence, self-directedness, and cooperativeness. In addition, higher scores in this latent measure were associated with a worse psychopathological state, and it was also a mediational link in the relationships between sex and psychopathology.

The remaining significant associations in the diagram indicated that younger age was a predictor of higher bets per gambling episode and higher GD severity levels, while older age predicted higher debts. Finally, strategic gambling was associated with higher bets.

Figure 2 includes the results of the path diagram of an additional SEM, which allows assessing specific associations between the genetic variables with each personality dimension (the TCI-R variables retained in the model because of significant structural coefficients were novelty seeking, harm avoidance, and cooperativeness). Adequate goodness of fit was achieved: $\chi2 = 76.16$ ($p = 0.123$), RMSEA = 0.038 (95% confidence interval: 0.001 to 0.066), CFI = 0.907, TLI = 0.901, and SRMR = 0.062. The global predictive capacity was CD = 0.372. This new model showed a mediational link between genetic variables with personality and psychopathology: carrying the non-protective variant of haplotype 2 was related to a lower level in the cooperativeness factor, and lower values in this personality dimension were a predictor of greater psychopathological problems.

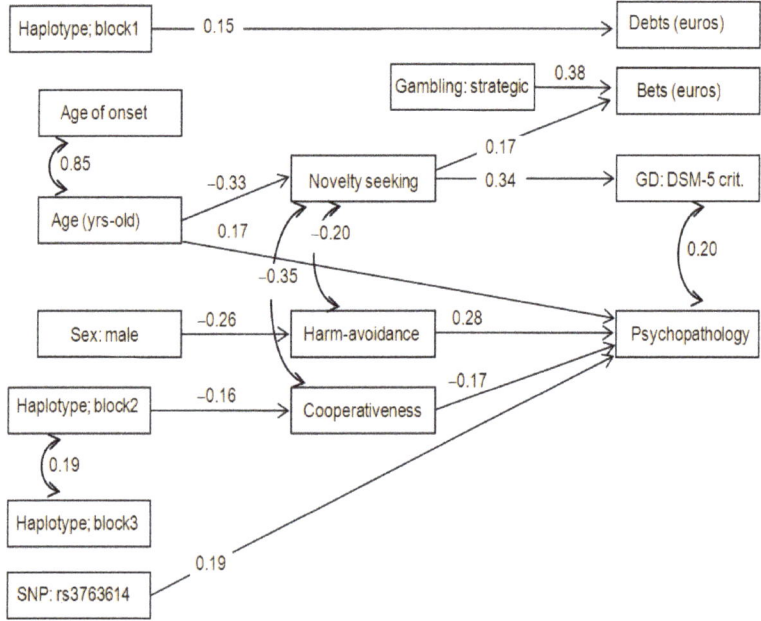

Figure 2. Path diagram: standardized coefficients ($n = 146$). Note: Only significant parameter estimates were retained in the final model. SNP: single nucleotide polymorphism. GD: Gambling Disorder.

4. Discussion

Most of the evidence accumulated suggests that the development and maintenance of GD is associated with multiple biopsychosocial variables (e.g., genetics, psychological features, socio-demographics, etc.) [18]. Apart from being identified as vulnerability factors, elucidating the relationship between these genotypic and phenotypic features could allow to define vulnerability profiles of GD [28,54]. Despite its potential clinical and therapeutic implications, analyses based on the interaction between genotypic and phenotypic factors in GD are lacking since there are difficulties in defining the associations between variables under an integrative theoretical model as well as considering the complexity of the interplay by the measurement of direct and mediational links between them.

Therefore, we aimed to assess whether NTF genetic variants previously associated with the development of GD [36] were also associated with GD severity in terms of their interaction with other different biopsychosocial variables. As we hypothesized, through SEM analysis, we found that the presence of these genetic variants predicted a higher GD severity, highlighting the mediational role of socio-demographic (e.g., sex, age), psychological (e.g., personality, and general psychopathology), and clinical variables related to gambling activity (e.g., age of GD onset).

Overall, the socio-demographic and clinical characteristics of the patients agreed with those described in previous studies by our group [28,69]. The diagrams showed a strong correlation between the chronological age and the age of GD onset. Compared to individuals with a later age of onset, those who started gambling earlier in adolescence had more severe gambling problems (e.g., higher bets) [70]. In this line, younger age as well as an early age of GD onset have been bidirectionally linked to higher novelty seeking, which appears as a mediational factor in the pathogenesis and severity of GD [13,20]. Moreover, this profile (i.e., younger individuals with an earlier age of onset and higher novelty seeking) has been associated with lower levels of harm avoidance and cooperativeness, as we shown when we individually analyzed personality dimensions [20]. Notably, this trend is probably being accentuated by the advent of new technologies and changes in gambling availability [71]. On the other hand, a worse psychopathological state was related to older individuals with GD, which also predicted higher GD severity. Previous studies have reported higher general psychopathology and higher frequency of psychiatric comorbidities among older individuals with GD, previous to the development of this disorder [20,21]. Likewise, greater physical and psychological symptoms have also been described because of GD, possibly contributing to amplifying this maladaptive behavior [72]. According to our results, the multifactorial networks that mediate GD severity could be associated with the patients' age. That is, higher GD severity was positively related to higher novelty seeking scores in younger patients, who were also characterized by early age of GD onset and higher bets. In contrast, a worse psychopathological state predicted GD severity among older individuals with GD, who tended to develop GD later in life but to take on more debt [21]. All these aspects support the heterogeneity of the disorder and the existence of subtypes based on different phenotypes and endophenotypes of GD patients [54,73,74].

Analyzing the contribution of sex on the underlying mechanisms of GD severity, a recent study showed that the complex links mediating GD severity were strongly related to sex [75]. Thus, while higher GD severity was directly related to a higher cognitive bias and a younger age of GD onset in men, GD severity was directly increased by younger age of onset, higher cognitive bias, and lower self-directedness among women. In this subgroup, lower socio-economic positions and higher levels in harm avoidance had an indirect effect on GD severity, mediated by the distortions related to the gambling activity. Going one step further, women generally seek treatment when they are older, and they commonly show higher levels of associated psychopathology, especially depression and anxiety, in comparison with men [76,77]. Along this line, although we failed to find a significant association between age and sex, our SEM showed that being female was positively associated with higher GD severity, and that this relationship appears to be mediated by a latent personality variant. Higher scores in this latent variant were translated into higher harm avoidance and lower self-directedness, among other personality measured dimensions. Furthermore, this latent variant predicted a worse psychopathological state. Considering both SEM analyses, we hypothesize that being a woman with higher levels of harm avoidance and a worse psychopathological state, despite lower scores in novelty seeking, would predict higher GD severity. Although our findings could partially be supported by the results of other studies, gender-specific studies focused on GD are scarce, and women with GD have been understudied. Therefore, further work is needed to better understand the differences between both sexes regarding GD severity and its biological correlates.

Regarding the psychological profile of patients with GD, the final SEM exhibited an already cited latent personality variable that directly predicted higher GD severity. Although our latent variable did not allow us to individually estimate the association of each personality dimension with the severity of GD, the whole picture was in agreement with previous research [21,78]. Regardless of the differences that may exist by sex or age, individuals with GD have been characterized as highly impulsive and usually show high scores in novelty seeking and harm avoidance [79–81]. In addition, a previous study by our group reported that novelty seeking and harm avoidance were positively and directly associated with GD severity, and also that sensitivity to reward and to punishment were meditational factors between these personality traits and GD severity [82]. In the case of general psychopathology, a worse psychopathological state has been reported among individuals with GD in comparison with the general population [83]. Interestingly, psychological distress has been considered a trigger for developing GD as a maladaptive strategy to regulate negative emotions [84]. Thus, the mediational role of these clinical features between biological variables and GD severity further emphasizes the complex and multifactorial etiology of GD [54,73,74].

While the results derived from the analysis of variables other than genetic traits are in line with the existing literature, one of the strengths of this work lies in its analysis of the associations between genetic risk variants for GD and the severity of the disorder. Regarding haplotype block 1, the risk group predicted higher debts due to gambling behavior in both SEM analysis. Although our study failed to find significant associations between debts that were caused by gambling activity and GD severity, other studies have reported a positive link [19].

Within the haplotype block 2, both SEM analyses suggested that the group carrying the non-protective allele "CAG" is indirectly and positively associated with higher GD severity. One the one hand, carrying the non-protective allele predicted higher bets in the gambling episodes, which was, in turn, correlated with higher severity of GD. In addition, younger age and strategic gambling were also related to higher bets per episode of gambling, emphasizing the existence of complex interrelations between the different variables. On the other hand, the non-protective allele was linked to lower cooperativeness, which predicted higher general psychopathology. These clinical interactions were in line with the results of previous studies. For example, a recent study based on cluster analysis showed that the group of patients with higher gambling severity was characterized by higher bets, younger age, early GD onset, a more dysfunctional personality profile, and greater psychopathological distress [19]. Although no direct links were observed for the risk group in haplotype block 3, it was significantly correlated with haplotype block 2, which are both found in the BDNF receptor's gene (NTRK2). As they are known to be involved in some addictive-related disorders such as EDs [85,86], it is not surprising that genetic variants on this gene would be associated with GD severity. To summarize, the presence of haplotype block 2, interrelated with haplotype block 3, was associated with a more dysfunctional personality profile and a worse psychopathological state, which, in turn, had a direct link with GD severity.

Finally, the presence of a particular CNTFR variant (rs3763614) was indirectly linked to GD severity through higher general psychopathology. At a molecular level, CNTF (i.e., CTNFR ligand) was shown to have an important effect on appetite and energy expenditure [87,88]. Thus, in line with previous studies, our findings suggest the existence of a common genetic pathway that could validate the NTF hypothesis role in some disorders related to impulsivity, such as EDs and GD [50].

Even though our study adds value to explorations of the interactions between already described phenotypic variables and genotypic features, genetic associations should be considered cautiously. Thus, the present work has an exploratory nature, and a causal relationship should not be established between these genetic markers and GD severity. Since the multifactorial pathogenesis of GD is complex, further functional analysis that includes larger samples, a wide range of genetic variants, and epigenetic influences, are needed to understand their biological impact on GD severity. However, the identification of genetic variants associated with the severity of a disorder, especially in the era of genomics, could be interesting from a clinical perspective to improve treatment approaches based on personalized medicine.

A deeper knowledge about the complex pathophysiology of GD, as well as a better understanding of the biological factors underlying core clinical features in GD (e.g., genetics) and their modulatory interaction with other biopsychosocial variables could facilitate the identification of GD profiles with distinctive clinical implications in terms of, for example, the severity of the disorder. As a result, more individualized preventive and therapeutic strategies could be developed, which should be applied beginning in early clinical stages with the intent of ameliorating a more deleterious clinical course, overall, in patients with a more severe profile. Along this line, research based on biological therapeutic targets in GD is still preliminary and scarce, and no pyschopharmalogical drugs are officially approved for the treatment of GD [9,21]. Therefore, those studies that shed light on potential biological targets associated with the disorder would be opening the door to research into their treatment implications. According to previous literature, sharing risk factors between some disorders (e.g., addictive and impulsive related disorders) would not be uncommon [89,90]. This fact could also favor new avenues of treatment, such as through testing pyschopharmalogical drugs that are used in other disorders other than GD (e.g., substance use disorders), as these biological therapeutic targets may underlie transdiagnostic phenotypic features (e.g., impulsivity) [52,53].

5. Conclusions

The present study described an interesting vulnerability model based on potential interactions between genotypic (i.e., NTFs genes) and phenotypic features (i.e., sociodemographic, psychosocial, and clinical factors) through SEM analysis. These results provide a deeper insight into the biopsychosocial mechanisms underlying GD severity. According to the idea that GD is a complex multifactorial disorder, the presence of nonprotective NTF genetic variants predicted a higher GD severity, with a mediational role of variables such as age, sex, personality traits, general psychopathology, and clinical features related to gambling behavior. Bearing the phenotypic heterogeneity of the disorder in mind, this work also sheds new light regarding the existence of vulnerability profiles whose identification would have potential applications in terms of diagnostic, preventive, and therapeutic approaches. However, future research based on longitudinal designs, with larger sample sizes and further functional analysis that includes not only the assessment of other NTF genetic variants but also other genetic targets, or the assessments of a wide range of biopsychosocial variables, are needed to consolidate these preliminary and exploratory results.

Author Contributions: Conceptualization, N.S.-M., I.B., F.F.-A. and S.J.-M.; methodology, R.G. and N.R.; formal analysis, R.G. and N.R.; investigation, N.S.-M. and I.B.; data curation, N.S.-M. and I.B.; writing—original draft preparation, N.S.-M. and I.B.; writing—review and editing, M.E., R.G., M.G., C.B., M.G.-P., L.M., N.R., P.G., F.F.-A. and S.J.-M.; supervision, F.F.-A. and S.J.-M.; funding acquisition, F.F.-A. and S.J.-M. All authors have read and agreed to the published version of the manuscript.

Funding: The present project has been founded by CERCA Programme/Generalitat de Catalunya guaranteed institutional support. The work was also supported by grants from the Delegación del Gobierno para el Plan Nacional sobre Drogas (2019I47 and 2021I031), Ministerio de Ciencia e Innovación (PDI2021-124887OB-I00), and Instituto de Salud Carlos III (ISCIII) (PI20/00132), and co-funded by FEDER funds/European Regional Development Fund (ERDF), a way to build Europe. Additional support was received from EU Grant Eat2beNice (H2020-SFS-2016-2; Ref. 728018). CIBER-Obn is an initiative of ISCIII. IB was partially supported by a Post-Residency Grant from the Research Committee of the University Hospital (2020–2021). This study has also been funded by Instituto de Salud Carlos III through the grant CM21/00172 (IB) (Co-funded by European Social Fund. ESF investing in your future). RG is supported by the Catalan Institution for Research and Advanced Studies (ICREA-Academia, 2021-Programme).

Institutional Review Board Statement: The study procedures were carried out in accordance with the Declaration of Helsinki. The Ethics Committee of Clinical Research of the University of Barcelona and Bellvitge University Hospital (Catalonia, Spain) approved the study (reference: 307/06). All the participants provided voluntary-signed informed consent. They received no financial remuneration.

Informed Consent Statement: Informed consent was obtained from all subjects involved in the study.

Data Availability Statement: Individuals may inquire with the corresponding authors regarding availability of the data as there are ongoing studies using the data and to preserve patient confidentiality. Authors will consider requests on a case-by-case basis.

Acknowledgments: We thank CERCA Programme/Generalitat de Catalunya guaranteed institutional support. We also thank the Ministerio de Ciencia, Innovación y Universidades and the Delegación del Gobierno para el Plan Nacional sobre Drogas, Instituto de Salud Carlos III (ISCIII), CIBERobn (an initiative of ISCIII), FEDER funds/European Regional Development Fund (ERDF), a way to build Europe, and European Social Fund-ESF investing in your future. This study has also been funded by Instituto de Salud Carlos III through the grant CM21/00172 (IB) (Co-funded by European Social Fund. ESF investing in your future). RG is supported by The Catalan Institution for Research and Advanced Studies (ICREA-2021 Academia Program).

Conflicts of Interest: Fernando Fernández-Aranda and Susana Jiménez-Murcia received consultancy honoraria from Novo Nordisk, and Fernando Fernández-Aranda editorial honoraria as EIC from Wiley. The rest of the authors declare no conflict of interest. The rest of the authors declare no conflict of interest.

References

1. Ji, L.J.; McGeorge, K.; Li, Y.; Lee, A.; Zhang, Z. Culture and gambling fallacies. *Springerplus* **2015**, *4*, 510. [CrossRef]
2. Potenza, M.N.; Kosten, T.R.; Rounsaville, B.J. Pathological Gambling. *JAMA* **2001**, *286*, 141. [CrossRef] [PubMed]
3. American Psychiatric Association. *Diagnostic and Statistical Manual of Mental Disorders*, 5th ed.; American Psychiatric Association: Washington, DC, USA, 2013.
4. Abbott, M.W.; Romild, U.; Volberg, R.A. Gambling and Problem Gambling in Sweden: Changes between 1998 and 2009. *J. Gambl. Stud.* **2014**, *30*, 985–999. [CrossRef]
5. Abbott, M.; Romild, U.; Volberg, R. The prevalence, incidence, and gender and age-specific incidence of problem gambling: Results of the Swedish longitudinal gambling study (Swelogs). *Addiction* **2018**, *113*, 699–707. [CrossRef]
6. Calado, F.; Alexandre, J.; Griffiths, M.D. Prevalence of Adolescent Problem Gambling: A Systematic Review of Recent Research. *J. Gambl. Stud.* **2017**, *33*, 397–424. [CrossRef] [PubMed]
7. Calado, F.; Griffiths, M.D. Problem gambling worldwide: An update and systematic review of empirical research (2000–2015). *J. Behav. Addict.* **2016**, *5*, 592–613. [CrossRef]
8. Thomas, S.L.; Thomas, S.D. The big gamble: The need for a comprehensive research approach to understanding the causes and consequences of gambling harm in Australia. *Australas. Epidemiol.* **2015**, *22*, 39–42.
9. Potenza, M.N.; Balodis, I.M.; Deverensky, J.; Grant, J.E.; Petry, N.M.; Verdejo-Garcia, A.; Yip, S.W. Gambling disorder. *Nat. Rev. Dis. Prim.* **2019**, *5*, 51. [CrossRef]
10. Castrén, S.; Basnet, S.; Salonen, A.H.; Pankakoski, M.; Ronkainen, J.E.; Alho, H.; Lahti, T. Factors associated with disordered gambling in Finland. *Subst. Abus. Treat. Prev. Policy* **2013**, *8*, 24. [CrossRef]
11. Hing, N.; Russell, A.M.T.T.; Vitartas, P.; Lamont, M. Demographic, behavioural and normative risk factors for gambling problems amongst sports bettors. *J. Gambl. Stud.* **2016**, *32*, 625–641. [CrossRef]
12. Yücel, M.; Whittle, S.; Youssef, G.J.; Kashyap, H.; Simmons, J.G.; Schwartz, O.; Lubman, D.I.; Allen, N.B. The influence of sex, temperament, risk-taking and mental health on the emergence of gambling: A longitudinal study of young people. *Int. Gambl. Stud.* **2015**, *15*, 108–123. [CrossRef]

13. Jiménez-Murcia, S.; Granero, R.; Tárrega, S.; Angulo, A.; Fernández-Aranda, F.; Arcelus, J.; Fagundo, A.B.; Aymamí, N.; Moragas, L.; Sauvaget, A.; et al. Mediational Role of Age of Onset in Gambling Disorder, a Path Modeling Analysis. *J. Gambl. Stud.* **2016**, *32*, 327–340. [CrossRef] [PubMed]
14. Granero, R.; Penelo, E.; Martínez-Giménez, R.; Álvarez-Moya, E.; Gómez-Peña, M.; Aymamí, M.N.; Bueno, B.; Fernández-Aranda, F.; Jiménez-Murcia, S. Sex differences among treatment-seeking adult pathologic gamblers. *Compr. Psychiatry* **2009**, *50*, 173–180. [CrossRef]
15. Jiménez-Murcia, S.; Stinchfield, R.; Álvarez-Moya, E.; Jaurrieta, N.; Bueno, B.; Granero, R.; Aymamí, M.N.; Gómez-Peña, M.; Martínez-Giménez, R.; Fernández-Aranda, F.; et al. Reliability, validity, and classification accuracy of a spanish translation of a measure of DSM-IV diagnostic criteria for pathological gambling. *J. Gambl. Stud.* **2009**, *25*, 93–104. [CrossRef] [PubMed]
16. Grant, J.E.; Odlaug, B.L.; Chamberlain, S.R.; Schreiber, L.R.N. Neurocognitive dysfunction in strategic and non-strategic gamblers. *Prog. Neuro-Psychopharmacol. Biol. Psychiatry* **2012**, *38*, 336–340. [CrossRef]
17. Slutske, W.S.; Piasecki, T.M.; Deutsch, A.R.; Statham, D.J.; Martin, N.G. Telescoping and gender differences in the time course of disordered gambling: Evidence from a general population sample. *Addiction* **2015**, *110*, 144–151. [CrossRef] [PubMed]
18. Jiménez-Murcia, S. Trastornos del Control de Impulsos: Juego Patológico. In *Introducción a la Psicopatología y la Psiquiatría*; Ruiloba, J.V., Ed.; Elsevier Masson: Barcelona, Spain, 2015; pp. 433–453.
19. Granero, R.; Jiménez-Murcia, S.; del Pino-Gutiérrez, A.; Mora, B.; Mendoza-Valenciano, E.; Baenas-Soto, I.; Gómez-Peña, M.; Moragas, L.; Codina, E.; López-González, H.; et al. Gambling Phenotypes in Online Sports Betting. *Front. Psychiatry* **2020**, *11*, 482. [CrossRef]
20. Granero, R.; Penelo, E.; Stinchfield, R.; Fernandez-Aranda, F.; Savvidou, L.G.; Fröberg, F.; Aymamí, N.; Gómez-Peña, M.; Pérez-Serrano, M.; del Pino-Gutiérrez, A.; et al. Is Pathological Gambling Moderated by Age? *J. Gambl. Stud.* **2014**, *30*, 475–492. [CrossRef]
21. Jiménez-Murcia, S.; Giménez, M.; Granero, R.; López-González, H.; Gómez-Peña, M.; Moragas, L.; Baenas, I.; Del Pino-Gutiérrez, A.; Codina, E.; Mena-Moreno, T.; et al. Psychopathogical status and personality correlates of problem gambling severity in sports bettors undergoing treatment for gambling disorder. *J. Behav. Addict.* **2021**, *10*, 422–434. [CrossRef]
22. Brewer, J.A.; Potenza, M.N. The neurobiology and genetics of impulse control disorders: Relationships to drug addictions. *Biochem. Pharmacol.* **2008**, *75*, 63–75. [CrossRef]
23. Blain, B.; Richard Gill, P.; Teese, R. Predicting problem gambling in Australian adults using a multifaceted model of impulsivity. *Int. Gambl. Stud.* **2015**, *15*, 239–255. [CrossRef]
24. Vintró-Alcaraz, C.; Mestre-Bach, G.; Granero, R.; Gómez-Peña, M.; Moragas, L.; Fernández-Aranda, F.; Jiménez-Murcia, S. Do emotion regulation and impulsivity differ according to gambling preferences in clinical samples of gamblers? *Addict. Behav.* **2022**, *126*, 107176. [CrossRef] [PubMed]
25. Dowling, N.A.; Merkouris, S.S.; Greenwood, C.J.; Oldenhof, E.; Toumbourou, J.W.; Youssef, G.J. Early risk and protective factors for problem gambling: A systematic review and meta-analysis of longitudinal studies. *Clin. Psychol. Rev.* **2017**, *51*, 109–124. [CrossRef]
26. Lara-Huallipe, M.L.; Granero, R.; Fernández-Aranda, F.; Gómez-Peña, M.; Moragas, L.; del Pino-Gutierrez, A.; Valenciano-Mendoza, E.; Mora-Maltas, B.; Baenas, I.; Etxandi, M.; et al. Clustering Treatment Outcomes in Women with Gambling Disorder. *J. Gambl. Stud.* **2021**, *38*, 1469–1491. [CrossRef]
27. Ledgerwood, D.M.; Dyshniku, F.; McCarthy, J.E.; Ostojic-Aitkens, D.; Forfitt, J.; Rumble, S.C. Gambling-Related Cognitive Distortions in Residential Treatment for Gambling Disorder. *J. Gambl. Stud.* **2020**, *36*, 669–683. [CrossRef] [PubMed]
28. Jiménez-Murcia, S.; Granero, R.; Fernández-Aranda, F.; Stinchfield, R.; Tremblay, J.; Steward, T.; Mestre-Bach, G.; Lozano-Madrid, M.; Mena-Moreno, T.; Mallorquí-Bagué, N.; et al. Phenotypes in gambling disorder using sociodemographic and clinical clustering analysis: An unidentified new subtype? *Front. Psychiatry* **2019**, *10*, 173. [CrossRef]
29. Slutske, W.S.; Meier, M.H.; Zhu, G.; Statham, D.J.; Blaszczynski, A.; Martin, N.G. The Australian Twin Study of Gambling (OZ-GAM): Rationale, Sample Description, Predictors of Participation, and a First Look at Sources of Individual Differences in Gambling Involvement. *Twin Res. Hum. Genet.* **2009**, *12*, 63–78. [CrossRef]
30. Slutske, W.S.; Richmond-Rakerd, L.S. A closer look at the evidence for sex differences in the genetic and environmental influences on gambling in the National Longitudinal Study of Adolescent health: From disordered to ordered gambling. *Addiction* **2014**, *109*, 120–127. [CrossRef]
31. Tak, Y.G.; Farnham, P.J. Making sense of GWAS: Using epigenomics and genome engineering to understand the functional relevance of SNPs in non-coding regions of the human genome. *Epigenetics Chromatin* **2015**, *8*, 57. [CrossRef]
32. Lang, M.; Leménager, T.; Streit, F.; Fauth-Bühler, M.; Frank, J.; Juraeva, D.; Witt, S.H.; Degenhardt, F.; Hofmann, A.; Heilmann-Heimbach, S.; et al. Genome-wide association study of pathological gambling. *Eur. Psychiatry* **2016**, *36*, 38–46. [CrossRef]
33. Munguía, L.; Jiménez-Murcia, S.; Granero, R.; Baenas, I.; Agüera, Z.; Sánchez, I.; Codina, E.; Del Pino-Gutiérrez, A.; Testa, G.; Treasure, J.; et al. Emotional regulation in eating disorders and gambling disorder: A transdiagnostic approach. *J. Behav. Addict.* **2022**, *10*, 508–523. [CrossRef]
34. Koskela, M.; Bäck, S.; Võikar, V.; Richie, C.T.; Domanskyi, A.; Harvey, B.K.; Airavaara, M. Update of neurotrophic factors in neurobiology of addiction and future directions. *Neurobiol. Dis.* **2017**, *97*, 189–200. [CrossRef]
35. Castrén, E. Neurotrophins and Psychiatric Disorders. *Handb. Exp. Pharmacol.* **2014**, *220*, 461–479. [CrossRef]

36. Solé-Morata, N.; Baenas, I.; Etxandi, M.; Granero, R. The role of neurotrophin genes involved in the vulnerability to gambling disorder. *Sci. Rep.* **2022**, *12*, 6925. [CrossRef] [PubMed]
37. Ernfors, P. Local and target-derived actions of neurotrophins during peripheral nervous system development. *Cell. Mol. Life Sci.* **2001**, *58*, 1036–1044. [CrossRef] [PubMed]
38. Linnet, J. The anticipatory dopamine response in addiction: A common neurobiological underpinning of gambling disorder and substance use disorder? *Prog. Neuro-Psychopharmacol. Biol. Psychiatry* **2020**, *98*, 109802. [CrossRef] [PubMed]
39. Pettorruso, M.; Zoratto, F.; Miuli, A.; De Risio, L.; Santorelli, M.; Pierotti, A.; Martinotti, G.; Adriani, W.; di Giannantonio, M. Exploring dopaminergic transmission in gambling addiction: A systematic translational review. *Neurosci. Biobehav. Rev.* **2020**, *119*, 481–511. [CrossRef]
40. Gratacòs, M.; Escaramís, G.; Bustamante, M.; Saus, E.; Agüera, Z.; Bayés, M.; Cellini, E.; de Cid, R.; Fernández-Aranda, F.; Forcano, L.; et al. Role of the neurotrophin network in eating disorders' subphenotypes: Body mass index and age at onset of the disease. *J. Psychiatr. Res.* **2010**, *44*, 834–840. [CrossRef]
41. Mercader, J.M.; Fernández-Aranda, F.; Gratacòs, M.; Ribasés, M.; Badía, A.; Villarejo, C.; Solano, R.; González, J.R.; Vallejo, J.; Estivill, X. Blood levels of brain-derived neurotrophic factor correlate with several psychopathological symptoms in anorexia nervosa patients. *Neuropsychobiology* **2008**, *56*, 185–190. [CrossRef]
42. Angelucci, F.; Martinotti, G.; Gelfo, F.; Righino, E.; Conte, G.; Caltagirone, C.; Bria, P.; Ricci, V. Enhanced BDNF serum levels in patients with severe pathological gambling. *Addict. Biol.* **2013**, *18*, 749–751. [CrossRef]
43. Choi, S.-W.; Shin, Y.-C.; Mok, J.Y.; Kim, D.-J.; Choi, J.-S.; Hwang, S.S.-H. Serum BDNF levels in patients with gambling disorder are associated with the severity of gambling disorder and Iowa Gambling Task indices. *J. Behav. Addict.* **2016**, *5*, 135–139. [CrossRef]
44. Geisel, O.; Banas, R.; Hellweg, R.; Müller, C.A. Altered Serum Levels of Brain-Derived Neurotrophic Factor in Patients with Pathological Gambling. *Eur. Addict. Res.* **2012**, *18*, 297–301. [CrossRef]
45. Kim, H.S.; von Ranson, K.M.; Hodgins, D.C.; McGrath, D.S.; Tavares, H. Demographic, psychiatric, and personality correlates of adults seeking treatment for disordered gambling with a comorbid binge/purge type eating disorder. *Eur. Eat. Disord. Rev.* **2018**, *26*, 508–518. [CrossRef] [PubMed]
46. Haniu, M.; Talvenheimo, J.; Le, J.; Katta, V.; Welcher, A.; Rohde, M.F. Extracellular domain of neurotrophin receptor trkB: Disulfide structure, N-glycosylation sites, and ligand binding. *Arch. Biochem. Biophys.* **1995**, *322*, 256–264. [CrossRef]
47. Otsuki, K.; Uchida, S.; Watanuki, T.; Wakabayashi, Y.; Fujimoto, M.; Matsubara, T.; Funato, H.; Watanabe, Y. Altered expression of neurotrophic factors in patients with major depression. *J. Psychiatr. Res.* **2008**, *42*, 1145–1153. [CrossRef]
48. Cho, S.C.; Kim, H.W.; Kim, B.N.; Kim, J.W.; Shin, M.S.; Cho, D.Y.; Chung, S.; Jung, S.W.; Yoo, H.J.; Chung, I.W.; et al. Neurotrophin-3 gene, intelligence, and selective attention deficit in a Korean sample with attention-deficit/hyperactivity disorder. *Prog. Neuro-Psychopharmacol. Biol. Psychiatry* **2010**, *34*, 1065–1069. [CrossRef]
49. Ceccarini, M.R.; Tasegian, A.; Franzago, M.; Patria, F.F.; Albi, E.; Codini, M.; Conte, C.; Bertelli, M.; Ragione, L.D.; Stuppia, L.; et al. 5-HT2AR and BDNF gene variants in eating disorders susceptibility. *Am. J. Med. Genet. B Neuropsychiatr. Genet.* **2020**, *183*, 155–163. [CrossRef] [PubMed]
50. Mercader, J.M.; Saus, E.; Agüera, Z.; Bayés, M.; Boni, C.; Carreras, A.; Cellini, E.; de Cid, R.; Dierssen, M.; Escaramís, G.; et al. Association of NTRK3 and its interaction with NGF suggest an altered cross-regulation of the neurotrophin signaling pathway in eating disorders. *Hum. Mol. Genet.* **2008**, *17*, 1234–1244. [CrossRef]
51. Retz, W.; Ringling, J.; Retz-Junginger, P.; Vogelgesang, M.; Rösler, M. Association of attention-deficit/hyperactivity disorder with gambling disorder. *J. Neural Transm.* **2016**, *123*, 1013–1019. [CrossRef] [PubMed]
52. Fatséas, M.; Hurmic, H.; Serre, F.; Debrabant, R.; Daulouède, J.P.; Denis, C.; Auriacombe, M. Addiction severity pattern associated with adult and childhood Attention Deficit Hyperactivity Disorder (ADHD) in patients with addictions. *Psychiatry Res.* **2016**, *246*, 656–662. [CrossRef] [PubMed]
53. Chowdhury, N.S.; Livesey, E.J.; Blaszczynski, A.; Harris, J.A. Pathological Gambling and Motor Impulsivity: A Systematic Review with Meta-Analysis. *J. Gambl. Stud.* **2017**, *33*, 1213–1239. [CrossRef] [PubMed]
54. Ledgerwood, D.M.; Petry, N.M. Subtyping pathological gamblers based on impulsivity, depression, and anxiety. *Psychol. Addict. Behav.* **2010**, *24*, 680–688. [CrossRef] [PubMed]
55. First, M.B.; Williams, J.B.W.; Karg, R.S.; Spitzer, R.L. *Structured Clinical Interview for DSM-5 Research Version*; American Psychiatric Association: Arlington, VA, USA, 2015.
56. Stinchfield, R. Reliability, Validity, and Classification Accuracy of a Measure of DSM-IV Diagnostic Criteria for Pathological Gambling. *Am. J. Psychiatry* **2003**, *160*, 180–182. [CrossRef]
57. American Psychiatric Association. *DSM-IV-TR. Diagnostic and Statistical Manual of Mental Disorders*, 4th ed.; American Psychiatric association (APA): Washington, DC, USA, 2000; ISBN 0-89042-334-2.
58. Lesieur, H.R.; Blume, S.B. The South Oaks Gambling Screen (SOGS): A new instrument for the identification of Pathological gamblers. *Am. J. Psychiatry* **1987**, *144*, 1184–1188. [CrossRef]
59. Echeburúa, E.; Báez, C.; Fernández-Montalvo, J.; Páez, D.; Baez, C.; Fernández-Montalvo, J.; Páez, D. Cuestionario de Juego Patológico de South Oaks (SOGS): Validación española. *Análisis Modif. Conduct.* **1994**, *20*, 769–791.
60. Derogatis, L.R. *SCL-90-R: Symptom Checklist-90-R. Administration, Scoring and Procedures Manuall—II for the Revised Version*; Clinical Psychometric Research: Towson, MD, USA, 1994.
61. Derogatis, L. *SCL-90-R. Cuestionario de 90 Síntomas-Manual*; TEA: Madrid, Spain, 2002.

62. Cloninger, C.R. *The Temperament and Character Inventory Revised*; Center for Psychobiology of Personality, Washington University: St Louis, MO, USA, 1999.
63. Gutiérrez-Zotes, J.A.; Bayón, C.; Montserrat, C.; Valero, J.; Labad, A.; Cloninger, C.R.; Fernández-Aranda, F. Temperament and Character Inventory Revised (TCI-R). Standardization and normative data in a general population sample. *Actas Españolas Psiquiatr.* **2004**, *32*, 8–15.
64. Jimenez-Murcia, S.; Aymamí-Sanromà, N.M.; Gómez-Peña, M.; Álvarez-Moya, E.M.; Vallejo, J. *Protocols de Tractament Cognitivo-conductual Pel Joc Patològic i D'altres Addiccions no Tòxiques*; Hospital Universitary de Bellvitge: Barcelona, Spain, 2006.
65. Kline, R.B. *Principles and Practice of Structural Equation Modeling*, 2nd ed.; The Guilford Press: New York, NY, USA, 2005.
66. Oertzen, T. Power equivalence in structural equation modelling. *Br. J. Math. Stat. Psychol.* **2010**, *63*, 257–272. [CrossRef] [PubMed]
67. Borsboom, D.; Mellenbergh, G.J.; van Heerden, J. The theoretical status of latent variables. *Psychol. Rev.* **2003**, *110*, 203–219. [CrossRef]
68. Barrett, P. Structural equation modelling: Adjudging model fit. *Pers. Individ. Dif.* **2007**, *42*, 815–824. [CrossRef]
69. Jiménez-Murcia, S.; Granero, R.; Fernández-Aranda, F.; Arcelus, J.; Aymamí, M.N.; Gómez-Peña, M.; Tárrega, S.; Moragas, L.; Del Pino-Gutiérrez, A.; Sauchelli, S.; et al. Predictors of outcome among pathological gamblers receiving cognitive behavioral group therapy. *Eur. Addict. Res.* **2015**, *21*, 169–178. [CrossRef] [PubMed]
70. Sharman, S.; Murphy, R.; Turner, J.; Roberts, A. Psychosocial correlates in treatment seeking gamblers: Differences in early age onset gamblers vs later age onset gamblers. *Addict. Behav.* **2019**, *97*, 20–26. [CrossRef] [PubMed]
71. Volberg, R.A.; Gupta, R.; Griffiths, M.D.; Olason, D.T.; Delfabbro, P. An international perspective on youth gambling prevalence studies. *Int. J. Adolesc. Med. Health* **2010**, *22*, 3–38. [CrossRef] [PubMed]
72. Kim, S.W.; Grant, J.E.; Eckert, E.D.; Faris, P.L.; Hartman, B.K. Pathological gambling and mood disorders: Clinical associations and treatment implications. *J. Affect. Disord.* **2006**, *92*, 109–116. [CrossRef] [PubMed]
73. Álvarez-Moya, E.M.; Jiménez-Murcia, S.; Aymamí, M.N.; Gómez-Peña, M.; Granero, R.; Santamaría, J.; Menchón, J.M.; Fernández-Aranda, F. Subtyping Study of a Pathological Gamblers Sample. *Can. J. Psychiatry* **2010**, *55*, 498–506. [CrossRef]
74. Granero, R.; Jiménez-Murcia, S.; del Pino-Gutiérrez, A.; Mena-Moreno, T.; Mestre-Bach, G.; Gómez-Peña, M.; Moragas, L.; Aymamí, N.; Giroux, I.; Grall-Bronnec, M.; et al. Gambling Phenotypes in Older Adults. *J. Gambl. Stud.* **2020**, *36*, 809–828. [CrossRef]
75. Jiménez-Murcia, S.; Granero, R.; Giménez, M.; del Pino-Gutiérrez, A.; Mestre-Bach, G.; Mena-Moreno, T.; Moragas, L.; Baño, M.; Sánchez-González, J.; de Gracia, M.; et al. Contribution of sex on the underlying mechanism of the gambling disorder severity. *Sci. Rep.* **2020**, *10*, 18722. [CrossRef]
76. Khanbhai, Y.; Smith, D.; Battersby, M. Gender by Preferred Gambling Activity in Treatment Seeking Problem Gamblers: A Comparison of Subgroup Characteristics and Treatment Outcomes. *J. Gambl. Stud.* **2017**, *33*, 99–113. [CrossRef]
77. Grant, J.E.; Chamberlain, S.R.; Schreiber, L.R.N.; Odlaug, B.L. Gender-related clinical and neurocognitive differences in individuals seeking treatment for pathological gambling. *J. Psychiatr. Res.* **2012**, *46*, 1206–1211. [CrossRef]
78. Odlaug, B.L.; Chamberlain, S.R. Gambling and Personality Dimensions. *Curr. Behav. Neurosci. Rep.* **2014**, *1*, 13–18. [CrossRef]
79. Janiri, L.; Martinotti, G.; Dario, T.; Schifano, F.; Bria, P. The Gamblers' Temperament and Character Inventory (TCI) Personality Profile. *Subst. Use Misuse* **2007**, *42*, 975–984. [CrossRef]
80. Lobo, D.S.S.; Quilty, L.C.; Martins, S.S.; Tavares, H.; Vallada, H.; Kennedy, J.L.; Bagby, R.M. Pathological gambling subtypes: A comparison of treatment-seeking and non-treatment-seeking samples from Brazil and Canada. *Addict. Behav.* **2014**, *39*, 1172–1175. [CrossRef] [PubMed]
81. Moragas, L.; Granero, R.; Stinchfield, R.; Fernández-Aranda, F.; Fröberg, F.; Aymamí, N.; Gómez-Peña, M.; Fagundo, A.B.; Islam, M.A.; del Pino-Gutiérrez, A.; et al. Comparative analysis of distinct phenotypes in gambling disorder based on gambling preferences. *BMC Psychiatry* **2015**, *15*, 86. [CrossRef]
82. Jiménez-Murcia, S.; Fernández-Aranda, F.; Mestre-Bach, G.; Granero, R.; Tárrega, S.; Torrubia, R.; Aymamí, N.; Gómez-Peña, M.; Soriano-Mas, C.; Steward, T.; et al. Exploring the Relationship between Reward and Punishment Sensitivity and Gambling Disorder in a Clinical Sample: A Path Modeling Analysis. *J. Gambl. Stud.* **2017**, *33*, 579–597. [CrossRef] [PubMed]
83. Lorains, F.K.; Cowlishaw, S.; Thomas, S.A. Prevalence of comorbid disorders in problem and pathological gambling: Systematic review and meta-analysis of population surveys. *Addiction* **2011**, *106*, 490–498. [CrossRef]
84. Atkinson, J.; Sharp, C.; Schmitz, J.; Yaroslavsky, I. Behavioral Activation and Inhibition, Negative Affect, and Gambling Severity in a Sample of Young Adult College Students. *J. Gambl. Stud.* **2012**, *28*, 437–449. [CrossRef] [PubMed]
85. Kernie, S.G.; Liebl, D.J.; Parada, L.F. BDNF regulates eating behavior and locomotor activity in mice. *EMBO J.* **2000**, *19*, 1290–1300. [CrossRef]
86. Xu, B.; Goulding, E.H.; Zang, K.; Cepoi, D.; Cone, R.D.; Jones, K.R.; Tecott, L.H.; Reichardt, L.F. Brain-derived neurotrophic factor regulates energy balance downstream of melanocortin-4 receptor. *Nat. Neurosci.* **2003**, *6*, 736–742. [CrossRef] [PubMed]
87. Sleeman, M.W.; Garcia, K.; Liu, R.; Murray, J.D.; Malinova, L.; Moncrieffe, M.; Yancopoulos, G.D.; Wiegand, S.J. Ciliary neurotrophic factor improves diabetic parameters and hepatic steatosis and increases basal metabolic rate in db/db mice. *Proc. Natl. Acad. Sci. USA* **2003**, *100*, 14297–14302. [CrossRef]
88. Kokoeva, M.V.; Yin, H.; Flier, J.S. Neurogenesis in the Hypothalamus of Adult Mice: Potential Role in Energy Balance. *Science* **2005**, *310*, 679–683. [CrossRef]

89. Fauth-Bühler, M.; Mann, K.; Potenza, M.N. Pathological gambling: A review of the neurobiological evidence relevant for its classification as an addictive disorder. *Addict. Biol.* **2017**, *22*, 885–897. [CrossRef]
90. Griffiths, M.D. Behavioural addiction and substance addiction should be defined by their similarities not their dissimilarities. *Addiction* **2017**, *112*, 1718–1720. [CrossRef] [PubMed]

Disclaimer/Publisher's Note: The statements, opinions and data contained in all publications are solely those of the individual author(s) and contributor(s) and not of MDPI and/or the editor(s). MDPI and/or the editor(s) disclaim responsibility for any injury to people or property resulting from any ideas, methods, instructions or products referred to in the content.

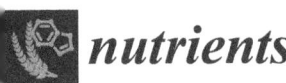

Review

Potential Biological Markers and Treatment Implications for Binge Eating Disorder and Behavioral Addictions

Gemma Mestre-Bach [1] and Marc N. Potenza [2,3,4,5,6,7],*

[1] Facultad de Ciencias de la Salud, Universidad Internacional de La Rioja, 26006 Logroño, Spain
[2] Department of Psychiatry, School of Medicine, Yale University, New Haven, CT 06510, USA
[3] Connecticut Mental Health Center, New Haven, CT 06519, USA
[4] Connecticut Council on Problem Gambling, Wethersfield, CT 06109, USA
[5] Wu Tsai Institute, Yale University, New Haven, CT 06510, USA
[6] Yale Child Study Center, School of Medicine, Yale University, New Haven, CT 06510, USA
[7] Department of Neuroscience, School of Medicine, Yale University, New Haven, CT 06510, USA
* Correspondence: marc.potenza@yale.edu

Abstract: The reward system is highly relevant to behavioral addictions such as gambling disorder (GD), internet gaming disorder (IGD), and food addiction/binge eating disorder (FA/BED). Among other brain regions, the ventral striatum (VS) has been implicated in reward processing. The main objective of the present state-of-the-art review was to explore in depth the specific role of the VS in GD, IGD and FA/BED, understanding it as a possible biomarker of these conditions. Studies analyzing brain changes following interventions for these disorders, and especially those that had explored possible treatment-related changes in VS, are discussed. More evidence is needed on how existing treatments (both pharmacological and psychobehavioral) for behavioral addictions affect the activation of the VS and related circuitry.

Keywords: reward system; ventral striatum; craving; internet gaming disorder; gambling disorder; binge eating disorder; food addiction

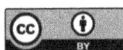

1. Introduction

The reward system is relevant to addictions, both substance and behavioral. Sex differences across neurobehavioral levels have been reported. It has been suggested that men may be more sensitive to the behavioral relevance (salience) of incentive stimuli, and that women and men show no differences in stimulus valence (e.g., losing versus winning money) [1]. Further, sex differences in motivations for engaging in addictive behaviors (positive reinforcement motivations for men and negative reinforcement motivations for women) may be linked to these neurobehavioral relationships [2,3].

This circuit includes structures such as the ventral tegmental area (VTA; a main brain area involved in the production and projected transmission of dopamine) and the ventral striatum (VS; a VTA projection site) and other areas (i.e., cortical regions including the ventromedial prefrontal cortex (vmPFC) and orbitofrontal cortex (OFC) comprising mesocortical pathways) [4].

The VS encompasses the nucleus accumbens (NAc), together with regions of the medial caudate nucleus and the rostroventral putamen. The VS receives dopaminergic input from the midbrain, as well as cortical input from the anterior cingulate cortex (ACC) and OFC. In turn, the VS projects output to the VTA and the ventral pallidum. These, via the medial dorsal nucleus of the thalamus, project output back to the prefrontal cortex (PFC) [5]. A figure including some of the key reward-related brain regions is included (Figure 1).

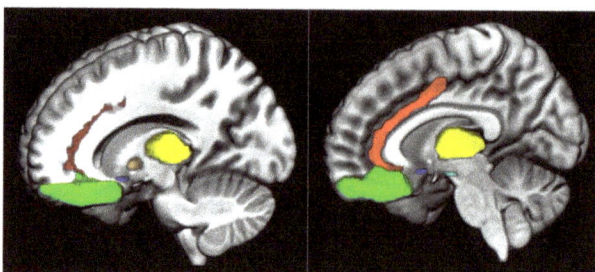

Figure 1. Main brain areas of the reward system anterior cingulate cortex: red; globus pallidus: orange; nucleus accumbens: royal blue; orbitofrontal cortex: neon green; thalamus: yellow; ventral tegmental area: cyan.

The VS, and especially the NAc, contribute importantly to reward processing, being activated by the anticipation and reception of different types of rewards. More specifically, the VS generates predictions about possible gains and establishes a comparison with actual outcomes [6]. In fact, it has been observed that the VS shows a higher activation to positive reward outcomes [7–10], and this activation seems to decrease if possible losses increase [11]. Moreover, different neurohormones, such as oxytocin, have been linked to reward systems and social behaviors. Oxytocin may influence dopamine and anandamide signaling [12] and relates importantly to sexual arousal and orgasm [13,14] and aspects of maternal bonding [15]. Oxytocin has also been implicated in addictive behaviors and disorders [16–18]. Dopamine is a relevant reward-related neurotransmitter [19], and it may influence potentially rewarding behaviors, including food intake [20].

As previously described [21], two complementary theoretical models of addictions associate the roles of the VS with the development and maintenance of addictions: the incentive salience [22] and reward deficiency syndrome theories [23,24]. On the one hand, the incentive salience theory [22] divides motivated behavior into two components: liking (associated with the experienced value of the reward, usually carried by an unconditional stimulus) and wanting (associated with the experienced value of the reward, usually carried by a conditional stimulus/cue). It has been observed that the conditioned cues related to addiction generate increased responses in the VS in individuals with addictions, as well as greater motivated behavior. On the other hand, the reward deficiency syndrome theory [23,24] postulates that individuals with addictions present with alterations in reward pathways and, in particular, a hypoactivation of these brain regions, together with a reduced pleasurable experience derived from non-addiction-related rewards. Therefore, addictive behaviors are used to stimulate the reward circuitry and, consequently, to compensate for reward deficiencies.

In this context, VS-cortical circuitry has been considered relevant to craving [25], and alterations in VS-cortical connectivity have been observed in both substance use disorders (SUDs) [26,27] and behavioral addictions [28,29]. The behavioral addictions most studied at the neurobiological level and accepted in the Diagnostic and Statistical Manual of Mental Disorders, Fifth Edition [30] or the International Classification of Diseases, 11th Revision [31] have been gambling disorder (GD) and internet gaming disorder (IGD; termed gaming disorder in the International Classification of Diseases, 11th Revision). GD is characterized by a maladaptive pattern of gambling behavior that persists despite negative consequences in major areas of life functioning [30]. IGD is characterized by difficulties in controlling excessive/interfering levels of videogaming, often with the presence of tolerance, withdrawal, and negative consequences in major life domains [30]. Likewise, food addiction (FA; typically to highly processed, hyperpalatable and densely caloric foods) has been proposed as another possible addiction, although it has been debated and FA is neither in the Diagnostic and Statistical Manual of Mental Disorders Fifth Edition, nor the International Classification of Diseases, 11th Revision. FA may have overlapping neurobiological systems, particularly when highly palatable foods activate reward circuitry as do substances in SUDs, and these processes may be particularly relevant in people with binge eating disorder (BED) [32]. For example, both in individuals with SUDs and in animal models focused on food intake/binge eating, decreased striatal dopaminergic release has been observed, as well as increased reward thresholds [33]. There is a high co-occurrence of FA with BED and similarities between the two constructs (e.g., although BED has been diagnosed as an eating disorder in the Diagnostic and Statistical Manual of Mental Disorders Fifth Edition [30], it has also been considered an addiction-like behavior [34]); however, they do not completely overlap [35]. Some authors have suggested that individuals with BED who present with FA have greater clinical impairment, possibly due to the impact of an addictive process [35] and, among individuals with BED, those with FA have demonstrated poorer treatment outcomes [36]. Epigenetic mechanisms, including with respect to early life food intake, may contribute to FA and other addictive behaviors [37,38].

The main objective of the present state-of-the-art review was to explore in depth the specific role of the VS in GD, IGD and FA/BED, considering it as a possible biomarker of behavioral addictions with treatment relevance. The aim was to review studies that had analyzed changes at the brain level after the application of interventions for these disorders, and especially those that had explored possible changes in the VS related to these treatments.

2. Materials and Methods

The present state-of-the-art review aimed to provide a comprehensive review of the existing literature and to describe the main findings in a narrative format. For this purpose, both PubMed and Google Scholar were searched for scientific articles that had been published in peer-reviewed international journals up to 20 December 2022. Both reviews and original studies with human samples of one or more participants were considered. Articles in both adolescent and adult populations with a diagnosis of GD, IGD or FA/BED were considered. Articles published in both English and Spanish were included. The different searches used terms such as functional magnetic resonance imaging (fMRI), ventral striatum, gambling, gaming, binge eating disorder, food addiction, cognitive behavioral therapy (CBT), treatment, intervention, pharmacotherapy and recovery, among others.

3. Results

3.1. Ventral Striatal Activation and GD

The VS has been implicated in urges in GD, as well as behavioral and physiological responses to rewards, and it has been hypothesized that differences in VS function may predispose individuals to develop addictions [39]. More specifically, greater gray-matter volume in the right VS has been described in individuals with (versus without) GD [40]. Alterations in dopaminergically innervated regions associated with reward, risk and motivation, such as the VS and vmPFC, have been described in individuals with GD [41–43]. Activity in the VS, together with the vmPFC, may reflect both probabilities and magnitudes of potential wins related to risky choices, so that these brain regions could present a coordinated representation of both decisional parameters [44]. However, some authors have been critical of the simplicity of theories of the neurobiological basis of GD, given that both hypersensitivity and hyposensitivity of the VS and other ventral regions of the reward system, such as the vmPFC, have been described [28,45–48].

Some studies have analyzed the role of VS in the processing of different types of stimuli in individuals with GD. For example, some have observed a blunted activation of the VS and the ventral PFC of individuals with GD in the processing of monetary rewards [49–51]. In one study, individuals with (versus without) GD presented differential responses to erotic versus monetary stimuli and, in particular, a reduced sensitivity toward erotic stimuli [52]. Considering the role of VS in instrumental motivation and in the context of imbalance hypotheses, the authors suggest that this asymmetric response pattern may be evidence of a neurophysiological mechanism in which monetary stimuli overpower other types of stimuli in terms of incentive salience. The extent of this differential response between both types of stimuli has been statistically predicted by the severity of GD, so that differential cue reactivity may be a defining feature of GD. Increased VS, dorsolateral prefrontal cortex (DLPFC) and ACC activation have also been described in individuals with GD, compared to controls, when presented with gambling-related cues versus neutral stimuli [53]. Differences in the response to gambling versus food cues have also been explored in individuals with GD. Individuals with (versus without) GD presented greater reactivity to gambling cues, but not to food cues [54]. Likewise, in the GD group, a positive association was observed between gambling-related craving and gambling cue-related activity in the VS, as well as a negative association with functional connectivity (FC) between the VS and the medial PFC [54]. However, other studies have reported relatively blunted VS activation in GD during simulated gambling, with the degree of activation inversely associated with problem gambling severity. Similarly, during the presentation of complex video cues that elicited gambling urges, individuals with (versus without) GD showed blunted VS activation, with similar findings in people with (versus without) cocaine use disorder noted in response to comparable cocaine-related cues. Thus, not all stimuli elicit increased brain responses in the reward-related circuitry in individuals with GD.

Relationships between near-misses (e.g., when 2 reels on a slot machine match but the third does not) and the VS have also been explored. It has been suggested that near-misses activate brain areas similar to wins. In fact, near-misses may lead to greater VS activity compared to non-winning full-miss events [55–57]. Neural signaling in the VS (involved in reinforcement learning) may be explained by near-misses being close to wins, so they may be erroneously considered as a sign of skill acquisition and enhance motivations for gambling [58]. This may explain why some studies have observed amplified VS responses to near-misses in individuals with (versus without) GD [58].

3.1.1. Neural Mechanisms of Recovery in GD
Pharmacological Interventions for GD

Currently, no pharmacological intervention has been approved by regulatory bodies with an indication for GD, and the study of pharmacotherapies for GD is thus needed. However, the efficacy of different medications for the treatment of GD has been explored, with mixed or negative evidence for lithium, serotonergic antidepressants, catechol-O-methyltransferase inhibitors (e.g., tolcapone), glutamatergic agents, neuroleptics, opioid receptor antagonists and dopamine-1-receptor and dopamine-2-receptor antagonists [59]. The efficacy of these drugs at the neuronal level warrants more examination and, to the best of our knowledge, to date there are no studies that focus on the specific effects of these medications on the VS.

Bupropion. Brain measures were obtained from three groups: 15 participants with online GD, 16 participants with IGD and 15 control participants with neither disorder [60]. In the online GD group, after 12 weeks of pharmacotherapy with bupropion, there was a reduction in FC in the default mode network, whereas there was an increase in FC in a cognitive control network. In addition, compared to the IGD group, individuals with online GD showed greater FC in the cognitive control network. Theoretically, pro-dopaminergic effects related to bupropion could stimulate activity of top-down circuitry and impact cognitive control networks, promoting more advantageous decision-making.

Tolcapone. A study explored the efficacy of 8 weeks of oral tolcapone, a catechol-O-methyltransferase inhibitor, in 12 individuals with GD through fMRI and an executive-planning task [61]. At baseline, patients with GD, compared to controls, showed fronto-parietal under-activation during the executive-planning task. After pharmacological intervention a reduction of IGD symptomatology was observed, which correlated significantly with the increase in fronto-parietal engagement. Treatment response was also related to a functional allelic variant of the gene coding for the catechol-O-methyltransferase protein, suggesting that personalized medicine approaches may be warranted.

Fluvoxamine. A case study explored brain activations with respect to fluvoxamine administration [62]. The individual with GD showed frontal, occipital and parietal activations at baseline with the presentation of playing cards. A decrease in the activated brain areas was observed after fluvoxamine, which was linked to a reduction in the desire to gamble. However, as it is a case report and there was no placebo control, more empirical evidence is needed.

Lithium. The efficacy of lithium has been tested in individuals with GD and co-occurring bipolar-spectrum disorders. Positron emission tomography was used to explore mechanisms related to treatment efficacy [63,64]. Lithium may increase the relative glucose metabolic rate in the ventral caudate, albeit not to a statistically significant level, in individuals with GD and bipolar-spectrum disorders. Moreover, lithium may increase the relative glucose metabolic rate in the OFC, DLPFC and posterior cingulate cortex [64].

Psychobehavioral Interventions for GD

Cognitive behavioral therapy (CBT). A proof-of-concept fMRI study [65] aimed to examine neural mechanisms related to treatment outcomes for GD. Seven treatment-seeking individuals with GD (with co-occurring tobacco use disorder) performed the Stroop task during fMRI before initiating treatment for GD. The treatment consisted of six weeks of CBT, and also included imaginal desensitization motivational interviewing, smoking cessation instruction, and either the amino-acid dietary supplement N-acetyl cysteine or placebo. N-acetyl cysteine is a nutraceutical that can influence VS dopaminergic function through glutamatergic mechanisms. The authors hypothesized that VS activation during the Stroop task would inversely correlate with pretreatment GD severity. It was further hypothesized that VS activity during the pretreatment Stroop task would correlate with improvements in post-treatment GD symptomatology. A positive correlation was found between GD symptomatology and activation of the right VS, including the NAc, thus providing some support for a role for the VS in treatment outcomes for GD.

Neuromodulatory Interventions for GD

Repetitive transcranial magnetic stimulation (rTMS) is a neuromodulatory approach to modify brain circuit function, including those related to control over craving [8,9]. However, studies on this non-invasive procedure in GD are relatively scarce. Thus, it may be relevant to focus on neurobiological similarities between gambling urges and drug craving in SUDs to facilitate advances [66,67]. Existing studies in addictions have considered stimulation of the DLPFC [68–71]. Through its connections with the VS and the VTA, the DLPFC may influence the function of mesostriatal and mesolimbic pathways. Therefore, stimulation of the DLPFC could potentially increase cognitive control over craving [68]. While this may involve dopaminergic circuits, some authors have suggested that stimulation of the DLPFC may have an impact on GABA and glutamate levels in this brain region and connected circuitry, which includes the VS. This may theoretically facilitate dopamine release indirectly in the mesocortical pathway, reducing levels of craving, impulsivity and reward-seeking [72].

3.2. Ventral Striatal Activation and IGD

A tripartite neurocognitive model has been proposed for IGD [73]. This would include a dual process that suggests that both the development and maintenance of this disorder may involve hyperactivity of the reward system (amygdala-VS-dependent) in response to gaming-related cues, together with the weakening of inhibition (DLPFC-dependent). The third system could refer to the interoceptive awareness system (insula-dependent), which may involve converting somatic signals of reward obtained with video games into subjective desire. Based on this theoretical model, it was hypothesized that IGD severity scores among people who played *League of Legends* would be positively related to the activation of the reward system and that, in turn, they would be negatively linked to the activation of prefrontal areas [74]. It was observed that the VS was more strongly activated in people who played *League of Legends* in response to gaming-related cues, and that the left frontal pole and DLPFC were more weakly activated compared to comparison subjects (who did not play *League of Legends*). Stronger activations of the VS have been reported in individuals with (versus without) IGD in other studies [75,76], as well as less activation in the DLPFC and inferior parietal lobe during the evaluation of potential losses and the risk perception [76]. This increased activation of the VS in the face of addiction-related cues appears to be a shared factor between IGD, GD and SUDs [77].

Data provide insights into the negative associations between craving and cue-induced activations in the VS [78], as well as the positive relationship between both factors in the dorsal striatum [79,80] in the case of individuals with SUDs. In this context, in individuals with IGD, brain activity in the left VS was inversely related to gaming-cue induced craving, which may suggest that in IGD there is a decreased involvement of the VS in cue processing [81]. A positive association between activation of the dorsal striatum and IGD duration was noted. In individuals with IGD, a negative association was observed between right VS volumes and cue-induced activity in the left putamen. Abnormal resting-state FC within a dorsal striatum network and VS network (i.e., reduced caudate–DLPFC and NAc–OFC resting-state FC strength) in individuals with IGD has also been described [82]. It has been suggested that the VS has an essential role in the early stages of addictions, while in later stages the dorsal striatum may be more involved in the compulsive aspects of addictions, highlighting a relevant shift [83,84].

The frequent use of video games has been associated with dopamine release in the VS [85], as well as with an increased volume of the left VS [86], which may reflect an alteration in reward processing [87]. Similarly, in individuals with IGD, larger volumes of the VS, specifically the NAc, as well as the dorsal striatum, specifically the caudate, have been observed [88]. However, other studies have obtained opposite results, suggesting that individuals with (versus without) IGD may have reduced striatal volumes, especially in the VS [89,90].

Some studies have highlighted an association between the VS and the left OFC (associated with cue reactivity in individuals with IGD) and the right inferior frontal gyrus (associated with inhibition processing) in individuals with IGD [91]. Other studies have found that, in the VS, individuals with IGD, compared to those with recreational game use, exhibited lower FC with the middle frontal gyrus, especially on the left and mostly in the supplementary motor area (involved in motor planning and execution) [92]. Therefore, considering that the VS is associated with the learning values of stimuli, the lower FC with the middle frontal gyrus may suggest that individuals with IGD present a possible disconnection between stimulus evaluation and behavioral responses in domains such as response inhibition [92]. Likewise, during response inhibition under high-load tasks, individuals with IGD present an increased inefficient engagement of the VS and DLPFC, which may highlight their vulnerability to inappropriate response inhibition with higher-level cognitive skills [93].

Taking into account specific aspects of IGD, it has been suggested that greater IGD severity may increase the effective connectivity between the VS bilaterally [94]. IGD severity has also been associated with VS bias for monetary rewards [95], and has been negatively associated with FC between frontal and striatal brain areas [96]. Furthermore, the number of IGD symptoms appears to be negatively associated with dorsal-ACC-VS resting-state FC, suggesting that it may be considered as a biomarker of IGD, as well as an important target for interventions addressing this disorder [97]. The functional coupling between dorsal ACC and VS may be involved in feedback learning. Therefore, the alterations presented by individuals with IGD may imply difficulties in representing value signals attached to action outcome relationships and, consequently, learning problems [98].

3.2.1. Neural Mechanisms of Recovery in IGD

Several studies have explored neural mechanisms involved in the recovery of individuals with IGD. For example, Dong et al. [99] hypothesized that brain regions involved in craving, such as the striatum, may show less activation in those individuals recovered from IGD (without formal intervention), compared to those with active IGD, when exposed to gaming cues. The authors observed decreased craving responses to gaming-related cues at both subjective and neural levels in individuals with IGD in recovery. More specifically, individuals recovered from IGD showed relatively diminished AAC activation and decreased gaming-cue related activations in the vmPFC/OFC and lentiform nucleus, thus possibly presenting a lower motivation to perform gaming. Likewise, cue-elicited activation of the lentiform nucleus has also been related to the development of IGD in individuals with regular videogame use [100]. Therefore, in both the emergence and recovery of IGD, gaming-cue elicited lentiform activity should be considered. Therefore, these authors highlighted the need to consider craving reduction in IGD as a potential neural target for interventions such as neuromodulation or behavioral approaches [99].

Pharmacological Interventions for IGD

Several pharmacological options have been suggested for IGD. Drugs used for treating depression (bupropion and escitalopram) and attention deficit/hyperactivity disorder (methylphenidate and atomoxetine), conditions that frequently co-occur with IGD, have been evaluated in IGD treatment [60,101–104]. However, no pharmacological intervention has a formal indication for the treatment of IGD, and none of the proposed options have been sufficiently evaluated for their efficacy and tolerability [105].

Few studies have explored the neural effects of pharmacological interventions in individuals with IGD, and of these, to the best of our knowledge, none have specifically examined the effect on the VS. In one study of IGD, GD and control comparison subjects [60], a reduction in FC in the posterior default mode network and between the posterior default mode network and the cognitive control network was observed in individuals with IGD after 12 weeks of bupropion treatment. Furthermore, the authors noted that FC in the default mode network was positively correlated with changes in IGD symptomatology after pharmacological intervention. A 12-week double blind prospective trial compared bupropion and escitalopram in 30 individuals with IGD and major depressive disorder (15 in each group) [106]. In the case of bupropion, a significant reduction in FC was observed in the salience network and between the salience network and the default mode network. In contrast, in the escitalopram group, only a reduction of FC in the default mode network was found. Speculatively, bupropion may show greater efficiency than escitalopram in reducing impulsivity and attentional symptoms, while both drugs may reduce depressive and IGD symptoms.

Psychobehavioral Interventions for IGD

Following behavioral interventions in patients with addictions (both substance and behavioral), changes in cortico-striatal function have been observed. In studies of individuals with SUDs, cortico-striatal circuitry has been a proposed mechanism underlying different treatments, such as cognitive therapy [107], mindfulness-oriented recovery enhancement [108], and cue-exposure based extinction training [109]. This may imply that cortico-striatal circuitry may also be altered in IGD, and the improvement of the functionality of this circuitry may be a mechanism underlying psychobehavioral interventions.

CBT. Han et al. [110] compared 26 individuals with IGD and 30 comparison subjects without, and examined the efficacy of CBT in 20 individuals with IGD. The CBT consisted of 12 group sessions lasting 1.5–2 h each in which topics such as emotion recognition, impulse control, and recognition and control of addictive behaviors were addressed. The authors hypothesized that individuals with IGD would present abnormal brain connectivity in prefrontal-striatal areas and that CBT would be effective in regulating this abnormal function. The results of the study suggested that CBT may regulate the abnormal low-frequency fluctuations in prefrontal-striatal areas of individuals with IGD and, consequently, improve IGD symptomatology.

The efficacy of CBT was contrasted with the efficacy of virtual reality in a study involving 36 individuals with IGD, 24 of whom were randomly assigned to the CBT group, while the remaining 12 were assigned to the virtual reality group [111]. The virtual reality program, lasting eight sessions, was designed to increase balanced activation of the brain reward circuitry with stimulation of the limbic system. More specifically, the intervention aimed to stimulate both the striatum (linked to craving) and the temporal lobe (linked to aversion), as well as to facilitate limbic-regulated responses to reward stimuli. The process was tested by pairing scenes of aversive consequences of gaming behavior and craving-inducing game-related stimuli. Both CBT and the virtual reality program showed similar effects on the reduction of IGD symptomatology. Likewise, the virtual reality program improved balance in the cortico-striatal-limbic circuit. Therefore, the authors suggested that virtual reality may be an effective tool for the facilitation of limbic-regulated responses to rewarding stimuli. Studies exploring the specific effects of CBT on VS activity are needed.

Family therapy. Han et al. [112] observed a change of striatal activity after family therapy in adolescents with IGD. The family therapy consisted of five sessions to increase family cohesion, along with two assessment sessions. Those adolescents with IGD and a poor family relationship may use video games as a compensatory strategy for reward deficits (potentially related to VS activity) relating to poor parental support. Both romantic and maternal love may influence activation of the striatum, as part of reward circuitry.

Craving behavioral intervention (CBI). Several studies have explored the impact of CBI on the VS of individuals with IGD. CBI is an intervention focused on reducing craving levels. The different studies that have used this intervention have used it in a group format (between 8–9 individuals) and organized in 6 weekly sessions in which topics such as perception and recognition of craving and training in coping skills and mindfulness to reduce craving are addressed [113].

Zhang et al. [113] evaluated effects of CBI on the resting-state FC of the VS. More specifically, the authors compared 76 individuals with IGD with 41 control participants, assessing resting-state FC of the VS. Of the individuals with IGD, 25 received CBI while 19 did not. Individuals with (versus without) IGD showed a significantly higher resting-state FC of VS to the left middle frontal gyrus, the left inferior parietal lobule and the right inferior frontal gyrus. When comparing the posttest with the pretest of IGD individuals who had received CBI, a significant reduction of the strength of VS-left inferior parietal lobule connectivity was observed ($p = 0.001$). However, the group of IGD individuals who had not undergone CBI showed no change between pretest and posttest ($p = 0.73$). In the light of these findings, the authors suggested that VS-left inferior parietal lobule FC may be considered as a stable biomarker for CBI efficacy in IGD. However, VS-left middle frontal gyrus, and especially VS-right inferior frontal gyrus connectivity, may not be regarded as specific markers of CBI efficacy, since they decreased significantly in both groups (the one that had undergone CBI and the one that had not). Considering this potential biomarker, non-invasive techniques, such as transcranial magnetic stimulation and transcranial direct current stimulation (tDCS) may be considered for treatment of IGD.

In a subsequent publication, Zhang et al. [114] hypothesized that individuals with (versus without) IGD may have greater activation of reward-related areas, including the VS, involved in cue-induced craving. The authors analyzed the efficacy of CBI by comparing a group of 23 individuals with IGD who received the intervention with a group of 17 individuals with IGD who did not. At a behavioral level, CBI reduced cue-induced craving and IGD severity. However, the intervention, at the neural level, did not "normalize" IGD-related cue-induced brain activation identified at baseline. Therefore, CBI may not have impacted the reward system and, specifically, the VS. However, CBI appeared to have impacted another brain region, the anterior insula, which at baseline had shown no differences between individuals with and without IGD. Therefore, the authors suggested that this intervention, rather than directly altering regions involved in reinforcement, may modulate brain areas involved in higher-level cognitive functioning. Thus, it was suggested that future studies may test combinations of CBI with other interventions that have a direct effect on the VS and other regions involved in cue reactivity, such as pharmacological interventions, non-invasive procedures such as transcranial magnetic stimulation or invasive procedures such as deep-brain stimulation.

Wang et al. [115], who also administered CBI to individuals with IGD, observed that some reward-related brain areas, especially the ventral and dorsal striatum, were not involved in their classification analysis. These findings are consistent with previous studies, which found that these specific areas did not show differences in activation to cue reactivity tasks [116]. One explanation suggested by the authors is that the individuals included in their study were in later stages of the addiction process, so it is possible that videogame-related stimuli may be evoking less robust responses than the gaming behavior itself.

Finally, Liu et al. [117] observed an association between changes in craving levels and IGD severity at six months after CBI and connectivity differences in the left angular gyrus and vmPFC. However, given that most previous studies have focused on the VS and other regions involved in reward processing, such as the vmPFC, the specific role of the angular gyrus in craving warrants direct examination.

Equine-assisted therapy. Kang et al. [118] explored the neural correlates of equine-assisted therapy and insecure attachment in 15 adolescents with and 15 without IGD. This intervention included 12 × 60-min therapeutic riding sessions. Although the authors did not specifically focus on examining the VS, they observed that the intervention reduced IGD severity and increased FC in an affective network, which was associated with attachment in both adolescents with and without IGD.

Neuromodulatory Interventions for IGD

Some studies have used transcranial magnetic stimulation in individuals with IGD [119–121]. Most of these studies, as with GD, have focused on the DLPFC. Cue-induced craving may involve automatic responses to addiction-related cues that may be difficult to attenuate [120]. TDCS of the DLPFC may enhance control over both negative emotions and craving [121] and have effects on control and reward systems [120]. Hyperactivation of reward networks (including the striatum) may induce neuroadaptations in craving, in response to addiction-related stimuli [120]. Therefore, weakening the neural-processes related behaviors linked to craving may require improving executive control in individuals with IGD [120]. RTMS may also augment activity in frontostriatal circuits and, consequently, reduce craving and improve cognitive functioning [122].

3.3. Ventral Striatal Activation and BED/FA

FA models are based in part on neurobiological evidence in individuals with obesity, although this approach has been debated. Individuals with obesity may demonstrate greater cue-evoked activation of the VS and other cortical-striatal areas that encode food-related reward cues [123–125]. Furthermore, this food-cue evoked activation has been associated with subjective assessments of craving [126,127]. However, the specific role of the VS in individuals with FA warrants further consideration. FA has shown similarities with SUDs with respect to ventral striatal sensitization, but arguably not dorsal striatal alterations [128]. FA scores have been associated with VS activity [129]. Fasting has been associated with greater sensitivity of VS to the reward value of food, and this relationship may be modulated by FA [128]. At a theoretical level, FA has been associated with a reduced responsivity of a dorsal striatum network to changes in the reward value of food following satiety [130,131]. Similarly, individuals with BED may present a greater sensitivity to rewarding stimuli, associated with increased activity in the VS and other reward-related brain regions, such as the insula or the OFC, during the presentation of food cues [132].

3.3.1. Neural Mechanisms of Recovery in BED/FA
Pharmacological Interventions for BED/FA

As described previously [133], pharmacological treatments have been examined for BED including monoamine stimulants; monoamine reuptake inhibitors; 5-HT2C and trace amine receptor agonists; mu opioid, NOP, orexin 1, cannabinoid and receptor antagonists;

glutamate N-methyl-D-aspartate receptor antagonists; Sigma$_1$ ligands; and GABA$_B$ receptor agonists. However, although the efficacy of these options has been explored to a greater or lesser extent, there is an evident lack of studies examining the specific impact of these drugs on the VS.

Sibutramine. Few studies have tested the efficacy of pharmacological interventions at a neurobiological level. Balodis et al. [134] tested 19 patients with obesity and BED over 4 months of treatment with sibutramine and cognitive behavioral-self-help interventions, alone or in combination. Together with findings from their previous study [135], the authors suggested that individuals with BED have relatively diminished activation of reward circuitry, including the VS, to monetary cues. Further, among individuals with BED, those who exhibited persistent bingeing behaviors following treatment demonstrated less activation of reward circuitry (including the VA) to monetary cues at baseline. The reduced frontostriatal responses to non-food rewards seem to be relevant to treatment outcome, which suggest a certain pathophysiology of BED [133] that is similar to those of SUDs and their treatment responses, including in tobacco and cocaine use disorders.

Lisdexamfetamine. The effects of lisdexamfetamine at the neurobiological level have also been tested in individuals with BED [136]. Fleck et al. [137] observed that, at baseline, 20 women with BED had greater activation of the striatum, ventrolateral PFC and globus pallidus during the presentation of food images. This activation was related to treatment outcome. After 12 weeks of treatment, women with BED showed significant reductions in globus pallidus activation. Likewise, reductions in vmPFC correlated with reductions in binge eating behaviors. Other studies have associated lisdexamfetamine with reduced activity bilaterally in the thalamus in individuals with BED when viewing food pictures [138]. Likewise, lisdexamfetamine appears to reduce motor impulsivity, but does not appear to have an effect on working memory or emotional bias [138]. Lisdexamfetamine is currently the only drug with formal regulatory approval for treating BED.

Mu opioid receptor antagonist. The effects of GSK1521498, a mu opioid receptor antagonist, have also been tested in individuals with BED [139]. Twenty-eight days of treatment were associated with a significant reduction in pallidatum/putamen responses to high-calorie food images. However, subjective liking toward these images increased after pharmacological treatment.

Psychobehavioral Interventions for BED/FA

Reward re-training (RTT). The efficacy of RTT has been explored at a neurobiological level. RRT is a 10-session group-based behavioral treatment that aims to augment standard CBT [140]. It focuses on the identification and implementation of activities to increase responses to monetary and sustained rewards. RRT appears to have an impact on the hypo- and hyper-reward response of individuals with BED, as assessed by self-report and fMRI [140]. However, empirical evidence about the specific impact of different psychobehavioral interventions on the VS in individuals with BED/FA is needed.

CBT. Thirty-five studies that have used CBT to treat individuals with BED were identified in a meta-analysis [141]. However, there is a lack of studies assessing CBT in relation to the reward system. To the best of our knowledge, only the study by Balodis et al. [134] (mentioned above) examined brain relationships with multiple treatments including CBT. More research is needed to examine brain measures related to CBT specifically and its putative active ingredients, as is the case for other disorders like GD [65].

Neuromodulatory Interventions for BED/FA

A proof-of-concept study examined tDCS in individuals with BED (Burgess et al., 2016). Thirty individuals with BED were administered tDCS to DLPFC areas. However, the mechanisms of tDCS on the DLPFC in BED are unclear. On the one hand, stimulation may disrupt reward neurocircuitry from signaling. On the other hand, it may accelerate satiety signaling, thereby decreasing food consumption. These findings suggested different recovery processes in BED.

Dunlop et al. [142] administered 20–30 sessions of rTMS in 28 subjects with anorexia nervosa, binge-purge subtype or bulimia nervosa. Individuals were stratified into responder and non-responder groups regarding ≥50% reduction in weekly binge/purge frequency. Enhanced frontostriatal connectivity was linked in responders to dmPFC-repetitive TMS for binge/purge behaviors. In the non-responder group, rTMS generated paradoxical suppression of frontostriatal connectivity. However, studies exploring effects of non-invasive procedures on the VS in individuals with BED/FA are needed.

4. Limitations and Future Studies

First, it should be noted that the narrative nature of the present state-of-the art review has potential biases that future studies could resolve by conducting systematic reviews following PRISMA standards. Second, few studies have evaluated possible biomarkers in behavioral addictions and the effect of treatments on them. Even fewer studies have focused on the impact of both pharmacological and psychobehavioral interventions on the VS and the reward system. Moreover, studies that currently exist have typically used very small samples and heterogeneous treatments, making the results difficult to generalize and compare. Finally, the lack of clinical recognition of an FA construct makes its evaluation and treatment difficult and promotes heterogeneous study methodologies. Future studies could explore the specific role of the VS in behavioral addictions and the impacts of different treatments on them using large samples and less biased study designs.

5. Conclusions

The VS has been suggested as a relevant biomarker in behavioral addictions including GD, IGD and FA/BED due to its role in reward processing. However, more evidence is needed on how existing treatments for these behavioral addictions (pharmacological, psychobehavioral and neuromodulatory) may impact the activation of this specific brain area and its connectivity with others.

Author Contributions: Conceptualization, G.M.-B. and M.N.P.; methodology, G.M.-B. and M.N.P.; writing—original draft preparation, G.M.-B.; writing—review and editing, M.N.P.; visualization, M.N.P.; supervision, M.N.P. All authors have read and agreed to the published version of the manuscript.

Funding: Potenza's involvement was supported by the Connecticut Council on Problem Gambling and the National Institutes of Health (RF1 MH128614, NIDDK R01 DK121551). Mestre-Bach was supported by a FUNCIVA postdoctoral grant.

Institutional Review Board Statement: Not applicable.

Informed Consent Statement: Not applicable.

Data Availability Statement: Not applicable.

Conflicts of Interest: The authors declare no conflict of interest. Potenza has consulted for Opiant Pharmaceuticals, Idorsia Pharmaceuticals, AXA, Game Day Data, Baria-Tek and the Addiction Policy Forum; has been involved in a patent application with Yale University and Novartis; has received research support (to Yale) from Mohegan Sun Casino and the Connecticut Council on Problem Gambling; has participated in surveys, mailings or telephone consultations related to drug addiction, impulse control disorders or other health topics; has consulted for and/or advised gambling and legal entities on issues related to impulse control/addictive disorders; has provided clinical care in a problem gambling services program; has performed grant reviews for research-funding agencies; has edited journals and journal sections; has given academic lectures in grand rounds, CME events and other clinical or scientific venues; and has generated books or book chapters for publishers of mental health texts.

Glossary

ACC	anterior cingulate cortex
BED	binge eating disorder
CBT	cognitive behavioral therapy
CBI	craving behavioral intervention
DLPFC	dorsolateral prefrontal cortex
FA	food addiction
FC	functional connectivity
fMRI	functional magnetic resonance imaging
GD	gambling disorder
IGD	internet gaming disorder
NAc	nucleus accumbens
OFC	orbitofrontal cortex
PFC	prefrontal cortex
rTMS	repetitive transcranial magnetic stimulation
SUDs	substance use disorders
tDCS	transcranial direct current stimulation
VS	ventral striatum
VTA	ventral tegmental area
vmPFC	ventromedial prefrontal cortex

References

1. Warthen, K.G.; Boyse-Peacor, A.; Jones, K.G.; Sanford, B.; Love, T.M.; Mickey, B.J. Sex differences in the human reward system: Convergent behavioral, autonomic and neural evidence. *Soc. Cogn. Affect. Neurosci.* **2020**, *15*, 789–801. [CrossRef]
2. Potenza, M.N.; Hong, K.A.; Lacadie, C.M.; Fulbright, R.K.; Tuit, K.L.; Sinha, R. Neural correlates of stress-induced and cue-induced drug craving: Influences of sex and cocaine dependence. *Am. J. Psychiatry* **2012**, *169*, 406–414. [CrossRef] [PubMed]
3. Nia, A.B.; Mann, C.; Kaur, H.; Ranganathan, M. Cannabis Use: Neurobiological, Behavioral, and Sex/Gender Considerations. *Curr. Behav. Neurosci. Rep.* **2018**, *5*, 271–280.
4. Arias-Carrión, O.; Stamelou, M.; Murillo-Rodríguez, E.; Menéndez-González, M.; Pöppel, E. Dopaminergic reward system: A short integrative review. *Int. Arch. Med.* **2010**, *3*, 24. [CrossRef]
5. Haber, S.N.; Knutson, B. The reward circuit: Linking primate anatomy and human imaging. *Neuropsychopharmacology* **2010**, *35*, 4–26. [CrossRef]
6. Camara, E.; Rodriguez-Fornells, A.; Münte, T.F. Functional connectivity of reward processing in the brain. *Front. Hum. Neurosci.* **2008**, *2*, 19. [CrossRef]
7. Delgado, M.R.; Nystrom, L.E.; Fissell, C.; Noll, D.C.; Fiez, J.A. Tracking the hemodynamic responses to reward and punishment in the striatum. *J. Neurophysiol.* **2000**, *84*, 3072–3077. [CrossRef] [PubMed]
8. Delgado, M.R.; Locke, H.M.; Stenger, V.A.; Fiez, J.A. Dorsal striatum responses to reward and punishment: Effects of valence and magnitude manipulations. *Cogn. Affect. Behav. Neurosci.* **2003**, *3*, 27–38. [CrossRef]
9. May, J.C.; Delgado, M.R.; Dahl, R.E.; Stenger, V.A.; Ryan, N.D.; Fiez, J.A.; Carter, C.S. Event-related functional magnetic resonance imaging of reward-related brain circuitry in children and adolescents. *Biol. Psychiatry* **2004**, *55*, 359–366. [CrossRef]
10. Riba, J.; Krämer, U.M.; Heldmann, M.; Richter, S.; Münte, T.F. Dopamine agonist increases risk taking but blunts reward-related brain activity. *PLoS ONE* **2008**, *3*, e2479. [CrossRef]
11. Tom, S.M.; Fox, C.R.; Trepel, C.; Poldrack, R.A. The neural basis of loss aversion in decision-making under risk. *Science* **2007**, *315*, 515–518. [CrossRef]
12. Wei, D.; Lee, D.; Cox, C.D.; Karsten, C.A.; Peñagarikano, O.; Geschwind, D.H.; Gall, C.M.; Piomelli, D. Endocannabinoid signaling mediates oxytocin-driven social reward. *Proc. Natl. Acad. Sci. USA* **2015**, *112*, 14084–14089. [CrossRef]
13. Filippi, S.; Luconi, M.; Granchi, S.; Vignozzi, L.; Bettuzzi, S.; Tozzi, P.; Ledda, F.; Forti, G.; Maggi, M. Estrogens, but not androgens, regulate expression and functional activity of oxytocin receptor in rabbit epididymis. *Endocrinology* **2002**, *143*, 4271–4280. [CrossRef]
14. Vignozzi, L.; Filippi, S.; Luconi, M.; Morelli, A.; Mancina, R.; Marini, M.; Vannelli, G.B.; Granchi, S.; Orlando, C.; Gelmini, S.; et al. Oxytocin Receptor Is Expressed in the Penis and Mediates an Estrogen-Dependent Smooth Muscle Contractility. *Endocrinology* **2004**, *145*, 1823–1834. [CrossRef]
15. Galbally, M.; Lewis, A.J.; van Ijzendoorn, M.; Permezel, M. The role of oxytocin in mother-infant relations: A systematic review of human studies. *Harv. Rev. Psychiatry* **2011**, *19*, 1–14. [CrossRef] [PubMed]
16. Kor, A.; Djalovski, A.; Potenza, M.N.; Zagoory-Sharon, O.; Feldman, R. Alterations in oxytocin and vasopressin in men with problematic pornography use: The role of empathy. *J. Behav. Addict.* **2022**, *11*, 116–127. [CrossRef] [PubMed]
17. Kim, S.; Kwok, S.; Mayes, L.C.; Potenza, M.N.; Rutherford, H.J.V.; Strathearn, L. Early adverse experience and substance addiction: Dopamine, oxytocin, and glucocorticoid pathways. *Ann. N. Y. Acad. Sci.* **2017**, *1394*, 74–91. [CrossRef] [PubMed]

18. Alvarez-Monjaras, M.; Mayes, L.C.; Potenza, M.N.; Rutherford, H.J. A developmental model of addictions: Integrating neurobiological and psychodynamic theories through the lens of attachment. *Attach. Hum. Dev.* **2019**, *21*, 616–637. [CrossRef]
19. Baik, J.-H. Dopamine signaling in reward-related behaviors. *Front. Neural. Circuits* **2013**, *7*, 152. [CrossRef]
20. Volkow, N.D.; Wang, G.-J.; Baler, R.D. Reward, dopamine and the control of food intake: Implications for obesity. *Trends Cogn. Sci.* **2011**, *15*, 37–46. [CrossRef]
21. Gola, M.; Draps, M. Ventral Striatal Reactivity in Compulsive Sexual Behaviors. *Front. Psychiatry* **2018**, *9*, 546. [CrossRef] [PubMed]
22. Robinson, T.E.; Berridge, K.C. The neural basis of drug craving: An incentive-sensitization theory of addiction. *Brain Res. Brain Res. Rev.* **1993**, *18*, 247–291. [CrossRef] [PubMed]
23. Blum, K.; Gardner, E.; Oscar-Berman, M.; Gold, M. "Liking" and "wanting" linked to Reward Deficiency Syndrome (RDS): Hypothesizing differential responsivity in brain reward circuitry. *Curr. Pharm. Des.* **2012**, *18*, 113–118. [CrossRef]
24. Comings, D.E.; Blum, K. Reward deficiency syndrome: Genetic aspects of behavioral disorders. *Prog. Brain Res.* **2000**, *126*, 325–341. [CrossRef]
25. Volkow, N.D.; Fowler, J.S.; Wang, G.-J.; Swanson, J.M. Dopamine in drug abuse and addiction: Results from imaging studies and treatment implications. *Mol. Psychiatry* **2004**, *9*, 557–569. [CrossRef] [PubMed]
26. Schmidt, A.; Denier, N.; Magon, S.; Radue, E.-W.; Huber, C.G.; Riecher-Rossler, A.; Wiesbeck, G.A.; Lang, U.E.; Borgwardt, S.; Walter, M. Increased functional connectivity in the resting-state basal ganglia network after acute heroin substitution. *Transl. Psychiatry* **2015**, *5*, e533. [CrossRef] [PubMed]
27. Forbes, E.E.; Rodriguez, E.E.; Musselman, S.; Narendran, R. Prefrontal response and frontostriatal functional connectivity to monetary reward in abstinent alcohol-dependent young adults. *PLoS ONE* **2014**, *9*, e94640. [CrossRef]
28. Gelskov, S.V.; Madsen, K.H.; Ramsøy, T.Z.; Siebner, H.R. Aberrant neural signatures of decision-making: Pathological gamblers display cortico-striatal hypersensitivity to extreme gambles. *Neuroimage* **2016**, *128*, 342–352. [CrossRef]
29. Hong, S.-B.; Harrison, B.J.; Dandash, O.; Choi, E.-J.; Kim, S.-C.; Kim, H.-H.; Shim, D.-H.; Kim, C.-D.; Kim, J.-W.; Yi, S.-H. A selective involvement of putamen functional connectivity in youth with internet gaming disorder. *Brain Res.* **2015**, *1602*, 85–95. [CrossRef]
30. APA. *Diagnostic and Statistical Manual of Mental Disorders 5 Edition (DSM-5) 5*; American Psychiatric Association: Washington, DC, USA, 2013.
31. World Health Organization. *International Classification of Diseases 11th Revision*; ICD-11; WHO: Geneva, Switzerland, 2019.
32. Schulte, E.M.; Joyner, M.A.; Potenza, M.N.; Grilo, C.M.; Gearhardt, A.N. Current considerations regarding food addiction. *Curr. Psychiatry Rep.* **2015**, *17*, 563. [CrossRef]
33. Kessler, R.M.; Hutson, P.H.; Herman, B.K.; Potenza, M.N. The neurobiological basis of binge-eating disorder. *Neurosci. Biobehav. Rev.* **2016**, *63*, 223–238. [CrossRef] [PubMed]
34. Novelle, M.G.; Diéguez, C. Food Addiction and Binge Eating: Lessons Learned from Animal Models. *Nutrients* **2018**, *10*, 71. [CrossRef] [PubMed]
35. Gearhardt, A.N.; White, M.A.; Potenza, M.N. Binge eating disorder and food addiction. *Curr. Drug Abus. Rev.* **2011**, *4*, 201–207. [CrossRef]
36. Wiedemann, A.A.; Ivezaj, V.; Gueorguieva, R.; Potenza, M.N.; Grilo, C.M. Examining Self-Weighing Behaviors and Associated Features and Treatment Outcomes in Patients with Binge-Eating Disorder and Obesity with and without Food Addiction. *Nutrients* **2020**, *13*, 29. [CrossRef] [PubMed]
37. Georgel, P.T.; Georgel, P. Where Epigenetics Meets Food Intake: Their Interaction in the Development/Severity of Gout and Therapeutic Perspectives. *Front. Immunol.* **2021**, *12*, 752359. [CrossRef]
38. Nestler, E.J.; Lüscher, C. The Molecular Basis of Drug Addiction: Linking Epigenetic to Synaptic and Circuit Mechanisms. *Neuron* **2019**, *102*, 48–59. [CrossRef]
39. Bullock, S.A.; Potenza, M.N. Pathological Gambling: Neuropsychopharmacology and Treatment. *Curr. Psychopharmacol.* **2012**, *1*, 67–85. [CrossRef]
40. Koehler, S.; Hasselmann, E.; Wüstenberg, T.; Heinz, A.; Romanczuk-Seiferth, N. Higher volume of ventral striatum and right prefrontal cortex in pathological gambling. *Brain Struct. Funct.* **2015**, *220*, 469–477. [CrossRef]
41. Van Holst, R.J.; van den Brink, W.; Veltman, D.J.; Goudriaan, A.E. Brain imaging studies in pathological gambling. *Curr. Psychiatry Rep.* **2010**, *12*, 418–425. [CrossRef]
42. Limbrick-Oldfield, E.H.; van Holst, R.J.; Clark, L. Fronto-striatal dysregulation in drug addiction and pathological gambling: Consistent inconsistencies? *NeuroImage. Clin.* **2013**, *2*, 385–393. [CrossRef]
43. Potenza, M.N. The neural bases of cognitive processes in gambling disorder. *Trends Cogn. Sci.* **2014**, *18*, 429–438. [CrossRef] [PubMed]
44. Studer, B.; Apergis-Schoute, A.M.; Robbins, T.W.; Clark, L. What are the Odds? The Neural Correlates of Active Choice during Gambling. *Front. Neurosci.* **2012**, *6*, 46. [CrossRef] [PubMed]
45. Koehler, S.; Ovadia-Caro, S.; van der Meer, E.; Villringer, A.; Heinz, A.; Romanczuk-Seiferth, N.; Margulies, D. Increased functional connectivity between prefrontal cortex and reward system in pathological gambling. *PLoS ONE* **2013**, *8*, e84565. [CrossRef] [PubMed]

46. Clark, L.; Boileau, I.; Zack, M. Neuroimaging of reward mechanisms in Gambling disorder: An integrative review. *Mol. Psychiatry* **2019**, *24*, 674–693. [CrossRef] [PubMed]
47. Brevers, D.; Noël, X.; He, Q.; Melrose, J.A.; Bechara, A. Increased ventral-striatal activity during monetary decision making is a marker of problem poker gambling severity. *Addict. Biol.* **2016**, *21*, 688–699. [CrossRef]
48. Raimo, S.; Cropano, M.; Trojano, L.; Santangelo, G. The neural basis of gambling disorder: An activation likelihood estimation meta-analysis. *Neurosci. Biobehav. Rev.* **2021**, *120*, 279–302. [CrossRef] [PubMed]
49. Reuter, J.; Raedler, T.; Rose, M.; Hand, I.; Gläscher, J.; Büchel, C. Pathological gambling is linked to reduced activation of the mesolimbic reward system. *Nat. Neurosci.* **2005**, *8*, 147–148. [CrossRef] [PubMed]
50. de Ruiter, M.B.; Veltman, D.J.; Goudriaan, A.E.; Oosterlaan, J.; Sjoerds, Z.; van den Brink, W. Response perseveration and ventral prefrontal sensitivity to reward and punishment in male problem gamblers and smokers. *Neuropsychopharmacology* **2009**, *34*, 1027–1038. [CrossRef] [PubMed]
51. Balodis, I.M.; Kober, H.; Worhunsky, P.D.; Stevens, M.C.; Pearlson, G.D.; Potenza, M.N. Diminished frontostriatal activity during processing of monetary rewards and losses in pathological gambling. *Biol. Psychiatry* **2012**, *71*, 749–757. [CrossRef]
52. Sescousse, G.; Barbalat, G.; Domenech, P.; Dreher, J.-C. Imbalance in the sensitivity to different types of rewards in pathological gambling. *Brain* **2013**, *136*, 2527–2538. [CrossRef] [PubMed]
53. van Holst, R.J.; van Holstein, M.; van den Brink, W.; Veltman, D.J.; Goudriaan, A.E. Response inhibition during cue reactivity in problem gamblers: An fMRI study. *PLoS ONE* **2012**, *7*, e30909. [CrossRef]
54. EH, L.-O.; Mick, I.; RE, C.; McGonigle, J.; SP, S.; AP, G.; PR, S.; Waldman, A.; Erritzoe, D.; Bowden-Jones, H.; et al. Neural substrates of cue reactivity and craving in gambling disorder. *Transl. Psychiatry* **2017**, *7*, e992. [CrossRef]
55. Chase, H.W.; Clark, L. Gambling severity predicts midbrain response to near-miss outcomes. *J. Neurosci.* **2010**, *30*, 6180–6187. [CrossRef]
56. Clark, L.; Lawrence, A.J.; Astley-Jones, F.; Gray, N. Gambling near-misses enhance motivation to gamble and recruit win-related brain circuitry. *Neuron* **2009**, *61*, 481–490. [CrossRef]
57. Worhunsky, P.D.; Malison, R.T.; Rogers, R.D.; Potenza, M.N. Altered neural correlates of reward and loss processing during simulated slot-machine fMRI in pathological gambling and cocaine dependence. *Drug Alcohol. Depend.* **2014**, *145*, 77–86. [CrossRef]
58. Sescousse, G.; Janssen, L.K.; Hashemi, M.M.; Timmer, M.H.M.; Geurts, D.E.M.; Ter Huurne, N.P.; Clark, L.; Cools, R. Amplified Striatal Responses to Near-Miss Outcomes in Pathological Gamblers. *Neuropsychopharmacology* **2016**, *41*, 2614–2623. [CrossRef]
59. Potenza, M.N.; Balodis, I.M.; Derevensky, J.; Grant, J.E.; Petry, N.M.; Verdejo-Garcia, A.; Yip, S.W. Gambling disorder. *Nat. Rev. Dis. Prim.* **2019**, *5*, 51. [CrossRef]
60. Bae, S.; Hong, J.S.; Kim, S.M.; Han, D.H. Bupropion shows different effects on brain functional connectivity in patients with Internet-based gambling disorder and internet gaming disorder. *Front. Psychiatry* **2018**, *9*, 130. [CrossRef]
61. Grant, J.E.; Odlaug, B.L.; Chamberlain, S.R.; Hampshire, A.; Schreiber, L.R.N.; Kim, S.W. A proof of concept study of tolcapone for pathological gambling: Relationships with COMT genotype and brain activation. *Eur. Neuropsychopharmacol.* **2013**, *23*, 1587–1596. [CrossRef]
62. Chung, S.K.; You, I.H.; Cho, G.H.; Chung, G.H.; Shin, Y.C.; Kim, D.J.; Choi, S.W. Changes of functional MRI findings in a patient whose pathological gambling improved with fluvoxamine. *Yonsei Med. J.* **2009**, *50*, 441–444. [CrossRef]
63. Pallanti, S.; Haznedar, M.M.; Hollander, E.; Licalzi, E.M.; Bernardi, S.; Newmark, R.; Buchsbaum, M.S. Basal ganglia activity in pathological gambling: A fluorodeoxyglucose- positron emission tomography study. *Neuropsychobiology* **2010**, *62*, 132–138. [CrossRef] [PubMed]
64. Hollander, E.; Buchsbaum, M.S.; Haznedar, M.M.; Berenguer, J.; Berlin, H.A.; Chaplin, W.; Goodman, C.R.; LiCalzi, E.M.; Newmark, R.; Pallanti, S. FDG-PET study in pathological gamblers: 1. Lithium increases orbitofrontal, dorsolateral and cingulate metabolism. *Neuropsychobiology* **2008**, *58*, 37–47. [CrossRef] [PubMed]
65. Potenza, M.N.; Balodis, I.M.; Franco, C.A.; Bullock, S.; Xua, J.; Chung, T.; Grant, J.E. Neurobiological considerations in understanding behavioral treatments for pathological gambling. *Psychol. Addict Behav* **2013**, *27*, 380–392. [CrossRef]
66. Spagnolo, P.A.; Gómez Pérez, L.J.; Terraneo, A.; Gallimberti, L.; Bonci, A. Neural correlates of cue- and stress-induced craving in gambling disorders: Implications for transcranial magnetic stimulation interventions. *Eur. J. Neurosci.* **2019**, *50*, 2370–2383. [CrossRef]
67. Gay, A.; Boutet, C.; Sigaud, T.; Kamgoue, A.; Sevos, J.; Brunelin, J.; Massoubre, C. A single session of repetitive transcranial magnetic stimulation of the prefrontal cortex reduces cue-induced craving in patients with gambling disorder. *Eur. Psychiatry* **2017**, *41*, 68–74. [CrossRef]
68. Gay, A.; Cabe, J.; De Chazeron, I.; Lambert, C.; Defour, M.; Bhoowabul, V.; Charpeaud, T.; Tremey, A.; Llorca, P.-M.; Pereira, B.; et al. Repetitive Transcranial Magnetic Stimulation (rTMS) as a Promising Treatment for Craving in Stimulant Drugs and Behavioral Addiction: A Meta-Analysis. *J. Clin. Med.* **2022**, *11*, 624. [CrossRef]
69. Soyata, A.Z.; Aksu, S.; Woods, A.J.; İşçen, P.; Saçar, K.T.; Karamürsel, S. Effect of transcranial direct current stimulation on decision making and cognitive flexibility in gambling disorder. *Eur. Arch. Psychiatry Clin. Neurosci.* **2019**, *269*, 275–284. [CrossRef]
70. Pettorruso, M.; Di Giuda, D.; Martinotti, G.; Cocciolillo, F.; De Risio, L.; Montemitro, C.; Camardese, G.; Di Nicola, M.; Janiri, L.; di Giannantonio, M.; et al. Dopaminergic and clinical correlates of high-frequency repetitive transcranial magnetic stimulation in gambling addiction: A SPECT case study. *Addict. Behav.* **2019**, *93*, 246–249. [CrossRef]

71. Martinotti, G.; Chillemi, E.; Lupi, M.; De Risio, L.; Pettorruso, M.; Giannantonio, M. Di Gambling disorder and bilateral transcranial direct current stimulation: A case report. *J. Behav. Addict.* **2018**, *7*, 834–837. [CrossRef]
72. Dickler, M.; Lenglos, C.; Renauld, E.; Ferland, F.; Edden, R.; Leblond, J.; Fecteau, S. Online effects of transcranial direct current stimulation on prefrontal metabolites in gambling disorder. *Neuropharmacology* **2018**, *131*, 51–57. [CrossRef]
73. Wei, L.; Zhang, S.; Turel, O.; Bechara, A.; He, Q. A tripartite neurocognitive model of internet gaming disorder. *Front. Psychiatry* **2017**, *8*, 285. [CrossRef]
74. Turel, O.; He, Q.; Wei, L.; Bechara, A. The role of the insula in internet gaming disorder. *Addict. Biol.* **2021**, *26*, e12894. [CrossRef]
75. Liu, Z.; Huang, P.; Gong, Y.; Wang, Y.; Wu, Y.; Wang, C.; Guo, X. Altered neural responses to missed chance contribute to the risk-taking behaviour in individuals with Internet gaming disorder. *Addict. Biol.* **2022**, *27*, e13124. [CrossRef]
76. Liu, L.; Xue, G.; Potenza, M.N.; Zhang, J.T.; Yao, Y.W.; Xia, C.C.; Lan, J.; Ma, S.S.; Fang, X.Y. Dissociable neural processes during risky decision-making in individuals with Internet-gaming disorder. *NeuroImage Clin.* **2017**, *14*, 741–749. [CrossRef]
77. Young, K.S.; Brand, M. Merging theoretical models and therapy approaches in the context of internet gaming disorder: A personal perspective. *Front. Psychol.* **2017**, *8*, 1853. [CrossRef]
78. Vollstädt-Klein, S.; Wichert, S.; Rabinstein, J.; Bühler, M.; Klein, O.; Ende, G.; Hermann, D.; Mann, K. Initial, habitual and compulsive alcohol use is characterized by a shift of cue processing from ventral to dorsal striatum. *Addiction* **2010**, *105*, 1741–1749. [CrossRef]
79. Volkow, N.D.; Wang, G.-J.; Telang, F.; Fowler, J.S.; Logan, J.; Childress, A.-R.; Jayne, M.; Ma, Y.; Wong, C. Cocaine cues and dopamine in dorsal striatum: Mechanism of craving in cocaine addiction. *J. Neurosci.* **2006**, *26*, 6583–6588. [CrossRef]
80. Volkow, N.D.; Wang, G.-J.; Telang, F.; Fowler, J.S.; Logan, J.; Childress, A.-R.; Jayne, M.; Ma, Y.; Wong, C. Dopamine increases in striatum do not elicit craving in cocaine abusers unless they are coupled with cocaine cues. *Neuroimage* **2008**, *39*, 1266–1273. [CrossRef]
81. Liu, L.; Yip, S.W.; Zhang, J.-T.; Wang, L.-J.; Shen, Z.-J.; Liu, B.; Ma, S.-S.; Yao, Y.-W.; Fang, X.-Y. Activation of the ventral and dorsal striatum during cue reactivity in Internet gaming disorder. *Addict. Biol.* **2017**, *22*, 791–801. [CrossRef]
82. Yuan, K.; Yu, D.; Cai, C.; Feng, D.; Li, Y.; Bi, Y.; Liu, J.; Zhang, Y.; Jin, C.; Li, L.; et al. Frontostriatal circuits, resting state functional connectivity and cognitive control in internet gaming disorder. *Addict. Biol.* **2017**, *22*, 813–822. [CrossRef]
83. Wang, M.; Zheng, H.; Zhou, W.; Jiang, Q.; Dong, G.-H. Persistent dependent behaviour is accompanied by dynamic switching between the ventral and dorsal striatal connections in internet gaming disorder. *Addict. Biol.* **2021**, *26*, e13046. [CrossRef]
84. Brand, M.; Wegmann, E.; Stark, R.; Müller, A.; Wölfling, K.; Robbins, T.W.; Potenza, M.N. The Interaction of Person-Affect-Cognition-Execution (I-PACE) model for addictive behaviors: Update, generalization to addictive behaviors beyond internet-use disorders, and specification of the process character of addictive behaviors. *Neurosci. Biobehav. Rev.* **2019**, *104*, 1–10. [CrossRef]
85. Weinstein, A.M. Computer and video game addiction-a comparison between game users and non-game users. *Am. J. Drug Alcohol. Abus.* **2010**, *36*, 268–276. [CrossRef]
86. Kühn, S.; Romanowski, A.; Schilling, C.; Lorenz, R.; Mörsen, C.; Seiferth, N.; Banaschewski, T.; Barbot, A.; Barker, G.J.; Büchel, C.; et al. The neural basis of video gaming. *Transl. Psychiatry* **2011**, *1*, e53. [CrossRef]
87. Weinstein, A.; Livny, A.; Weizman, A. New developments in brain research of internet and gaming disorder. *Neurosci. Biobehav. Rev.* **2017**, *75*, 314–330. [CrossRef]
88. Cai, C.; Yuan, K.; Yin, J.; Feng, D.; Bi, Y.; Li, Y.; Yu, D.; Jin, C.; Qin, W.; Tian, J. Striatum morphometry is associated with cognitive control deficits and symptom severity in internet gaming disorder. *Brain Imaging Behav.* **2016**, *10*, 12–20. [CrossRef]
89. Hou, H.; Jia, S.; Hu, S.; Fan, R.; Sun, W.; Sun, T.; Zhang, H. Reduced striatal dopamine transporters in people with internet addiction disorder. *J. Biomed. Biotechnol.* **2012**, *2012*, 854524. [CrossRef]
90. Palaus, M.; Marron, E.M.; Viejo-Sobera, R.; Redolar-Ripoll, D. Neural basis of video gaming: A systematic review. *Front. Hum. Neurosci.* **2017**, *11*, 248. [CrossRef]
91. Lorenz, R.C.; Krüger, J.-K.; Neumann, B.; Schott, B.H.; Kaufmann, C.; Heinz, A.; Wüstenberg, T. Cue reactivity and its inhibition in pathological computer game players. *Addict. Biol.* **2013**, *18*, 134–146. [CrossRef]
92. Dong, G.-H.; Dong, H.; Wang, M.; Zhang, J.; Zhou, W.; Du, X.; Potenza, M.N. Dorsal and ventral striatal functional connectivity shifts play a potential role in internet gaming disorder. *Commun. Biol.* **2021**, *4*, 866. [CrossRef]
93. Shin, Y.B.; Kim, H.; Kim, S.J.; Kim, J.J. A neural mechanism of the relationship between impulsivity and emotion dysregulation in patients with Internet gaming disorder. *Addict. Biol.* **2021**, *26*, e12916. [CrossRef]
94. Chun, J.W.; Park, C.H.; Kim, J.Y.; Choi, J.; Cho, H.; Jung, D.J.; Ahn, K.J.; Choi, J.S.; Kim, D.J.; Choi, I.Y. Altered core networks of brain connectivity and personality traits in internet gaming disorder. *J. Behav. Addict.* **2020**, *9*, 298–311. [CrossRef] [PubMed]
95. Kim, J.; Kim, H.; Kang, E. Impaired Feedback Processing for Symbolic Reward in Individuals with Internet Game Overuse. *Front. Psychiatry* **2017**, *8*, 195. [CrossRef]
96. Dong, H.; Wang, M.; Zhang, J.; Hu, Y.; Potenza, M.N.; Dong, G.-H. Reduced frontostriatal functional connectivity and associations with severity of Internet gaming disorder. *Addict. Biol.* **2021**, *26*, e12985. [CrossRef]
97. Gong, L.; Zhou, H.; Su, C.; Geng, F.; Xi, W.; Teng, B.; Yuan, K.; Zhao, M.; Hu, Y. Self-control impacts symptoms defining Internet gaming disorder through dorsal anterior cingulate-ventral striatal pathway. *Addict. Biol.* **2022**, *27*, e13210. [CrossRef]
98. Kim, J.; Kang, E. Internet Game Overuse Is Associated With an Alteration of Fronto-Striatal Functional Connectivity During Reward Feedback Processing. *Front. Psychiatry* **2018**, *9*, 371. [CrossRef]

99. Dong, G.H.; Wang, M.; Zhang, J.; Du, X.; Potenza, M.N. Functional neural changes and altered cortical–subcortical connectivity associated with recovery from Internet gaming disorder. *J. Behav. Addict.* **2019**, *8*, 692–702. [CrossRef]
100. Dong, G.; Wang, M.; Liu, X.; Liang, Q.; Du, X.; Potenza, M.N. Cue-elicited craving-related lentiform activation during gaming deprivation is associated with the emergence of Internet gaming disorder. *Addict Biol.* **2020**, *25*, e12713. [CrossRef]
101. Zajac, K.; Ginley, M.K.; Chang, R. Treatments of internet gaming disorder: A systematic review of the evidence. *Expert Rev. Neurother.* **2020**, *20*, 85–93. [CrossRef] [PubMed]
102. Zajac, K.; Ginley, M.K.; Chang, R.; Petry, N.M. Treatments for Internet Gaming Disorder and Internet Addiction: A Systematic Review. *Psychol. Addict Behav.* **2017**, *31*, 979–994. [CrossRef]
103. Park, J.H.; Lee, Y.S.; Sohn, J.H.; Han, D.H. Effectiveness of atomoxetine and methylphenidate for problematic online gaming in adolescents with attention deficit hyperactivity disorder. *Hum. Psychopharmacol.* **2016**, *31*, 427–432. [CrossRef]
104. Han, D.H.; Hwang, J.W.; Renshaw, P.F. Bupropion sustained release treatment decreases craving for video games and cue-induced brain activity in patients with internet video game addiction. *Exp. Clin. Psychopharmacol.* **2010**, *18*, 297–304. [CrossRef]
105. Seo, E.H.; Yang, H.J.; Kim, S.G.; Park, S.C.; Lee, S.K.; Yoon, H.J. A Literature Review on the Efficacy and Related Neural Effects of Pharmacological and Psychosocial Treatments in Individuals With Internet Gaming Disorder. *Psychiatry Investig.* **2021**, *18*, 1149–1163. [CrossRef]
106. Nam, B.; Bae, S.; Kim, S.M.; Hong, J.S.; Han, D.H. Comparing the Effects of Bupropion and Escitalopram on Excessive Internet Game Play in Patients with Major Depressive Disorder. *Clin. Psychopharmacol. Neurosci.* **2017**, *15*, 361–368. [CrossRef]
107. Konova, A.B.; Moeller, S.J.; Goldstein, R.Z. Common and distinct neural targets of treatment: Changing brain function in substance addiction. *Neurosci. Biobehav. Rev.* **2013**, *37*, 2806–2817. [CrossRef]
108. Garland, E.L.; Froeliger, B.; Howard, M.O. Neurophysiological evidence for remediation of reward processing deficits in chronic pain and opioid misuse following treatment with Mindfulness-Oriented Recovery Enhancement: Exploratory ERP findings from a pilot RCT. *J. Behav. Med.* **2015**, *38*, 327–336. [CrossRef]
109. Vollstädt-Klein, S.; Loeber, S.; Kirsch, M.; Bach, P.; Richter, A.; Bhler, M.; Von Der Goltz, C.; Hermann, D.; Mann, K.; Kiefer, F. Effects of cue-exposure treatment on neural cue reactivity in alcohol dependence: A randomized trial. *Biol. Psychiatry* **2011**, *69*, 1060–1066. [CrossRef]
110. Han, X.; Wang, Y.; Jiang, W.; Bao, X.; Sun, Y.; Ding, W.; Cao, M.; Wu, X.; Du, Y.; Zhou, Y. Resting-state activity of prefrontal-striatal circuits in internet gaming disorder: Changes with cognitive behavior therapy and predictors of treatment response. *Front. Psychiatry* **2018**, *9*, 341. [CrossRef]
111. Park, S.Y.; Kim, S.M.; Roh, S.; Soh, M.A.; Lee, S.H.; Kim, H.; Lee, Y.S.; Han, D.H. The effects of a virtual reality treatment program for online gaming addiction. *Comput. Methods Programs Biomed.* **2016**, *129*, 99–108. [CrossRef]
112. Han, D.H.; Kim, S.M.; Lee, Y.S.; Renshaw, P.F. The effect of family therapy on the changes in the severity of on-line game play and brain activity in adolescents with on-line game addiction. *Psychiatry Res. Neuroimaging* **2012**, *202*, 126–131. [CrossRef]
113. Zhang, J.T.; Ma, S.S.; Li, C.S.R.; Liu, L.; Xia, C.C.; Lan, J.; Wang, L.-J.; Liu, B.; Yao, Y.W.; Fang, X.-Y. Craving Behavioral Intervention for Internet Gaming Disorder: Remediation of Functional Connectivity of the Ventral Striatum. *Addict Biol.* **2018**, *23*, 337–346. [CrossRef]
114. Zhang, J.T.; Yao, Y.W.; Potenza, M.N.; Xia, C.C.; Lan, J.; Liu, L.; Wang, L.J.; Liu, B.; Ma, S.S.; Fang, X.Y. Effects of craving behavioral intervention on neural substrates of cue-induced craving in Internet gaming disorder. *NeuroImage Clin.* **2016**, *12*, 591–599. [CrossRef]
115. Wang, Z.L.; Potenza, M.N.; Song, K.R.; Fang, X.Y.; Liu, L.; Ma, S.S.; Xia, C.C.; Lan, J.; Yao, Y.W.; Zhang, J.T. Neural classification of internet gaming disorder and prediction of treatment response using a cue-reactivity fMRI task in young men. *J. Psychiatr. Res.* **2020**, *145*, 309–316. [CrossRef]
116. Zheng, H.; Hu, Y.; Wang, Z.; Wang, M.; Du, X.; Dong, G. Meta-analyses of the functional neural alterations in subjects with Internet gaming disorder: Similarities and differences across different paradigms. *Prog. Neuropsychopharmacol. Biol. Psychiatry* **2019**, *94*, 109656. [CrossRef] [PubMed]
117. Liu, L.; Potenza, M.N.; Lacadie, C.M.; Zhang, J.T.; Yip, S.W.; Xia, C.C.; Lan, J.; Yao, Y.W.; Deng, L.Y.; Park, S.Q.; et al. Altered intrinsic connectivity distribution in internet gaming disorder and its associations with psychotherapy treatment outcomes. *Addict. Biol.* **2021**, *26*, e12917. [CrossRef]
118. Kang, K.D.; Jung, T.W.; Park, I.H.; Han, D.H. Effects of equine-assisted activities and therapies on the affective network of adolescents with internet gaming disorder. *J. Altern. Complement. Med.* **2018**, *24*, 841–849. [CrossRef]
119. Lee, J.; Jang, J.H.; Choi, A.R.; Chung, S.J.; Kim, B.; Park, M.; Oh, S.; Jung, M.H.; Choi, J. Neuromodulatory Effect of Transcranial Direct Current Stimulation on Resting-State EEG Activity in Internet Gaming Disorder: A Randomized, Double-Blind, Sham-Controlled Parallel Group Trial. *Cereb. Cortex Commun.* **2021**, *2*, tgaa095. [CrossRef] [PubMed]
120. Wu, L.L.; Potenza, M.N.; Zhou, N.; Kober, H.; Shi, X.H.; Yip, S.W.; Xu, J.H.; Zhu, L.; Wang, R.; Liu, G.Q.; et al. Efficacy of single-session transcranial direct current stimulation on addiction-related inhibitory control and craving: A randomized trial in males with internet gaming disorder. *J. Psychiatry Neurosci.* **2021**, *46*, E111–E118. [CrossRef] [PubMed]
121. Wu, L.; Potenza, M.N.; Zhou, N.; Kober, H.; Shi, X.; Yip, S.W.; Xu, J.; Zhu, L.; Liu, G.; Zhang, J.; et al. A Role for the Right Dorsolateral Prefrontal Cortex in Enhancing Regulation of both Craving and Negative Emotions in Internet Gaming Disorder: A Randomized Trial. *Eur. Neuropsychopharmacol.* **2021**, *36*, 29–37. [CrossRef]

122. Cuppone, D.; Perez, L.J.G.; Cardullo, S.; Cellini, N.; Sarlo, M.; Soldatesca, S.; Chindamo, S.; Madeo, G.; Gallimberti, L. The role of repetitive transcranial magnetic stimulation (rTMS) in the treatment of behavioral addictions: Two case reports and review of the literature. *J. Behav. Addict.* **2021**, *10*, 361–370. [CrossRef] [PubMed]
123. Potenza, M.N. Obesity, food, and addiction: Emerging neuroscience and clinical and public health implications. *Neuropsychopharmacology* **2014**, *39*, 249–250. [CrossRef]
124. Stoeckel, L.E.; Weller, R.E.; Cook, E.W.; Twieg, D.B.; Knowlton, R.C.; Cox, J.E. Widespread reward-system activation in obese women in response to pictures of high-calorie foods. *Neuroimage* **2008**, *41*, 636–647. [CrossRef] [PubMed]
125. Davids, S.; Lauffer, H.; Thoms, K.; Jagdhuhn, M.; Hirschfeld, H.; Domin, M.; Hamm, A.; Lotze, M. Increased dorsolateral prefrontal cortex activation in obese children during observation of food stimuli. *Int. J. Obes.* **2010**, *34*, 94–104. [CrossRef] [PubMed]
126. Pelchat, M.L.; Johnson, A.; Chan, R.; Valdez, J.; Ragland, J.D. Images of desire: Food-craving activation during fMRI. *Neuroimage* **2004**, *23*, 1486–1493. [CrossRef] [PubMed]
127. Hommer, R.E.; Seo, D.; Lacadie, C.M.; Chaplin, T.M.; Mayes, L.C.; Sinha, R.; Potenza, M.N. Neural correlates of stress and favorite-food cue exposure in adolescents: A functional magnetic resonance imaging study. *Hum. Brain Mapp.* **2013**, *34*, 2561–2573. [CrossRef]
128. Contreras-Rodriguez, O.; Burrows, T.; Pursey, K.M.; Stanwell, P.; Parkes, L.; Soriano-Mas, C.; Verdejo-Garcia, A. Food addiction linked to changes in ventral striatum functional connectivity between fasting and satiety. *Appetite* **2019**, *133*, 18–23. [CrossRef]
129. Romer, A.L.; Su Kang, M.; Nikolova, Y.S.; Gearhardt, A.N.; Hariri, A.R. Dopamine genetic risk is related to food addiction and body mass through reduced reward-related ventral striatum activity. *Appetite* **2019**, *133*, 24–31. [CrossRef]
130. Smith, D.G.; Robbins, T.W. The neurobiological underpinnings of obesity and binge eating: A rationale for adopting the food addiction model. *Biol. Psychiatry* **2013**, *73*, 804–810. [CrossRef]
131. Tomasi, D.; Volkow, N.D. Striatocortical pathway dysfunction in addiction and obesity: Differences and similarities. *Crit. Rev. Biochem. Mol. Biol.* **2013**, *48*, 1–19. [CrossRef]
132. Romei, A.; Voigt, K.; Verdejo-Garcia, A. A Perspective on Candidate Neural Underpinnings of Binge Eating Disorder: Reward and Homeostatic Systems. *Curr. Pharm. Des.* **2020**, *26*, 2327–2333. [CrossRef]
133. Hutson, P.H.; Balodis, I.M.; Potenza, M.N. Binge-eating disorder: Clinical and therapeutic advances. *Pharmacol. Ther.* **2018**, *182*, 15–27. [CrossRef] [PubMed]
134. Balodis, I.M.; Grilo, C.M.; Kober, H.; Worhunsky, P.D.; White, M.A.; Stevens, M.C.; Pearlson, G.D.; Potenza, M.N. A pilot study linking reduced fronto-Striatal recruitment during reward processing to persistent bingeing following treatment for binge-eating disorder. *Int. J. Eat. Disord.* **2014**, *47*, 376–384. [CrossRef]
135. Balodis, I.M.; Kober, H.; Worhunsky, P.D.; White, M.A.; Stevens, M.C.; Pearlson, G.D.; Sinha, R.; Grilo, C.M.; Potenza, M.N. Monetary reward processing in obese individuals with and without binge eating disorder. *Biol. Psychiatry* **2013**, *73*, 877–886. [CrossRef]
136. Griffiths, K.R.; Yang, J.; Touyz, S.W.; Hay, P.J.; Clarke, S.D.; Korgaonkar, M.S.; Gomes, L.; Anderson, G.; Foster, S.; Kohn, M.R. Understanding the neural mechanisms of lisdexamfetamine dimesylate (LDX) pharmacotherapy in Binge Eating Disorder (BED): A study protocol. *J. Eat. Disord.* **2019**, *7*, 23. [CrossRef]
137. Fleck, D.E.; Eliassen, J.C.; Guerdjikova, A.I.; Mori, N.; Williams, S.; Blom, T.J.; Beckwith, T.; Tallman, M.J.; Adler, C.M.; DelBello, M.P.; et al. Effect of lisdexamfetamine on emotional network brain dysfunction in binge eating disorder. *Psychiatry Res. Neuroimaging* **2019**, *286*, 53–59. [CrossRef] [PubMed]
138. Schneider, E.; Martin, E.; Rotshtein, P.; Qureshi, K.L.; Chamberlain, S.R.; Spetter, M.S.; Dourish, C.T.; Higgs, S. The effects of lisdexamfetamine dimesylate on eating behaviour and homeostatic, reward and cognitive processes in women with binge-eating symptoms: An experimental medicine study. *Transl. Psychiatry* **2022**, *12*, 9. [CrossRef]
139. Cambridge, V.C.; Ziauddeen, H.; Nathan, P.J.; Subramaniam, N.; Dodds, C.; Chamberlain, S.R.; Koch, A.; Maltby, K.; Skeggs, A.L.; Napolitano, A.; et al. Neural and behavioral effects of a novel mu opioid receptor antagonist in binge-eating obese people. *Biol. Psychiatry* **2013**, *73*, 887–894. [CrossRef] [PubMed]
140. Juarascio, A.S.; Presseller, E.K.; Wilkinson, M.L.; Kelkar, A.; Srivastava, P.; Chen, J.Y.; Dengler, J.; Manasse, S.M.; Medaglia, J. Correcting the reward imbalance in binge eating: A pilot randomized trial of reward re-training treatment. *Appetite* **2022**, *176*, 106103. [CrossRef]
141. Linardon, J.; Wade, T.D.; de la Piedad Garcia, X.; Brennan, L. The efficacy of cognitive-behavioral therapy for eating disorders: A systematic review and meta-analysis. *J. Consult. Clin. Psychol.* **2017**, *85*, 1080–1094. [CrossRef] [PubMed]
142. Dunlop, K.; Woodside, B.; Lam, E.; Olmsted, M.; Colton, P.; Giacobbe, P.; Downar, J. Increases in frontostriatal connectivity are associated with response to dorsomedial repetitive transcranial magnetic stimulation in refractory binge/purge behaviors. *NeuroImage Clin.* **2015**, *8*, 611–618. [CrossRef] [PubMed]

Disclaimer/Publisher's Note: The statements, opinions and data contained in all publications are solely those of the individual author(s) and contributor(s) and not of MDPI and/or the editor(s). MDPI and/or the editor(s) disclaim responsibility for any injury to people or property resulting from any ideas, methods, instructions or products referred to in the content.

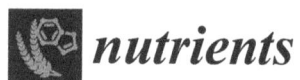

Article

Impact of Impulsivity and Therapy Response in Eating Disorders from a Neurophysiological, Personality and Cognitive Perspective

Giulia Testa [1,2,*], Roser Granero [2,3], Alejandra Misiolek [4], Cristina Vintró-Alcaraz [2,4,5], Núria Mallorqui-Bagué [2,6,7], Maria Lozano-Madrid [4], Misericordia Veciana De Las Heras [8], Isabel Sánchez [2,4,5], Susana Jiménez-Murcia [2,4,5,9] and Fernando Fernández-Aranda [2,4,5,9,*]

1. Universidad Internacional de La Rioja, 26006 La Rioja, Spain
2. CIBER Physiology of Obesity and Nutrition (CIBEROBN), Carlos III Health Institute, 28029 Madrid, Spain
3. Department of Psychobiology and Methodology, Autonomous University of Barcelona, 08193 Barcelona, Spain
4. Psychoneurobiology of Eating and Addictive Behaviors Group, Institut d'Investigació Biomèdica de Bellvitge (IDIBELL), 08907 Barcelona, Spain
5. Department of Psychiatry, University Hospital of Bellvitge, 08907 Barcelona, Spain
6. Addictive Behaviours Unit, Department of Psychiatry, Hospital de la Santa Creu i Sant Pau, Biomedical Research Institute Sant Pau (IIB Sant Pau), 08041 Barcelona, Spain
7. Department of Psychology, University of Girona, 17004 Girona, Spain
8. Neurophysiology Unit, Neurology Department, Hospital Universitari de Bellvitge, 08908 L'Hospitalet de Llobregat, Spain
9. Department of Clinical Sciences, School of Medicine and Health Sciences, University of Barcelona, 08907 L'Hospitalet de Llobregat, Spain
* Correspondence: giulia.testa@unir.net (G.T.); ffernandez@bellvitgehospital.cat (F.F.-A.); Tel.: +34-604-377-326 (G.T.); +34-932-607-227 (F.F.-A.)

Abstract: Impulsivity, as a multidimensional construct, has been linked to eating disorders (EDs) and may negatively impact treatment response. The study aimed to identify the dimensions of impulsivity predicting poor remission of ED symptoms. A total of 37 ED patients underwent a baseline assessment of impulsive personality traits and inhibitory control, including the Stroop task and the emotional go/no-go task with event-related potentials (ERPs) analysis. The remission of EDs symptomatology was evaluated after 3 months of cognitive-behavioral therapy (CBT) and at a 2-year follow-up. Poor remission after CBT was predicted by poor inhibitory control, as measured by the Stroop task. At 2 years, the risk of poor remission was higher in patients with higher novelty seeking, lower inhibitory control in the Stroop and in ERPs indices (N2 amplitudes) during the emotional go/no-go task. The present results highlight inhibitory control negatively impacting both short- and long-term symptomatology remission in ED patients. On the other hand, high novelty seeking and ERPs indices of poor inhibition seem to be more specifically related to long-term remission. Therefore, a comprehensive assessment of the impulsivity dimension in patients with ED is recommended to tailor treatments and improve their efficacy.

Keywords: eating disorders; impulsivity traits; inhibitory control; event-related potentials; treatment outcome

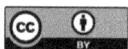

1. Introduction

Impulsivity is recognized as a multidimensional construct, reflecting multiple and separable psychological dimensions. An important contribution to this multidimensional conception has been provided by the UPPS model, which describes different personality traits that reflect impulsive behaviors [1].

From a neuropsychological perspective, the cognitive functions linked to impulsivity include inhibitory control and decision-making processes [2]. Inhibitory control refers to the ability to inhibit cognitive or motor responses [3–5]. Cognitive inhibition is usually measured by interference control tasks (e.g., Stroop Color–Word Task) in which effortful inhibition at a covert cognitive level is required to suppress the competing automatic response in favor of the correct response [6]. In contrast, inhibition of motor responses is assessed by go/no-go tasks, which measure the overt effortful expression of inhibition, involving the suppression of activated motor response [6].

Impulsivity has been proposed as a transdiagnostic feature of eating disorders (EDs) [7,8]. From a traditional view, impulsivity mainly characterizes the bulimic EDs spectrum, including binge eating disorder (BED) and bulimia nervosa (BN), whereas compulsivity would be more likely to be associated with anorexia nervosa (AN) [9,10]. However, evidence of impulsivity also exists in patients with AN [11,12], which is in line with the transdiagnostic approach of EDs [13,14].

Impulsivity plays a role in the etiology and maintenance of ED symptoms, which may have important implications for therapy response. Cognitive-behavioral therapy (CBT) is one of the most common and effective treatments, which have been shown to reduce EDs symptoms [15]. However, a considerable number of patients are at risk of dropping out of therapy, and others do not show complete remission of symptoms after CBT [16]. Identifying the factors that interfere with the optimal remission of EDs symptoms following CBT and at a longer follow-up is crucial to designing more personalized treatment approaches [17].

Although impulsivity is not necessarily dysfunctional in the nonclinical population [18], in individuals with mental disorders, impulsive personality traits predicted poor treatment outcomes [19,20]. Similarly, in individuals with EDs, impulsivity has been related to lower engagement with treatment and higher dropout rates [21–23]. Novelty seeking has been associated with a higher risk of dropout and not obtaining full remission [24]. Negative urgency, which reflects the tendency to rush impulsively in response to negative emotions, has also been shown to predict poor treatment outcomes in patients with BED [25].

Regarding inhibitory control, studies in patients with EDs have shown difficulties in both motor and cognitive inhibition [26–29], even though some discrepancies are present in the literature [30,31]. Furthermore, poor inhibition has been suggested to interfere with treatment remission in individuals with substance addictions [32] and behavioral addictions [33]. Similarly, low inhibitory control predicted poor weight loss after treatment in individuals with obesity [34–36].

Previous studies showed the association between poor decision making and treatment outcome in EDs [37,38]. However, the impact that inhibitory control may have on therapy response in EDs is heterogeneous and may need further research [25,39]. The recording of electroencephalographic (EEG) activity during response inhibition tasks gives more sensitive indices of inhibitory control through the analysis of event-related potentials (ERPs). Specifically, the ERP component classically associated with inhibition is the N2, which is a negative wave that emerges approximately 200–300 ms after stimulus presentation. The amplitude of the N2, which is usually enhanced in "no-go" compared to "go" stimuli, is a valuable measure of inhibitory control [40]. Lack of inhibitory control indexed by the N2 amplitude has been reported among clinical samples, including individuals with substance addiction [41,42], behavioral addiction [43] and BED [44]. However, further research is needed to determine whether a lack of inhibitory control is related to treatment response in individuals with EDs.

The present study aimed to analyze the impact of several facets of impulsivity in ED therapy response. Within this scope, multiple components of impulsivity were evaluated in a comprehensive perspective, including: (1) impulsive personality, measured by the UPPS dimensions and novelty seeking trait; (2) inhibitory control process, measuring cognitive inhibition with a Stroop task; and (3) motor inhibition, measured with an emotional go/no-go task with EEG recording.

This multidimensional impulsivity assessment was conducted at baseline, and regression models were adopted to identify which dimensions predicted ED symptomatologic remission after CBT treatment and at a longer follow-up (i.e., 2 years). We hypothesized that the most impulsive individuals would present partial or non-remission of EDs symptomatology, after CBT and at the longest follow-up. Different dimensions of impulsivity are expected to contribute to suboptimal remission of EDs symptoms, observed both immediately after treatment and in the medium term.

2. Materials and Methods

2.1. Participants

A total of 37 treatment-seeking individuals with ED were consecutively recruited at the ED Unit within the Department of Psychiatry at Bellvitge University Hospital (HUB)—a public health hospital certified as a tertiary care center with a highly specialized unit for the treatment of ED in Barcelona (Spain). To avoid the possible gender difference in impulsivity shown in the literature [45], recruitment was limited to female patients, which is the most representative gender in EDs. Patients were diagnosed with anorexia nervosa (AN; $n = 20$) and bulimic spectrum disorders (BSD $n = 17$), including bulimia nervosa (BN) and binge eating disorder (BED), according to DSM-5 criteria [46]. Patients voluntarily participated in the study, and their informed consent was obtained. They all underwent a baseline assessment before starting the CBT treatment. Remission of ED symptoms was analyzed after CBT and in a two-year follow-up. To that end, clinical records and online shared electronic medical records were analyzed retrospectively throughout Catalonia (Spain).

2.2. Measures

2.2.1. Baseline Assessment

The Temperament and Character Inventory-Revised (TCI-R) [47] validated for the Spanish population [48] is a questionnaire of 240 items answered on a 5-point Likert scale. The novelty seeking subscale of the TCI-R was adopted in the present study as a measure of impulsive temperament. The internal consistency of the subscale in the sample was $\alpha = 0.836$.

The UPPS-P Impulsivity Scale [49] is a 59-item scale that assesses impulsive behavior on 5 different scales: sensation seeking, lack of premeditation, lack of perseverance, negative and positive urgency. Positive urgency has been included more recently. All items are rated on a 4-point scale from 1 (strongly agree) to 4 (strongly disagree). The UPPS-P has satisfactory psychometric properties in terms of both convergent and discriminative validity. The Spanish version of the UPPS-P scale was obtained by a back-translation process, and its Spanish adaptation shows adequate psychometric properties [50]. The α values for the different UPPS-P scales in our sample are lack of premeditation (0.836), lack of perseverance (0.850), sensation seeking (0.827), positive urgency (0.941) and negative urgency (0.861). Total score (0.911).

The Eating Disorders Inventory (EDI-2) [51] was adopted to screen symptomatology related to eating disorders on a six-point Likert scale. EDI-2 is a self-report measure consisting of 91 items and provides scores on 11 subscales: drive for thinness, body dissatisfaction, bulimia, ineffectiveness, perfectionism, interpersonal distrust, interoceptive awareness, maturity fears, asceticism, impulse regulation and social insecurity. The sum of all subscales provides an eating disorder measure, which is considered a global scale of ED severity. The internal consistency of the global scale in the sample was $\alpha = 0.931$.

The Stroop Color–Word Test (SCWT) [52] is a paper and pencil test, which measures the ability to inhibit cognitive interference known as the Stroop effect. The task consists of reading 3 pages with 100 words each as fast as possible. The first 2 pages are called the "congruous condition", and the participants are asked to (1) read the color words printed in black and (2) name the colors of the printed "Xs" (red, green and blue). The last page (3) contains the names of colors printed in an incongruent color (i.e., the word "red" printed in blue ink), and the subjects are asked to name the color of the ink instead of reading the word. The subjects are given 45 s for each page, and when the time is over, the last named item is noted. The total score for each task is calculated from the number of items completed on each page. Higher scores in the incongruent task variable indicate a better capacity for inhibition response. The test has shown adequate reliability and construct validity for the assessment of inhibition and switching skills [52].

The emotional go/no-go task [8] is a computerized task for assessing response inhibition. Participants were presented with 600 images surrounded by a colored frame. They were asked to respond as quickly as possible to images within a blue frame (i.e., go cues) and to withhold the response to images within a yellow frame (i.e., no-go cues). The images were divided into three blocks presented in a randomized way and with different emotional valence: 200 pleasant images, 200 neutral images and 200 unpleasant images. Out of each block of 200 images, 75% were go cues, and 25% were no-go cues. The interstimulus interval was pseudorandomized from 1.500 to 1.700 ms to discourage anticipatory responses. The reaction times (RTs) in go trials and the accuracy in go and no-go trials were calculated for each emotional category.

The electroencephalogram (EEG) was recorded continuously throughout the emotional go/no-go task using PyCorder (BrainVision). In total, 60 active Ag/AgCl electrodes were placed into an EEG recording cap (EASYCAP GmbH), distributed according to the 10–20 system; additional 3 electrodes were adopted for recording the vertical and horizontal electrooculogram (EOG), and Cz was used as an online reference. Impedances were kept below 20 kΩ using the SuperVisc high-viscosity electrolyte gel for active electrodes. Signals from all channels were digitized with a sampling rate of 500 Hz and 24 bit/channel resolution and online filtered between 0.1 and 100 Hz. Offline EEG analyses were performed with Brain Vision Analyser consisting of the following steps: high pass filtering at 0.1 Hz, low pass filtering at 30 Hz (Butterworth zero-phase filter; 24 dB/octave slope) and a notch filter at 50 Hz; raw data inspection for manual detection of artifacts and screening for bad channels, semi-automatic eye-blink correction using independent component analysis (ICA); artifact rejection of trials with an amplitude exceeding ±80 µV; EEG data were segmented into 1500 ms epochs from 500 ms before to 1000 ms after stimulus onset. Data were baseline corrected against the mean voltage during the 200 ms pre-stimulus periods. Artifact-free epochs were separately averaged for each subject in each experimental condition (go, no-go) and stimulus type (positive, negative, neutral). Event-related potentials (ERPs) analyses were based on visual inspection of the grand average waveforms and the existing literature. Peak amplitudes for the N2 were analyzed in a frontocentral electrodes cluster (FC1, FC2, Fz, C3, C4, Cz), in time windows between 200 and 380 ms. Since N2 is a negative peak wave, the more negative the values, the greater its amplitude.

2.2.2. Treatment

Patients received cognitive-behavioral therapy (CBT) at HUB, which was carried out by clinical psychology experts in the field. Patients diagnosed with AN completed a day hospital treatment program, which included group CBT sessions, lasting 90 min each, for 15 weeks. Treatment for the other EDs diagnoses (BED, BN) consisted of 16 weekly outpatient group sessions of CBT lasting 90 min. All patients attended follow-up sessions for a period of about two years' duration. The goal of the treatment was to train patients to implement CBT strategies to reduce eating symptoms and to enable patients to acquire good healthy habits. Voluntary treatment discontinuation was categorized as dropout (i.e., not attending treatment for at least three consecutive sessions). Patients completing treatment were re-evaluated by their clinician to classify the remission of ED-related symptomatology. According to the DSM-5 criteria [46], full remission was considered as the total absence of ED symptoms meeting diagnostic criteria for at least 4 consecutive weeks. We considered full remission as an index of good treatment outcomes. By contrast, we considered the following as measures of "poor treatment" outcomes: voluntary treatment discontinuation or dropout (i.e., not attending treatment for at least three consecutive sessions); partial remission of EDs (i.e., symptomatic improvement with residual symptoms); and non-remission of EDs.

2.3. Statistical Analysis

Statistical analysis was carried out with Stata17 for Windows [53]. The comparison between the groups defined for the treatment outcome (good versus poor) was performed with an analysis of covariance (ANCOVA) adjusted for the ED subtype. Finner's method controlled the increase in type I error due to the multiple null-hypothesis tests [54], and the effect size of the mean differences was estimated with the standardized Cohen d-coefficient (mild–moderate effect size was considered for $|d| > 0.5$ and large–high effect size for $|d| > 0.8$) [55].

Two predictive models were obtained for the risk of poor treatment outcome (defined as the dependent variable, with values 1 = good outcome versus 0 = poor outcome) post-CBT and at 2-year follow-up, with logistic regression models adjusted for the ED subtype. The list of the potential predictors included the EEG measures registered during the emotional go/no-go task, the Stroop interference score and the impulsivity scores (obtained in the UPPS-P and the NS scales). Goodness of fit was assessed with the Hosmer–Lemeshow test ($p > 0.05$ is indicative of adequate fit) [56], predictive capacity with the Nagelkerke pseudo-R2 coefficient and global discriminative capacity with the area under the ROC curve (AUC).

3. Results

3.1. Characteristics of the Participants

The first block of Table 1 displays the description of the sociodemographic variables. Most participants were single (62.2%), with secondary education (51.4%), employed (54.1%) and within mean-low to low social position indices (75.7%). The mean age was 30.7 years (SD = 12.0); the mean age of onset of ED-related problems was 22.2 years (SD = 8.4); and the mean duration of the disease was 8.5 years (SD = 8.4).

Table 1. Description of the sample.

Sociodemographic	n	%	Clinical Profile	Mean	SD
Civil status			Age (years old)	30.73	12.00
Single	23	62.2%	Age of onset of ED (years old)	22.22	8.42
Married	12	32.4%	Duration of ED (years)	8.48	8.41
Divorced	2	5.4%	ED subtype	n	%
Education			Anorexia nervosa	20	54.1%
Primary	11	29.7%	Bulimia nervosa	17	45.9%
Secondary	19	51.4%	Treatment outcome: end treatment	n	%
University	7	18.9%	Dropout	8	21.6%
Employment			Non-remission	1	2.7%
Employed/student	20	54.1%	Partial remission	13	35.1%
Unemployed	17	45.9%	Full remission	15	40.5%
Social position			Treatment outcome: 2-year follow-up		
High	1	2.7%	Dropout	9	24.3%
Mean-high	5	13.5%	Non-remission	3	8.1%
Mean	3	8.1%	Partial remission	9	24.3%
Mean-low	9	24.3%	Full remission	16	43.2%
Low	19	51.4%			

Note. SD: standard deviation.

3.2. Variables Related to the CBT Outcome and Follow-Up

The second block of Table 1 displays the distribution of treatment outcomes during the CBT treatment and at 2-year follow-up. Good remission was achieved for 40.6% of the participants at the end of the treatment plan (the risk of poor outcome was 59.4%). At the

2-year follow-up, good remission was registered for 43.3% of the sample (the risk of poor outcome was 56.7%).

Table 2 shows the results of the ANCOVA exploring the relationships between the clinical variables measured at baseline (duration of the ED, EDI-2 scales, UPPS-P scales, TCI-R novelty seeking, go/no-go task and Stroop interference) and the treatment outcome (good/poor) measured at two time points—(1) at final treatment after CBT and (2) at 2-year follow-up. These analyses were adjusted–controlled for the ED subtype. At the end of the CBT (i.e., final treatment), patients with poor outcomes were characterized by higher scores in the EDI-2 bulimia and interpersonal distrust, higher values in UPPS-P sensation seeking, lower values in the accuracy go task and a lower average score in Stroop interference (these measures registered a difference in the significance test and/or effect size within the ranges mild to large).

Table 2. Variables related to the treatment outcome: ANCOVA adjusted for ED subtype.

	Final Treatment						2-Year Follow-Up					
	Good (n = 15)		Poor (n = 22)				Good (n = 16)		Poor (n = 21)			
	Mean	SD	Mean	SD	p	|d|	Mean	SD	Mean	SD	p	|d|
Duration of ED (years)	8.62	10.76	8.39	6.46	0.928	0.03	8.60	10.68	8.39	6.43	0.933	0.02
EDI-2 Drive for thinness	11.22	5.64	12.08	6.15	0.669	0.15	12.13	5.85	11.43	5.99	0.718	0.12
EDI-2 Body dissatisfaction	16.76	7.48	16.08	6.80	0.742	0.10	16.36	6.76	16.34	7.50	0.993	0.00
EDI-2 Interoceptive awareness	12.09	7.12	10.58	5.56	0.489	0.24	12.87	7.43	9.91	4.83	0.155	0.47
EDI-2 Bulimia	4.41	4.68	7.77	5.40	0.025 *	0.67 †	4.65	4.44	7.74	5.43	0.034 *	0.62 †
EDI-2 Interpersonal distrust	3.97	3.50	6.97	5.48	0.080	0.65 †	5.98	4.93	5.58	5.02	0.814	0.08
EDI-2 Ineffectiveness	11.95	6.98	9.81	5.69	0.333	0.34	10.99	6.36	10.44	6.30	0.799	0.09
EDI-2 Maturity fears	8.98	6.47	7.74	5.51	0.555	0.20	7.31	6.12	8.96	5.71	0.413	0.28
EDI-2 Perfectionism	5.48	4.38	6.22	4.59	0.631	0.17	6.15	4.57	5.74	4.53	0.786	0.09
EDI-2 Impulse regulation	4.45	5.01	4.55	4.41	0.951	0.02	2.82	2.32	5.80	5.47	0.043 *	0.71 †
EDI-2 Asceticism	6.14	3.71	5.81	3.21	0.786	0.09	6.33	3.61	5.65	3.25	0.557	0.20
EDI-2 Social insecurity	7.85	5.95	6.38	5.10	0.368	0.30	7.54	5.29	6.54	4.11	0.526	0.21
EDI-2 Total	93.27	41.29	93.95	31.78	0.957	0.02	93.13	37.95	94.09	34.29	0.936	0.03
UPPS-P Lack of premeditation	23.03	6.91	21.30	6.00	0.434	0.27	20.93	6.89	22.81	6.07	0.378	0.29
UPPS-P Lack of perseverance	24.29	5.89	21.76	6.45	0.212	0.41	21.83	6.06	23.51	6.77	0.394	0.26
UPPS-P Sensation seeking	22.89	6.15	26.39	7.84	0.172	0.50 †	24.26	7.37	25.52	7.46	0.617	0.17
UPPS-P Positive urgency	24.66	8.59	27.73	11.06	0.389	0.31	23.42	7.97	28.83	11.07	0.111	0.56 †
UPPS-P Negative urgency	32.70	8.06	34.07	7.27	0.584	0.18	31.22	7.93	35.26	6.91	0.088	0.54 †
UPPS-P Total score	127.59	21.85	131.37	24.78	0.634	0.16	121.66	17.87	136.07	25.65	0.044 *	0.65 †
TCI-R Novelty seeking	94.49	20.70	98.53	15.44	0.505	0.22	87.36	17.09	104.15	14.67	0.002 *	1.05 †
N2 Positive go	−4.00	2.72	−3.50	2.32	0.571	0.20	−4.69	2.71	−2.94	2.01	0.033 *	0.73 †
N2 Positive no-go	−5.08	2.46	−4.03	2.46	0.248	0.43	−5.15	2.47	−3.86	2.25	0.113	0.54 †
N2 Negative go	−4.53	2.53	−4.01	2.28	0.528	0.22	−5.05	2.32	−3.59	2.25	0.063	0.64 †
N2 Negative no-go	−5.12	2.12	−4.47	2.98	0.483	0.25	−5.89	2.58	−3.85	2.40	0.019 *	0.82 †
N2 Neutral go	−4.20	2.38	−3.73	2.06	0.542	0.21	−4.80	2.08	−3.25	2.04	0.031 *	0.75 †
N2 Neutral no-go	−5.48	2.40	−4.43	2.69	0.251	0.41	−5.80	2.82	−4.13	2.19	0.054	0.66 †
Accuracy Negative go	0.99	0.02	0.96	0.06	0.110	0.59 †	0.97	0.04	0.97	0.06	0.904	0.04
Accuracy Negative no-go	0.79	0.12	0.81	0.12	0.663	0.15	0.80	0.10	0.80	0.13	0.956	0.02
Accuracy Positive go	0.99	0.02	0.96	0.06	0.071	0.68 †	0.97	0.06	0.97	0.05	0.656	0.15
Accuracy Positive no-go	0.80	0.11	0.81	0.12	0.827	0.08	0.80	0.09	0.80	0.13	0.981	0.01
Accuracy Neutral go	0.98	0.03	0.95	0.07	0.168	0.52 †	0.96	0.08	0.97	0.04	0.383	0.28
Accuracy Neutral no-go	0.76	0.11	0.80	0.13	0.355	0.33	0.77	0.08	0.80	0.15	0.571	0.20
Stroop interference	8.72	14.57	0.22	11.07	0.036 *	0.66 †	8.20	15.44	0.21	9.46	0.042 *	0.62 †

Note. Good outcome: full remission. Bad outcome: dropout, non-remission or partial remission. SD: standard deviation. * significant comparison. † Effect size in the ranges mild–moderate to high–large.

At the 2-year follow-up, poor outcome was related to higher mean scores in the EDI-2 bulimia and impulse regulation scales, higher personality traits related to impulsivity (in the UPPS-P total and TCI-R novelty seeking scales), lower mean in the Stroop interference score and lower amplitude of the N2 wave in positive go trials, negative no-go trials and neutral go trials (mean differences with a significant result and/or effect size within at least the mild range). The ERPs and the topographical maps for the no-go negative condition are presented in Figure 1, showing the lower N2 amplitude in patients with poor outcome at follow-up compared to those with good outcome. Figure 2 displays the radar charts with the results of the comparisons between the patients with good and poor treatment outcome (z-standardized means are plotted due to the different measurement scales of the variables analyzed in the study).

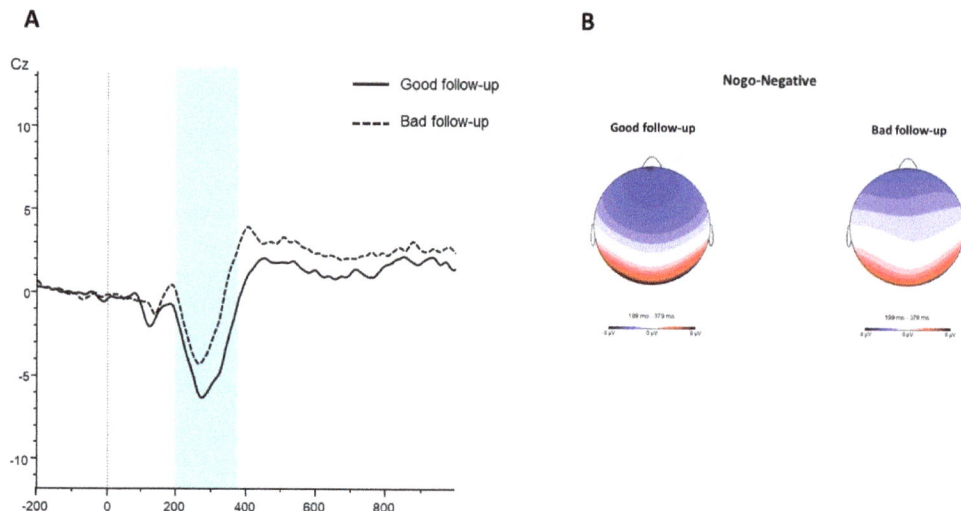

Figure 1. (**A**) Grand average ERPs waver for the no-go negative condition in the group of patients with good outcomes at follow-up (continuous line) and those showing bad outcomes at follow-up (dotted line). (**B**) Topographical maps (200–380 ms) for the no-go negative condition in patients with good outcomes at follow-up (**left panel**) and those with poor outcomes at follow-up (**right panel**).

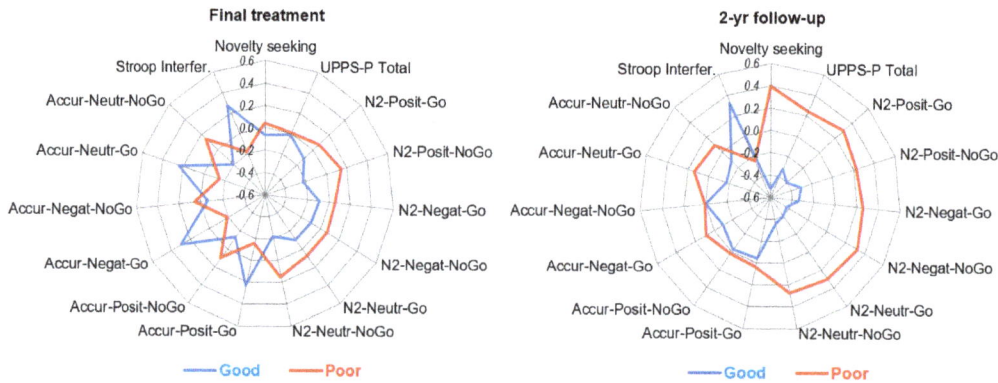

Figure 2. Radar charts with the z-standardized mean scores obtained among the groups with good and poor treatment outcomes.

The two logistic regression models displayed in Table 3 indicated that a lower score in the Stroop interference task increased the risk of poor outcomes post-CBT. At the 2-year follow-up, the risk of poor outcomes was increased for patients with higher scores in the TCI-R novelty seeking scale, lower amplitude of the N2 in negative no-go trials and lower scores in the Stroop interference.

Table 3. Predictive models for the risk of poor outcome: logistic regression adjusted for ED subtype.

	B	SE	p	OR	95%CI (OR)		HL	NR²	AUC
Poor outcome: final treatment									
Stroop interference	−0.076	0.041	0.027	0.927	0.855	0.998	0.941	0.230	0.718
Poor outcome: 2-year follow-up									
TCI-R Novelty seeking	0.078	0.032	0.003	1.082	1.017	1.150	0.090	0.405	0.872
N2 Negative no-go	0.394	0.206	0.027	1.484	1.001	2.220			
Stroop interference	−0.090	0.053	0.040	0.914	0.824	0.999			

Note. SE: standard error. OR: odds ratio. HL: Hosmer–Lemeshow test (p-Value). NR²: pseudo-R2 coefficient. AUC: area under ROC.

4. Discussion

The present study investigated the impact that impulsivity may have on therapy response in patients with EDs. Remission of ED symptomatology was evaluated after 3 months of CBT and at a 2-year follow-up. Multiple impulsivity dimensions were measured before treatment and significantly predicted poor treatment response, with more consistent evidence emerging at follow-up.

With regard to impulsive personality traits, patients with poor remission following CBT were characterized by higher sensation seeking, whereas those with poor remission at follow-up were characterized by higher novelty seeking and higher UPPS total score. Novelty seeking emerged as a predictor of poor ED remission at follow-up, suggesting its relation to long-term remission of ED symptomatology. Along this line, some of the previous studies in patients with EDs showed associations between novelty seeking and a higher risk of dropout and suboptimal remission following CBT [24,57].

At a neurocognitive level, lower cognitive control predicted CBT outcome and remission at follow-up. Thus, individuals with difficulties in controlling the interference in the Stroop task showed poor remission of EDs after 3 months of CBT and at 2 years from treatment. In contrast, a study in patients with BED did not show an association between cognitive inhibition and reduction in ED psychopathology after treatment [39]. The discrepant results are possibly related to the heterogeneity of the present sample, which includes various ED subtypes other than BED. Interestingly, reduced cognitive inhibition has been associated with longer EDs duration in AN [58], which in turn is a factor contributing to poor remission of EDs. The present results in a mixed sample of EDs suggest that cognitive inhibition is a relevant factor associated with both short-term and long-term remission. Future studies in larger samples would help detect and elucidate the differences across ED subtypes.

Regarding motor inhibition, the lower amplitude of the N2 was associated with poor ED remission at follow-up. By contrast, the behavioral measures of response accuracy in the go/no-go task did not predict EDs remission, in line with some previous findings [25]. It can be argued that the ERPs indexed, such as the N2, may be particularly sensitive in detecting alterations in inhibitory processes, as recently shown in patients with BN undergoing an odd-ball task [59]. So far, this is the first evidence of a relation between lower N2 amplitude and suboptimal remission of ED symptoms. Interestingly, this effect was shown to be maximal in the no-go trials with negative emotional stimuli. Affective versions of response inhibition tasks (e.g., emotional go/no-go) have been adopted to study how response inhibition is modulated by emotional stimuli [60]. In this case, the difficulties in inhibition (indexed by lower N2 amplitudes) when a negative emotional state is induced could be more strongly related to poor remission of EDs. This result may be explained by the fact that both impulsivity and emotion regulation difficulties have been proposed as central transdiagnostic phenomena across EDs [61,62].

Taken together, the present results highlighted the relevance of novelty seeking and inhibitory control in remission of EDs. A comprehensive assessment of impulsivity, including personality traits and neurocognitive indices of inhibitory control, may be particularly useful to improve treatment effectiveness. For instance, those individuals with a tendency to be more impulsive, excitable, dramatic and with intolerance to routine might benefit from treatment tailored to reduce their impulsive behaviors. To address the difficulties in inhibition, inhibitory control training with general or food-specific stimuli has been tested in individuals with EDs showing promising results [63,64]. Recently, the outcome of a food-specific inhibitory control training has been measured with ERPs indices [65]. The results of our emotional go/no-go task encourage testing the effectiveness of novel inhibitory training using emotional stimuli to target impulsivity and emotion regulation.

The present findings should be considered under some limitations. First, the small sample was not suitable for the analysis of different ED subtypes, even though this variable was controlled for by statistical adjustment. Nevertheless, it could be of interest to study in the future the relationship between impulsivity dimensions and remission in specific ED subgroups. The small sample size also impacts the ability to avoid type II errors, the power capacity to detect the existence of a true relationship and the accuracy of the results obtained in the multivariate analyses. In this sense, the empirical evidence of this work should be interpreted with caution, pending future studies with larger samples to confirm or refute it. In addition, it should be considered that the assessment conducted in this study is difficult to perform in clinical samples, and therefore, research in this area is scarce and with low sample sizes. A second limitation is related to the nature of the outcome measure. Specifically, ED remission was assessed by the clinician at the end of treatment and at follow-up, according to the DSM-5 criteria. It is important to remark that optimal remission included only those individuals who fully remitted from symptomatology. Although this is particularly relevant in clinical practice, the adoption of a quantitative measure to track the changes in ED symptoms (e.g., EDI-2) should be considered in future works. Finally, the absence of a control group of patients undergoing treatment other than CBT or untreated individuals limits the interpretation and generalization of these results.

Despite these limitations, several strengths of the study should be remarked on, such as the comprehensive assessment of impulsivity, which included personality, neuropsychological and neurophysiological measures. Thus, the multidimensional assessment enables a better characterization of impulsive profiles, which could interfere with treatment outcomes. Furthermore, remission of ED was not only considered immediately after treatment but also at a longer follow-up of 2 years, thus providing an opportunity to study the relationship between impulsivity and long-term recovery.

5. Conclusions

In conclusion, high novelty seeking and low inhibitory control in individuals with EDs, but also specific neurophysiological indices, seem to contribute to poor remission of ED symptomatology. In particular, cognitive inhibition emerged as the dimension of impulsivity that more consistently predicted both short-term and medium-term remission of ED symptoms, confirming the importance of conducting a comprehensive assessment.

From a clinical perspective, early detection of patients with a lack of inhibition is recommended to personalize treatments and improve their effectiveness. A replication of these results in individuals with different subtypes of EDs is needed in future studies assessing the response to treatment.

Author Contributions: Conceptualization, G.T., F.F.-A., N.M.-B. and S.J.-M.; methodology, F.F.-A., G.T., R.G., N.M.-B. and S.J.-M.; formal analysis, R.G.; data curation, G.T., A.M., C.V.-A., M.L.-M., I.S. and M.V.D.L.H.; writing—original draft preparation, G.T., R.G. and A.M.; writing—review and editing, F.F.-A., S.J.-M., N.M.-B. and G.T.; supervision, S.J.-M. and F.F.-A.; funding acquisition, S.J.-M. and F.F.-A. All authors have read and agreed to the published version of the manuscript.

Funding: We thank CERCA Program/Generalitat de Catalunya for institutional support. This manuscript and research were supported by grants from the Instituto de Salud Carlos III (ISCIII) [FIS PI14/00290, PI17/01167, PI20/132] and co-funded by FEDER funds/European Regional Development Fund (ERDF), a way to build Europe]. CIBER Fisiopatología de la Obesidad y Nutrición (CIBERobn) is an initiative of ISCIII. RG is supported by The Catalan Institution for Research and Advanced

Studies (ICREA-2021 Academia Program). M.L.-M. and C.V.-A. are supported by predoctoral grants of the Ministerio de Educación, Cultura y Deporte (FPU15/02911 and FPU16/01453).

Institutional Review Board Statement: The study was conducted in accordance with the Declaration of Helsinki and approved by the Ethics Committee of University Hospital of Bellvitge (ethical approval code: PR146/14). Informed Consent Statement: Informed consent was obtained from all subjects involved in the study.

Informed Consent Statement: Written informed consent has been obtained from the patients to publish this paper.

Data Availability Statement: Data are not available in any repository. Please contact the corresponding authors.

Conflicts of Interest: F.F.-A. received consultancy honoraria from Novo Nordisk and editorial honoraria as EIC from Wiley. The rest of the authors declare no conflict of interest. The funders had no role in the design of the study; in the collection, analyses, or interpretation of data; in the writing of the manuscript, or in the decision to publish the results.

References

1. Whiteside, S.P.; Lynam, D.R. The Five Factor Model and impulsivity: Using a structural model of personality to understand impulsivity. *Pers. Individ. Dif.* **2001**, *30*, 669–689. [CrossRef]
2. Rochat, L.; Billieux, J.; Gagnon, J.; Van der Linden, M. A multifactorial and integrative approach to impulsivity in neuropsychology: Insights from the UPPS model of impulsivity. *J. Clin. Exp. Neuropsychol.* **2017**, *40*, 45–61. [CrossRef] [PubMed]
3. Wu, M.; Hartmann, M.; Skunde, M.; Herzog, W.; Friederich, H.C. Inhibitory Control in Bulimic-Type Eating Disorders: A Systematic Review and Meta-Analysis. *PLoS ONE* **2013**, *8*, e83412. [CrossRef] [PubMed]
4. Lavagnino, L.; Arnone, D.; Cao, B.; Soares, J.C.; Selvaraj, S. Inhibitory control in obesity and binge eating disorder: A systematic review and meta-analysis of neurocognitive and neuroimaging studies. *Neurosci. Biobehav. Rev.* **2016**, *68*, 714–726. [CrossRef] [PubMed]
5. Bartholdy, S.; Dalton, B.; O'Daly, O.G.; Campbell, I.C.; Schmidt, U. A systematic review of the relationship between eating, weight and inhibitory control using the stop signal task. *Neurosci. Biobehav. Rev.* **2016**, *64*, 35–62. [CrossRef] [PubMed]
6. Nigg, J.T. On Inhibition/Disinhibition in Developmental Psychopathology: Views from Cognitive and Personality Psychology and a Working Inhibition Taxonomy. *Psychol. Bull.* **2000**, *126*, 220–246. [CrossRef]
7. Lavender, J.M.; Mitchell, J.E. Eating Disorders and Their Relationship to Impulsivity. *Curr. Treat. Options Psychiatry* **2015**, *2*, 394–401. [CrossRef]
8. Mallorquí-Bagué, N.; Testa, G.; Lozano-Madrid, M.; Vintró-Alcaraz, C.; Sánchez, I.; Riesco, N.; Granero, R.; Perales, J.C.; Navas, J.F.; Megías-Robles, A.; et al. Emotional and non-emotional facets of impulsivity in eating disorders: From anorexia nervosa to bulimic spectrum disorders. *Eur. Eat. Disord. Rev.* **2020**, *28*, 410–422. [CrossRef]
9. Atiye, M.; Miettunen, J.; Raevuori-Helkamaa, A. A Meta-Analysis of Temperament in Eating Disorders. *Eur. Eat. Disord. Rev.* **2015**, *23*, 89–99. [CrossRef]
10. Wolz, I.; Agüera, Z.; Granero, R.; Jiménez-Murcia, S.; Gratz, K.L.; Menchón, J.M.; Fernández-Aranda, F. Emotion regulation in disordered eating: Psychometric properties of the difficulties in emotion regulation scale among spanish adults and its interrelations with personality and clinical severity. *Front. Psychol.* **2015**, *6*, 907. [CrossRef]
11. Favaro, A.; Santonastaso, P. Suicidality in eating disorders: Clinical and psychological correlates. *Acta Psychiatr. Scand.* **1997**, *95*, 508–514. [CrossRef] [PubMed]
12. Favaro, A.; Zanetti, T.; Tenconi, E.; Degortes, D.; Ronzan, A.; Veronese, A.; Santonastaso, P. The relationship between temperament and impulsive behaviors in eating disordered subjects. *Eat. Disord.* **2005**, *13*, 61–70. [CrossRef] [PubMed]
13. Fairburn, C.G.; Cooper, Z.; Shafran, R. Cognitive behaviour therapy for eating disorders: A "transdiagnostic" theory and treatment. *Behav. Res. Ther.* **2003**, *41*, 509–528. [CrossRef] [PubMed]
14. Wade, T.D.; Bergin, J.L.; Martin, N.G.; Gillespie, N.A.; Fairburn, C.G. A transdiagnostic approach to understanding eating disorders. *J. Nerv. Ment. Dis.* **2006**, *194*, 510–517. [CrossRef]
15. Linardon, J.; Wade, T.D.; de la Piedad Garcia, X.; Brennan, L. The efficacy of cognitive-behavioral therapy for eating disorders: A systematic review and meta-analysis. *J. Consult. Clin. Psychol.* **2017**, *85*, 1080–1094. [CrossRef]
16. Nazar, B.P.; Gregor, L.K.; Albano, G.; Marchica, A.; Coco, G.L.; Cardi, V.; Treasure, J. Early Response to treatment in Eating Disorders: A Systematic Review and a Diagnostic Test Accuracy Meta-Analysis. *Eur. Eat. Disord. Rev.* **2017**, *25*, 67–79. [CrossRef]
17. Vintró-Alcaraz, C.; Munguía, L.; Granero, R.; Gaspar-Pérez, A.; Solé-Morata, N.; Sánchez, I.; Sánchez-González, J.; Menchón, J.M.; Jiménez-Murcia, S.; Fernández-Aranda, F. Emotion regulation as a transdiagnostic factor in eating disorders and gambling disorder: Treatment outcome implications. *J. Behav. Addict.* **2022**, *11*, 140–146. [CrossRef]
18. Stoyanova, S.; Ivantchev, N.; Giannuoli, V. Functional, Dysfunctional Impulsivity and Sensation Seeking in Medical Staff—PubMed. *Psychiatr. Danub.* **2021**, *33*, 25–29.

19. Hershberger, A.R.; Um, M.; Cyders, M.A. The relationship between the UPPS-P impulsive personality traits and substance use psychotherapy outcomes: A meta-analysis. *Drug Alcohol Depend.* **2017**, *178*, 408–416. [CrossRef]
20. Mallorquí-Bagué, N.; Mestre-Bach, G.; Lozano-Madrid, M.; Fernandez-Aranda, F.; Granero, R.; Vintró-Alcazaz, C.; Del Pino-Gutiérrez, A.; Steward, T.; Gómez-Peña, M.; Aymamí, N.; et al. Trait impulsivity and cognitive domains involving impulsivity and compulsivity as predictors of gambling disorder treatment response. *Addict. Behav.* **2018**, *87*, 169–176. [CrossRef]
21. Agras, W.S.; Crow, S.J.; Halmi, K.A.; Mitchell, J.E.; Wilson, G.T.; Kraemer, H.C. Outcome predictors for the cognitive behavior treatment of bulimia nervosa: Data from a multisite study. *Am. J. Psychiatry* **2000**, *157*, 1302–1308. [CrossRef]
22. Fassino, S.; Abbate-Daga, G.; Pierò, A.; Leombruni, P.; Rovera, G.G. Dropout from Brief Psychotherapy within a Combination Treatment in Bulimia nervosa: Role of Personality and Anger. *Psychother. Psychosom.* **2003**, *72*, 203–210. [CrossRef] [PubMed]
23. Fassino, S.; Pierò, A.; Tomba, E.; Abbate-Daga, G. Factors associated with dropout from treatment for eating disorders: A comprehensive literature review. *BMC Psychiatry* **2009**, *9*, 67. [CrossRef] [PubMed]
24. Agüera, Z.; Sánchez, I.; Granero, R.; Riesco, N.; Steward, T.; Martín-Romera, V.; Jiménez-Murcia, S.; Romero, X.; Caroleo, M.; Segura-García, C.; et al. Short-Term Treatment Outcomes and Dropout Risk in Men and Women with Eating Disorders. *Eur. Eat. Disord. Rev.* **2017**, *25*, 293–301. [CrossRef] [PubMed]
25. Manasse, S.M.; Espel, H.M.; Schumacher, L.M.; Kerrigan, S.G.; Zhang, F.; Forman, E.M.; Juarascio, A.S. Does impulsivity predict outcome in treatment for binge eating disorder? A multimodal investigation. *Appetite* **2016**, *105*, 172–179. [CrossRef]
26. Rosval, L.; Steiger, H.; Bruce, K.; Israël, M.; Richardson, J.; Aubut, M. Impulsivity in women with eating disorders: Problem of response inhibition, planning, or attention? *Int. J. Eat. Disord.* **2006**, *39*, 590–593. [CrossRef]
27. Kemps, E.; Wilsdon, A. Preliminary evidence for a role for impulsivity in cognitive disinhibition in bulimia nervosa. *J. Clin. Exp. Neuropsychol.* **2009**, *32*, 515–521. [CrossRef]
28. Fagundo, A.B.; de la Torre, R.; Jiménez-Murcia, S.; Agüera, Z.; Granero, R.; Tárrega, S.; Botella, C.; Baños, R.; Fernández-Real, J.M.; Rodríguez, R.; et al. Executive Functions Profile in Extreme Eating/Weight Conditions: From Anorexia Nervosa to Obesity. *PLoS ONE* **2012**, *7*, e43382. [CrossRef]
29. Carr, M.M.; Wiedemann, A.A.; Macdonald-Gagnon, G.; Potenza, M.N. Impulsivity and compulsivity in binge eating disorder: A systematic review of behavioral studies. *Prog. Neuropsychopharmacol. Biol. Psychiatry* **2021**, *110*, 110318. [CrossRef]
30. Claes, L.; Nederkoorn, C.; Vandereycken, W.; Guerrieri, R.; Vertommen, H. Impulsiveness and lack of inhibitory control in eating disorders. *Eat. Behav.* **2006**, *7*, 196–203. [CrossRef]
31. Van Den Eynde, F.; Samarawickrema, N.; Kenyon, M.; Dejong, H.; Lavender, A.; Startup, H.; Schmidt, U. A study of neurocognition in bulimia nervosa and eating disorder not otherwise specified–bulimia type. *J. Clin. Exp. Neuropsychol.* **2012**, *34*, 67–77. [CrossRef] [PubMed]
32. Krishnan-Sarin, S.; Reynolds, B.; Duhig, A.M.; Smith, A.; Liss, T.; McFetridge, A.; Cavallo, D.A.; Carroll, K.M.; Potenza, M.N. Behavioral impulsivity predicts treatment outcome in a smoking cessation program for adolescent smokers. *Drug Alcohol Depend.* **2007**, *88*, 79–82. [CrossRef] [PubMed]
33. Goudriaan, A.E.; Oosterlaan, J.; De Beurs, E.; Van Den Brink, W. The role of self-reported impulsivity and reward sensitivity versus neurocognitive measures of disinhibition and decision-making in the prediction of relapse in pathological gamblers. *Psychol. Med.* **2008**, *38*, 41–50. [CrossRef] [PubMed]
34. Anzman, S.L.; Birch, L.L. Low Inhibitory Control and Restrictive Feeding Practices Predict Weight Outcomes. *J. Pediatr.* **2009**, *155*, 651–656. [CrossRef] [PubMed]
35. Nederkoorn, C.; Jansen, E.; Mulkens, S.; Jansen, A. Impulsivity predicts treatment outcome in obese children. *Behav. Res. Ther.* **2007**, *45*, 1071–1075. [CrossRef]
36. Pauli-Pott, U.; Albayrak, Ö.; Hebebrand, J.; Pott, W. Does inhibitory control capacity in overweight and obese children and adolescents predict success in a weight-reduction program? *Eur. Child Adolesc. Psychiatry* **2009**, *19*, 135–141. [CrossRef]
37. Cavedini, P.; Zorzi, C.; Bassi, T.; Gorini, A.; Baraldi, C.; Ubbiali, A.; Bellodi, L. Decision-making functioning as a predictor of treatment outcome in anorexia nervosa. *Psychiatry Res.* **2006**, *145*, 179–187. [CrossRef]
38. Lucas, I.; Miranda-Olivos, R.; Testa, G.; Granero, R.; Sánchez, I.; Sánchez-González, J.; Jiménez-Murcia, S.; Fernández-Aranda, F.; Erzegovesi, S. Neuropsychological Learning Deficits as Predictors of Treatment Outcome in Patients with Eating Disorders. *Nutrients* **2021**, *13*, 2145. [CrossRef]
39. Dingemans, A.E.; van Son, G.E.; Vanhaelen, C.B.; van Furth, E.F. Depressive symptoms rather than executive functioning predict group cognitive behavioural therapy outcome in binge eating disorder. *Eur. Eat. Disord. Rev.* **2020**, *28*, 620–632. [CrossRef]
40. Falkenstein, M.; Hoormann, J.; Hohnsbein, J. ERP components in Go/Nogo tasks and their relation to inhibition. *Acta Psychol.* **1999**, *101*, 267–291. [CrossRef]
41. Luijten, M.; Machielsen, M.W.J.; Veltman, D.J.; Hester, R.; de Haan, L.; Franken, I.H.A. Systematic review of ERP and fMRI studies investigating inhibitory control and error processing in people with substance dependence and behavioural addictions. *J. Psychiatry Neurosci.* **2014**, *39*, 149–169. [CrossRef] [PubMed]
42. Zhang, Y.; Ou, H.; Yuan, T.F.; Sun, J. Electrophysiological indexes for impaired response inhibition and salience attribution in substance (stimulants and depressants) use disorders: A meta-analysis. *Int. J. Psychophysiol.* **2021**, *170*, 133–155. [CrossRef] [PubMed]
43. Dong, G.; Lu, Q.; Zhou, H.; Zhao, X. Impulse inhibition in people with Internet addiction disorder: Electrophysiological evidence from a Go/NoGo study. *Neurosci. Lett.* **2010**, *485*, 138–142. [CrossRef] [PubMed]

44. Leehr, E.J.; Schag, K.; Dresler, T.; Grosse-Wentrup, M.; Hautzinger, M.; Fallgatter, A.J.; Zipfel, S.; Giel, K.E.; Ehlis, A.-C. Food specific inhibitory control under negative mood in binge-eating disorder: Evidence from a multimethod approach. *Int. J. Eat. Disord.* 2018, *51*, 112–123. [CrossRef]
45. Stoyanova, S.; Giannouli, V. Bulgarian students' impulsivity differentiated by gender, age, and some scientific areas. *Psychol. Thought* 2018, *11*, 138–147. [CrossRef]
46. *American Psychiatric Association Diagnostic and Statistical Manual of Mental Disorders*; American Psychiatric Association: Washington, DC, USA, 2013; ISBN 0-89042-555-8.
47. Cloninger, C.R. (Ed.) *The Temperament and Character Inventory—Revised*; Center for Psychobiology of Personality, Washington University: Seattle, WA, USA, 1999.
48. Gutiérrez-Zotes, J.A.; Bayón, C.; Montserrat, C.; Valero, J.; Labad, A.; Cloninger, C.R.; Fernández-Aranda, F. Temperament and Character Inventory-Revised (TCI-R). Standardization and Normative Data in a General Population Sample. *Actas Esp. Psiquiatr.* 2004, *32*, 8–15. Available online: https://pubmed.ncbi.nlm.nih.gov/14963776/ (accessed on 2 November 2022).
49. Whiteside, S.P.; Lynam, D.R.; Miller, J.D.; Reynolds, S.K. Validation of the UPPS impulsive behaviour scale: A four-factor model of impulsivity. *Eur. J. Pers.* 2005, *19*, 559–574. [CrossRef]
50. Verdejo-García, A.; Lozano, Ó.; Moya, M.; Alcázar, M.Á.; Pérez-García, M. Psychometric properties of a spanish version of the UPPS-P impulsive behavior scale: Reliability, validity and association with trait and cognitive impulsivity. *J. Pers. Assess.* 2010, *92*, 70–77. [CrossRef]
51. Garner, D.M. Eating disorder inventory-2 manual. *Int. J. Eat Disord.* 1991, *14*, 59–64.
52. Golden, C.J. *Stroop Color and Word Test: A Manual for Clinical and Experimental Uses*; Stoelting: Chicago, IL, USA, 1978; pp. 1–46.
53. StataCorp *Stata Statistical Software, Release 17*; StataCorp LLC: College Station, TX, USA, 2021.
54. Finner, H.; Roters, M. On the False Discovery Rate and Expected Type I Errors. *J. Am. Stat. Assoc.* 2001, *88*, 920–923. [CrossRef]
55. Kelley, K.; Preacher, K.J. On effect size. *Psychol. Methods* 2012, *17*, 137–152. [CrossRef] [PubMed]
56. Hosmer, D.W.; Hosmer, T.; Le Cessie, S.; Lemeshow, S. A comparison of goodness-of-fit tests for the logistic regression model. *Stat. Med.* 1997, *16*, 965–980. [CrossRef]
57. Fernàndez-Aranda, F.; Álvarez-Moya, E.M.; Martínez-Viana, C.; Sànchez, I.; Granero, R.; Penelo, E.; Forcano, L.; Peñas-Lledó, E. Predictors of early change in bulimia nervosa after a brief psychoeducational therapy. *Appetite* 2009, *52*, 805–808. [CrossRef] [PubMed]
58. Miranda-Olivos, R.; Testa, G.; Lucas, I.; Sánchez, I.; Sánchez-González, J.; Granero, R.; Jiménez-Murcia, S.; Fernández-Aranda, F. Clinical factors predicting impaired executive functions in eating disorders: The role of illness duration. *J. Psychiatr. Res.* 2021, *144*, 87–95. [CrossRef] [PubMed]
59. Merlotti, E.; Mucci, A.; Volpe, U.; Montefusco, V.; Monteleone, P.; Bucci, P.; Galderisi, S. Impulsiveness in Patients with Bulimia Nervosa: Electrophysiological Evidence of Reduced Inhibitory Control. *Neuropsychobiology* 2013, *68*, 116–123. [CrossRef] [PubMed]
60. Schulz, K.P.; Fan, J.; Magidina, O.; Marks, D.J.; Hahn, B.; Halperin, J.M. Does the emotional go/no-go task really measure behavioral inhibition?: Convergence with measures on a non-emotional analog. *Arch. Clin. Neuropsychol.* 2007, *22*, 151–160. [CrossRef]
61. McDonald, C.E.; Rossell, S.L.; Phillipou, A. The comorbidity of eating disorders in bipolar disorder and associated clinical correlates characterised by emotion dysregulation and impulsivity: A systematic review. *J. Affect. Disord.* 2019, *259*, 228–243. [CrossRef]
62. Brockmeyer, T.; Skunde, M.; Wu, M.; Bresslein, E.; Rudofsky, G.; Herzog, W.; Friederich, H.-C.C. Difficulties in emotion regulation across the spectrum of eating disorders. *Compr. Psychiatry* 2014, *55*, 565–571. [CrossRef]
63. Turton, R.; Nazar, B.P.; Burgess, E.E.; Lawrence, N.S.; Cardi, V.; Treasure, J.; Hirsch, C.R. To Go or Not to Go: A Proof of Concept Study Testing Food-Specific Inhibition Training for Women with Eating and Weight Disorders. *Eur. Eat. Disord. Rev.* 2018, *26*, 11–21. [CrossRef]
64. Keeler, J.L.; Chami, R.; Cardi, V.; Hodsoll, J.; Bonin, E.; MacDonald, P.; Treasure, J.; Lawrence, N. App-based food-specific inhibitory control training as an adjunct to treatment as usual in binge-type eating disorders: A feasibility trial. *Appetite* 2022, *168*, 105788. [CrossRef]
65. Chami, R.; Treasure, J.; Cardi, V.; Lozano-Madrid, M.; Eichin, K.N.; McLoughlin, G.; Blechert, J. Exploring Changes in Event-Related Potentials After a Feasibility Trial of Inhibitory Training for Bulimia Nervosa and Binge Eating Disorder. *Front. Psychol.* 2020, *11*, 1056. [CrossRef] [PubMed]

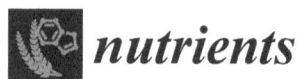 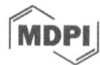

Article

Conditioning by a Previous Experience Impairs the Rewarding Value of a Comfort Meal

Adoracion Nieto [1,2,3,†], Dan M. Livovsky [1,4,*,†] and Fernando Azpiroz [1,2,3,*]

1. Digestive System Research Unit, University Hospital Vall d'Hebron, 08035 Barcelona, Spain
2. Departament de Medicina, Universitat Autònoma de Barcelona, Bellaterra, 08193 Cerdanyola del Vallès, Spain
3. Centro de Investigación Biomédica en Red de Enfermedades Hepáticas y Digestivas (Ciberehd), Instituto de Salud Carlos III, 28029 Madrid, Spain
4. Digestive Diseases Institute, Shaare Zedek Medical Center, Faculty of Medicine, Hebrew University of Jerusalem, Jerusalem 9103102, Israel

* Correspondence: danlivo@szmc.org.il (D.M.L.); azpiroz.fernando@gmail.com (F.A.); Tel.: +34-93-274-6259 (F.A.)
† These authors contributed equally to this work.

Abstract: Background. Meal ingestion induces a postprandial experience that involves homeostatic and hedonic sensations. Our aim was to determine the effect of aversive conditioning on the postprandial reward of a comfort meal. Methods: A sham-controlled, randomised, parallel, single-blind study was performed on 12 healthy women (6 per group). A comfort meal was tested before and after coupling the meal with an aversive sensation (conditioning intervention), induced by infusion of lipids via a thin naso-duodenal catheter; in the pre- and post-conditioning tests and in the control group, a sham infusion was performed. Participants were instructed that two recipes of a tasty humus would be tested; however, the same meal was administered with a colour additive in the conditioning and post-conditioning tests. Digestive well-being (primary outcome) was measured every 10 min before and 60 min after ingestion using graded scales. Results: In the aversive conditioning group, the comfort meal in the pre-conditioning test induced a pleasant postprandial experience, which was significantly lower in the post-conditioning test; the effect of aversive conditioning (change from pre- to post-conditioning) was significant as compared to sham conditioning in the control group, which showed no differences between study days. Conclusion: The hedonic postprandial response to a comfort meal in healthy women is impaired by aversive conditioning. ClinicalTrials.gov ID: NCT04938934.

Keywords: Pavlovian conditioning; aversive conditioning; eating behaviour; digestive sensations; postprandial symptoms; digestive well-being; food valence

Citation: Nieto, A.; Livovsky, D.M.; Azpiroz, F. Conditioning by a Previous Experience Impairs the Rewarding Value of a Comfort Meal. *Nutrients* 2023, 15, 2247. https://doi.org/10.3390/nu15102247

Academic Editors: Robyn M Brown, Roser Granero, Susana Jiménez-Murcia and Fernando Fernández-Aranda

Received: 28 February 2023
Revised: 16 April 2023
Accepted: 7 May 2023
Published: 9 May 2023

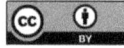

Copyright: © 2023 by the authors. Licensee MDPI, Basel, Switzerland. This article is an open access article distributed under the terms and conditions of the Creative Commons Attribution (CC BY) license (https://creativecommons.org/licenses/by/4.0/).

1. Introduction

The digestive process that follows meal ingestion is associated with a postprandial experience that involves homeostatic sensations (satiety, fullness) with a hedonic dimension (digestive well-being, mood) [1]. The postprandial experience depends on the characteristics of the meal (organoleptic, amount and composition) and of the individual, including digestive function, intestinal sensitivity and cognitive/emotive factors, which may be influenced by a variety of conditions [2]. Pavlovian conditioning, also known as classical conditioning, refers to the behavioural technique of pairing a physiological stimulus with a neutral stimulus; repeated exposure to the pairing induces a learning process, by which the biologic response to the physiological stimulus is triggered by the neutral stimulus alone. Pavlovian conditioning has been shown to magnify the expectation of aversive sensations and has been postulated as a mechanism of hypervigilance and visceral hypersensitivity [3–6]. Associative learning, understood as the learned association between two unrelated stimuli, has also been also shown to induce taste aversion and avoidance: e.g., a pleasant taste becomes disagreeable by previous association with an unpleasant experience [7].

We hypothesised that the postprandial experience, in particular the hedonic component (i.e., postprandial sensation of digestive well-being), may be modified by conditioning. Our specific aim was to determine the effect of aversive conditioning on the hedonic and homeostatic sensations in response to a comfort meal in healthy subjects.

The postprandial experience in humans is important because it may influence dietary decisions and habits. Moreover, a negative postprandial experience is a main complaint in patients with functional gut disorders, particularly in those with functional dyspepsia [8,9]; hence, aversive conditioning might be a mechanism of meal intolerance and postprandial symptoms in these patients.

2. Material and Methods

2.1. Experimental Design

A sham-controlled, randomised, parallel, single-blind study on the effect of aversive conditioning on the responses to a comfort meal in healthy women was performed in a tertiary referral centre between February and August 2021. The research was conducted according to the Declaration of Helsinki. The protocol for the study had been previously approved by the Institutional Review Board of the University Hospital Vall d'Hebron (Comitè d'Ètica d'Investigació Clinica, Vall d'Hebron Institut de Recerca; protocol number PR(AG)338/2016M approved 28 October 2016, revised 11 December 2020) and all participants provided written informed consent. The study protocol was registered with ClinicalTrials.gov NCT04938934.

2.2. Participants

Twelve, non-obese, non-dieting and weight-stable women (6 per group), without history of gastrointestinal symptoms were recruited by public advertising to participate in the study. For this pilot, proof-of-concept study, only women were included for the sake of homogeneity and because some data indicate that they are more susceptible to factors that modulate the postprandial experience than men [10]. Exclusion criteria were chronic health conditions, previous abdominal surgery (except appendectomy or hernia repair), use of medications (except occasional use of NSAIDs and antihistamines), alcohol abuse and use of recreational drugs. By specific questioning, candidates with a history of anosmia or ageusia, antecedents of obesity (defined as body mass index > 30 kg/m^2), current dieting or any pattern of selective eating, such as vegetarianism, were not included in the study to prevent potential biases on the responses to food ingestion. Candidates were asked whether they liked hummus, and those who did not were not included. Absence of current digestive symptoms was verified using a standard abdominal symptom questionnaire (no symptom > 2 on a 0–10 scale). Psychological and eating symptoms and/or traits were evaluated using the Hospital Anxiety and Depression Scale (HAD), Dutch Eating Behaviour Questionnaire (DEBQ—Emotional eating, External eating, Restrained eating) and Physical Anhedonia Scale (PAS); participants were not included if they scored >7 on the anxiety or depression subscales [11]; cut-offs for emotional eating (>2.83), external eating (>3.5) and restrained eating (>3.0) were adapted from a study in the local population [12]. Studies were performed during the follicular phase of the menstrual cycle (days 5–15). For this pilot proof-of-concept study, no a priori sample size calculation was performed; analysis of the data performed after 12 studies were completed indicated that a sample size of 8 subjects (i.e., 4 per group) was required to detect changes in the primary outcome with 90% power and a 5% significance threshold, and hence, no further participants were included. Thus, each group consisted of 6 participants.

2.3. Experimental Paradigm

Participants were informed that the aim of the study was to investigate the effect of meal composition on the postprandial responses and that a nasoduodenal tube was used to evaluate gastric outflow. Participants were informed that two recipes of a tasty humus with different compositions would be tested; however, the same meal (low-fat humus) without or with the addition of a colourant (i.e., non-coloured or coloured) was administered (Figure 1). Using a computerised random sequence generator, participants were allocated into aversive conditioning (intervention) or sham conditioning (control) groups. During meal ingestion, either lipids or sham infusion was simultaneously infused single-blind (without participants knowing which) into the duodenum via the nasoduodenal catheter (see below). Each participant underwent three experiments on consecutive days, as follows (Figure 1). First day—pre-conditioning exposure: non-coloured meal plus sham infusion in both groups. Second day—conditioning intervention: coloured meal in both groups plus (a) duodenal lipid infusion in the aversive conditioning group (to induce aversive sensations, e.g., a negative sensation of digestive well-being) or (b) sham infusion in the sham conditioning (control) group. Third day—post-conditioning exposure: coloured meal plus sham infusion in both groups. Primary outcome: effect of conditioning on digestive well-being measured by scales (difference in the area under the curve from pre-conditioning to post-conditioning, i.e., day 3 minus day 1) in aversive conditioning versus sham conditioning groups.

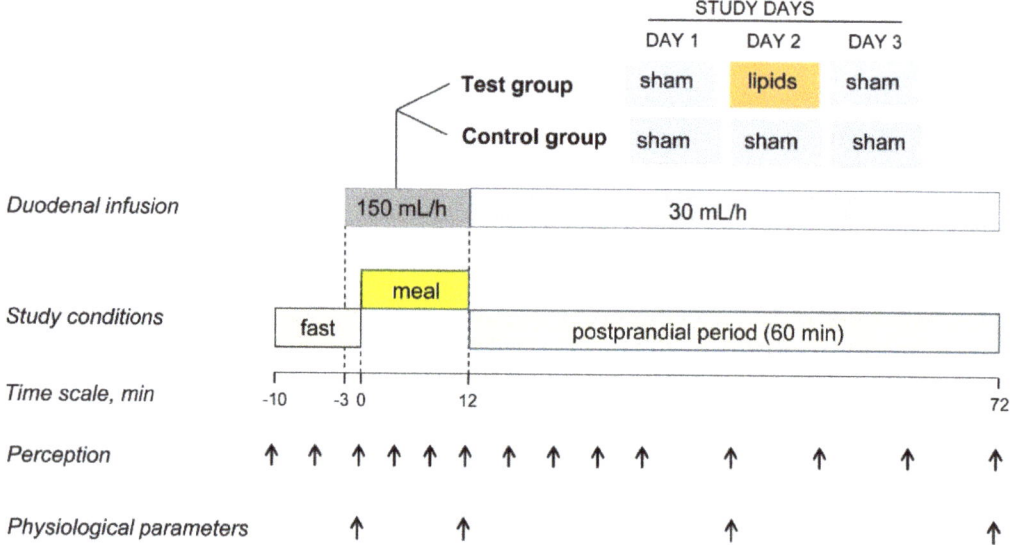

Figure 1. Experimental design and procedure. In a sham-controlled, parallel, randomised, blind study, a comfort meal was paired with duodenal lipid infusion to induce aversive conditioning (DAY 2) and the responses to the meal were compared before (DAY 1) and after conditioning (DAY 3).

2.4. General Procedure

During the 3 consecutive study days, participants were instructed to refrain from strenuous physical activity, to consume a standard dinner (100 g chicken, 50 g rice, 50 g white bread and one apple; 503 kcal, 7 g fat, 82 g carbohydrates, 30 g protein) the night before, to fast overnight and to eat a standard breakfast (200 mL coffee with semi-skimmed milk and a 50 g white bread sandwich with 30 g ham and 40 g cheese; 338 kcal, 11 g fat, 38 g carbohydrate, 24 g protein) 4 h before each study. After intubation per nose, the catheter (Flocare Bengmark NI Tube, Nutricia Medical, Hoofddorp, The Netherlands) was positioned into the duodenum under fluoroscopic control. Studies were conducted in a quiet, isolated room. Outcomes were measured 10 min before ingestion of the probe meal (pre-ingestion period), during the ingestion period and during the 60 min after ingestion (postprandial period) (Figure 1).

2.5. Interventions

2.5.1. Probe Meal

The probe meal consisted of 150 g low-fat hummus (219 Kcal; 12 g fat, 82 g carbohydrates, 13 g protein; Hummus Classic, Ametller Origen, Barcelona, Spain) served at a controlled temperature (20 °C), 20 g toasts (81 Kcal; 0.9 g fat, 15.2 g carbohydrates, 2.4 g protein; Mini Tostas, Bimbo, Barcelona, Spain) and 120 mL water. The probe meal was administered stepwise in 3 equal servings at a fixed rate: every 180 s one meal portion (50 g hummus plus a 6.6 g toast) was presented on a tray; after each serving, participants were allowed 60 s for evaluation of digestive sensations (see below); total ingestion time was 12 min, the water load (120 mL) was ingested ad libitum throughout the ingestion period. On the 1st study day, the original humus preparation (i.e., non-coloured) was served; on the 2nd and 3rd study days (conditioning and post-conditioning experiments, respectively), the humus was coloured by adding 1% fat-soluble, odourless and flavourless pink colourant (Decora, Karma, Salerno, Italy), to modify its appearance, but not its organoleptic characteristics or nutrient composition. The composition and meal load were established based on a series of preliminary feasibility studies.

2.5.2. Duodenal Infusion

Aversive conditioning (2nd study day in aversive conditioning group only) was produced by infusion of lipids (300 mg/mL purified soybean oil; Intralipid, Fresenius Kabi, Barcelona, Spain) into the duodenum via the nasoduodenal catheter. Lipids were continuously infused starting 3 min before, during and 60 min after ingestion of the probe meal (total infusion time = 75 min) using an infusion pump (Compat Ella Push, Nestle Health Science, Barcelona, Spain) at a rate of 150 mL/h during the first 15 min (3 min pre-ingestion period and 12 min ingestion period) and at 30 mL/h during the 60 min postprandial period (Figure 1). On the rest of the study days (i.e., 1st and 3rd days in the conditioning group, and the three study days in the control group), a sham infusion was performed following the same procedure, but diverting the lipid flow from the infusion line via a 3-way stopcock to a reservoir. Lipid and sham infusions were performed single-blind, i.e., without the participants knowing the type of infusion.

The aversive conditioning procedure (lipid load and delivery rate) was established by a series of preliminary studies in 3 additional participants so that the lipid infusion would induce a negative sensation of digestive well-being (below score -2 on a -5 to $+5$ scale, see below) without severe nausea, bloating or pain (score ≤ 2 on 0–10 scales; see below).

2.6. Outcomes

2.6.1. Perception of Homeostatic and Hedonic Sensations

Five 10-cm scales graded from -5 to $+5$ were used to measure: (a) meal wanting (impossible/eagerly), (b) meal liking (very disagreeable/very agreeable), (c) hunger/satiety (extremely hungry/completely satiated), (d) digestive well-being (extremely unpleasant sensation/extremely pleasant sensation) and (e) mood (negative/positive); three additional 10-cm scales graded from 0 (not at all) to 10 (very much) were used to measure (f) abdominal bloating–fullness, (g) discomfort–pain and (h) nausea. The wanting scale was scored at the presentation of each meal serving (how much would you like to eat this portion) and at the end of the meal (how much would you like to eat another portion). The liking scale was scored after each meal serving (how much did you like eating the previous portion). The rest of the scales were scored: (a) during the pre-ingestion period (10 min before the meal) at 5 min intervals, (b) during meal ingestion, after each meal serving, and (c) during the postprandial period at 5 min intervals during the first 20 min and at 10 min intervals up to 60 min after ingestion (Figure 1). It has been previously shown that these scales detect consistent and reproducible differences in post-prandial sensations induced by various conditioning factors [13–19] and that perception measurements correlate with changes in circulating metabolites [20,21] and with some objective parameters of brain function measured by functional magnetic resonance [22,23].

2.6.2. Physiological Parameters

The following physiological parameters were measured at 4 time points: before meal ingestion (baseline) and at the beginning, mid and end of the postprandial observation period (0 min, 30 min and 60 min after ingestion) (Figure 1).

Gastric emptying was measured by ultrasonography, as previously described [24,25]. In brief, ultrasound images of the gastric antrum were obtained using a Chison ultrasound scanner (ECO1; Chison, Wuxi, China) with an abdominal 3.5 Hz probe (C3A; Chison, Wuxi, China); images were obtained with the subjects seated and leaning slightly backwards in an ergonomic chair. Gastric images between antral contractions were obtained in triplicate; using the superior mesenteric vein and the aorta as landmarks, the outer profile and the cross-sectional area of the antrum were measured using the built-in calliper and measurement tool.

Changes in abdominal girth from pre-ingesta were measured by a tape measure placed over the umbilicus and the superior edge of the iliac crests [26]. The position of the tape was marked over the skin for subsequent measurements.

Changes in the position of the diaphragm from the pre-ingestion level were determined at each time point, as previously described [24]. Briefly, the position of the lower margin of the right liver lobe at the right anterior axillary line was identified by ultrasonography (Eco 1, Chison Medical Technologies, Wuxi, China) using a 3.5 MHz curved array transducer held over the edge of the costal wall in the coronal plane with the shaft held in a horizontal position and the head in an axial direction. At each time point, the position (averaged over 3 respiratory cycles) was marked over the skin.

2.7. Statistical Analysis

Calculations were performed using SPSS Statistics for Windows (Version 25.0, IBM Corp, Armonk, NY, USA). A significance level of 5% (two tails) was used for comparisons.

In each group, the means and standard errors of the measured variables were calculated. In each experiment, the effects of the intervention on sensation scores were analysed, measuring the area under the curve normalised for baseline (except for the wanting and liking scores, which were not normalised) as follows: for each observation interval, the area was calculated as duration (min) of the observation interval × normalised score (absolute score—mean premeal score); the area under the curve during ingestion and the postprandial period (expressed as score × min) was calculated as the sum of the area of all observation intervals.

In each participant, the effect of the aversive (or sham) stimulus was measured as the difference in the area under the curve on day 2 (duodenal lipids or sham infusion) minus day 1 (pre-conditioning); the effect of conditioning (previous exposure to aversive stimulus) was measured as the difference in day 3 (post-conditioning) minus day 1 (pre-conditioning). Mean values for the test group (lipid infusion) and control group (sham infusion) were calculated, and statistical analyses within groups and between groups were performed. The Shapiro–Wilk test was used to determine the normality of data distribution. Parametric normally distributed data were compared by Student's t-test for paired or unpaired data; otherwise, the Wilcoxon signed-rank test was used for paired data, and the Mann–Whitney U test was used for unpaired data. Differences were considered significant at a p value < 0.05.

All co-authors had access to the study data and reviewed and approved the final manuscript.

3. Results

3.1. Demographics

Participants were 30.9 ± 2.3 years of age (range 23–49 years), had a 21.3 ± 0.5 kg/m^2 body mass index (range 18.6–24.8 kg/m^2), scored 11.8 ± 2.1 in the physical anhedonia scale (range 2–23) and were non-smokers. No differences between the aversive conditioning and control groups were detected. Intubation was well tolerated without side effects; all participants completed the studies and were included for analysis.

3.2. Responses to the Probe Meal before Conditioning (Study Day 1)

Pre-ingestion. Before the probe meal (baseline fasting period), subjects reported hunger, neutral digestive well-being and positive mood without the sensations of abdominal fullness/bloating, discomfort/pain or nausea (Figures 2 and 3).

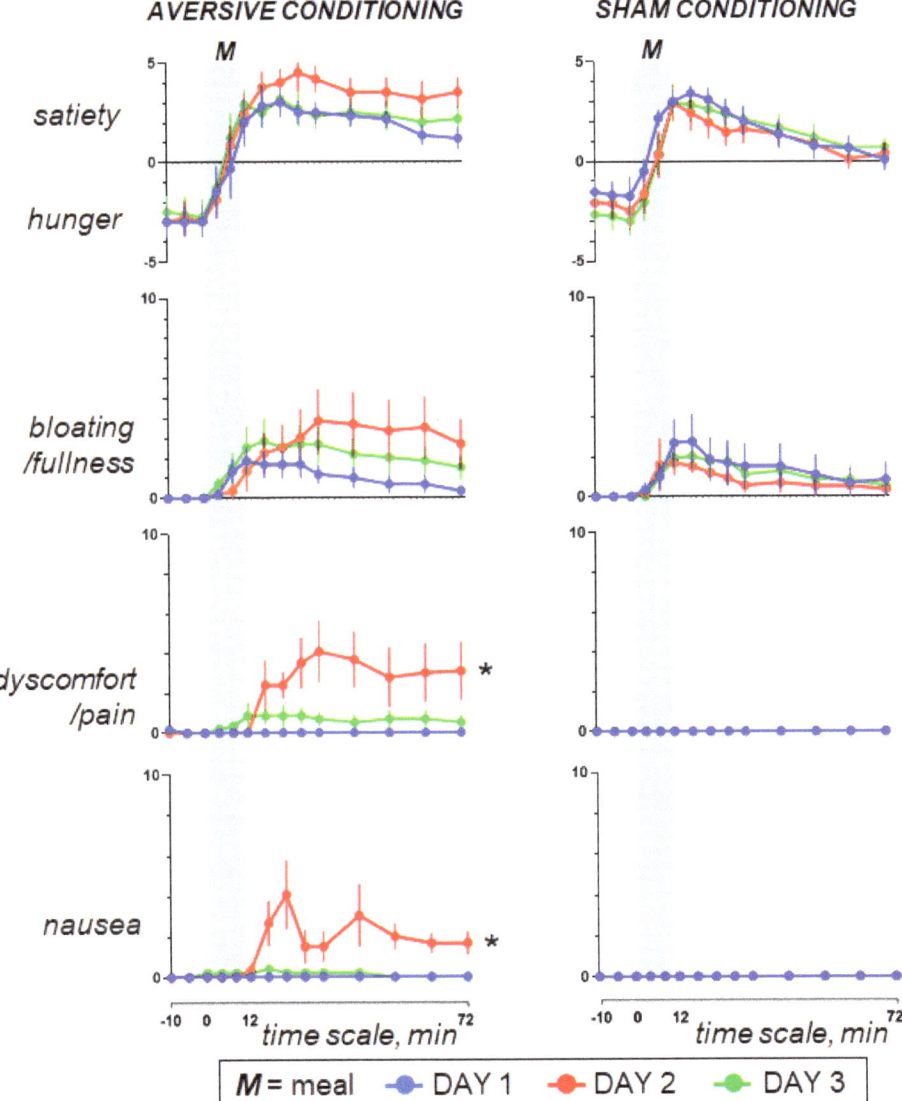

Figure 2. Homeostatic sensations. Concomitant duodenal lipid infusion on day 2 impaired the postprandial response and the effect was significant for abdominal discomfort and nausea (effect measured as the change in the area under the curve on day 2 minus day 1; * p = 0.002 vs. sham infusion). However, data on day 3 show that aversive conditioning in the test group (duodenal lipid infusion on the previous day) did not induce significant effects. Values represent mean ± SE.

Ingestion phase. All participants ingested the meal at a fixed rate (12 min). Participants found the meal attractive at the initial presentation and liked it (positive meal wanting and meal liking; Figure 4). During meal ingestion satiety progressively increased, associated with mild fullness sensation and positive sensations of digestive well-being and mood, without abdominal discomfort or nausea (Figures 2 and 3).

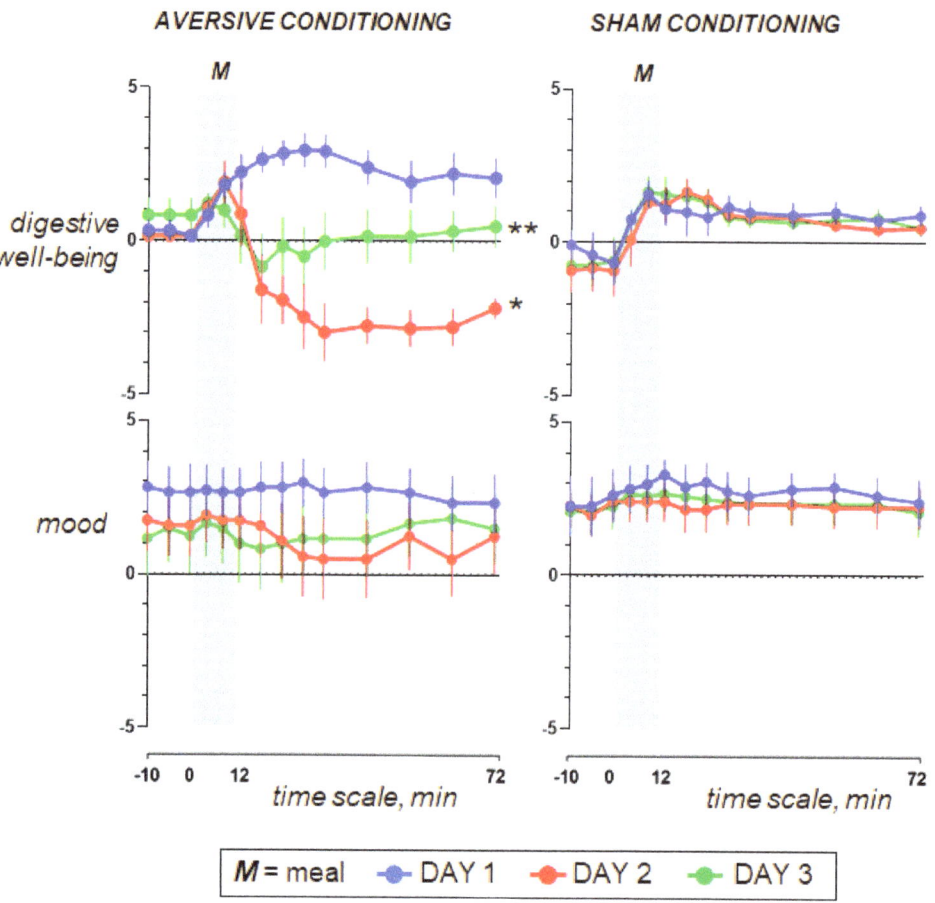

Figure 3. Hedonic sensations. Concomitant duodenal lipid infusion on day 2 impaired the postprandial response and the effect was significant for digestive well-being (effect measured as the change in the area under the curve on day 2 minus day 1; * $p < 0.001$ vs. sham infusion). Data on day 3 show that aversive conditioning in the test group (previous exposure to the aversive stimulus) significantly impaired postprandial well-being (effect measured as the change in the area under the curve on day 3 minus day 1; ** $p = 0.004$ vs. sham conditioning). Values represent mean ± SE.

Postprandial phase. During the postprandial phase, these sensations gradually decayed (Figures 2 and 3).

No significant differences in the sensations measured before, during and after ingestion were detected between groups.

3.3. Effect of Aversive Stimulation (Study Day 2 vs. Day 1)

Pre-ingestion and ingestion phase. The sensations measured before and during meal ingestion on the second study day were not different from those on the first day in both groups (Figures 2 and 3), except for meal wanting and meal liking (Figure 4), which were reduced by duodenal lipid infusion in the test group, but were unaffected by sham infusion in the control group; the effect of lipid infusion in the aversive conditioning group (measured as the change in the area under the curve for Day 2 minus Day 1) was significantly different from that of sham infusion in the control group both for meal wanting (change by −36 ± 16 vs. 5 ± 12 score × min in controls; $p = 0.041$) and meal liking (change by −27 ± 9 vs. 2 ± 6 score × min in controls; $p = 0.013$).

Postprandial phase. In the control group, sham infusion on the second study day did not modify the postprandial experience as compared to the first study day. By contrast, concomitant duodenal lipid infusion in the test group induced a marked change in postprandial sensations, with an increase in satiety and bloating, a decrease in digestive well-being and mood and some degree of abdominal discomfort and nausea (Figures 2 and 3). The effect of lipid infusion (measured as the change in the area under the curve on day 2 minus day 1) was significantly different from that of sham infusion for digestive well-being (change by −294 ± 34 vs. 25 ± 20 score × min in controls; $p < 0.001$), abdominal discomfort (change by 172 ± 65 vs. 0 ± 0 score × min in controls; $p = 0.002$) and nausea (change by 134 ± 28 vs. 0 ± 0 score × min; $p = 0.002$).

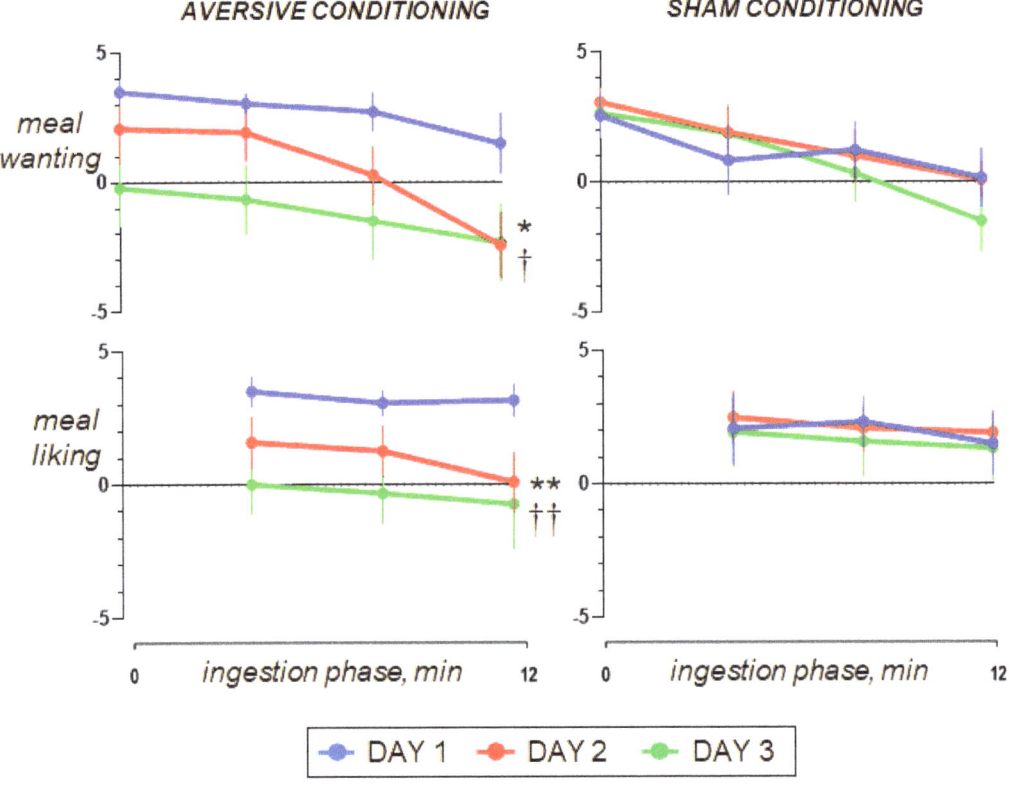

Figure 4. Reward value during meal ingestion. The comfort meal was served in 3 portions; meal wanting was measured before each serving and at the end of ingestion; meal liking was measured after each serving. On day 2, concomitant duodenal lipid infusion impaired the ingestive response (effect measured as the change in the area under the curve on day 2 minus day 1 vs. sham infusion; * $p = 0.041$ for meal wanting; ** $p = 0.013$ for meal liking). Data on Day 3 show that aversive conditioning in the test group (previous exposure to the aversive stimulus) significantly reduced the valence of the comfort meal (effect measured as the change in the area under the curve on day 3 minus day 1 vs. sham conditioning; † $p = 0.023$ for meal wanting; †† $p = 0.030$ for meal liking). Values represent mean ± SE.

3.4. Effect of Conditioning (Study Day 3 vs. Day 1)

Pre-ingestion and ingestion phase. No significant differences were detected in the sensations measured before and during meal ingestion on the study day 3 as compared to day 1 in both groups (Figures 2 and 3), except for meal wanting and meal liking (Figure 4). Meal wanting and liking were unaffected in the control group, but in the test group, previous exposure to the aversive stimulus (aversive conditioning) significantly reduced the valence of the comfort meal; the effect of conditioning (duodenal lipid or sham infusion on the previous study day), measured as the change in the area under the curve on day 3 minus day 1, was significantly decreased in the aversive conditioning group compared to the control group both for meal wanting (change by -62 ± 16 vs. -6 ± 9 score × min in controls; $p = 0.023$) and for meal liking (change by -43 ± 13 vs. -4 ± 5 score × min in controls; $p = 0.030$). Meal wanting and liking on day 3 were somewhat, but not significantly, lower than on day 2.

Postprandial phase. In the control group, sham conditioning (duodenal sham infusion on the previous day) did not modify the postprandial experience as compared to the first study day. By contrast, in the test group, aversive conditioning (duodenal lipid infusion on the previous day) significantly impaired postprandial well-being, and this was associated with a trend to increase in bloating and mild abdominal discomfort, without changes in satiety, nausea and mood (Figures 2 and 3). The effect of lipid infusion on the previous day (measured as the change in the area under the curve on day 3 minus day 1) was significantly different from that of sham infusion for digestive well-being (change by -186 ± 68 vs. 16 ± 19 score × min in controls; $p = 0.004$), but not for the rest of the sensations: bloating changed by 74 ± 67 vs. -16 ± 40 score × min in controls ($p = 0.235$), abdominal discomfort by 43 ± 23 vs. 0 ± 0 score × min in controls ($p = 0.074$), satiety by -2 ± 50 vs. 82 ± 43 score × min in controls ($p = 0.179$), nausea by 6 ± 4 vs. 0 ± 0 score × min in controls ($p = 0.181$) and mood by 8 ± 27 vs. -12 ± 31 score × min in controls ($p = 0.813$).

3.5. Physiological Parameters

3.5.1. Responses to the Probe Meal before Conditioning (Study Day 1)

Ingestion of the probe meal was associated with gastric filling (increase in antral cross-sectional area) and abdominal accommodation (elevation of the diaphragm with limited increase in girth) (Figure 5).

3.5.2. Effect of Aversive Stimulation (Study Day 2 vs. Day 1)

In the control group, sham infusion on the second study day had no effects on any of the physiological parameters as compared to the first study day. By contrast, in the test group, lipid infusion (effect measured as the change in the area under the curve in day 2 minus day 1 vs. sham infusion) was associated with gastric retention (more sustained increase in the antral cross-sectional area; $p < 0.001$) and abdominal accommodation (elevation of the diaphragm; $p = 0.002$), (Figure 5).

3.5.3. Effect of Conditioning (Study Day 3 vs. Day 1)

Neither aversive nor sham conditioning had consistent effects on the physiological response to meal ingestion (Figure 5).

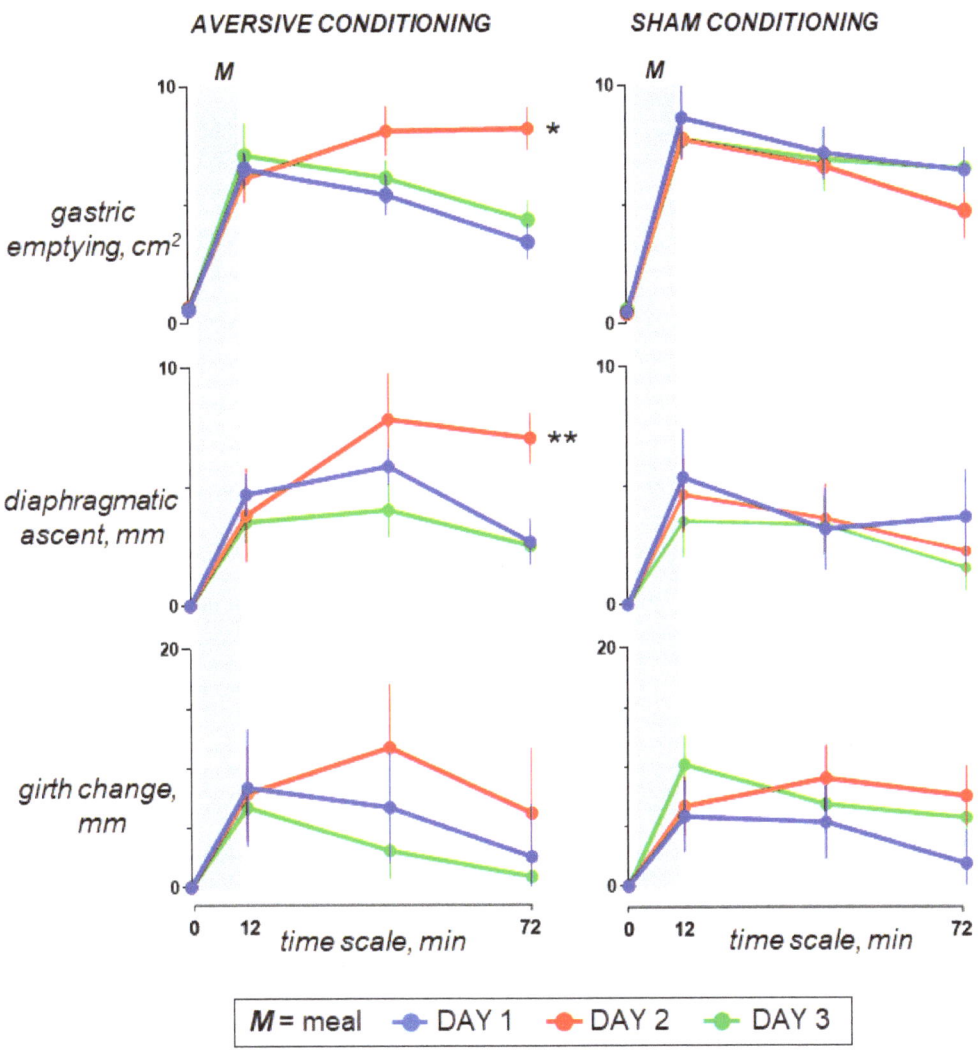

Figure 5. Digestive response to meal ingestion. On day 2, duodenal lipid infusion in the test group was associated with a sustained increase in antral cross-sectional area (delayed gastric emptying; * $p < 0.001$) and diaphragmatic ascent (prolonged abdominal accommodation; ** $p = 0.002$); effects measured as the changes in the area under the curve on day 2 minus day 1 vs. sham infusion. However, data for day 3 show that aversive conditioning in the test group (previous exposure to the aversive stimulus) did not induce significant effects. Values represent mean ± SE.

4. Discussion

Our study shows that pairing a pleasant meal with an experimentally-induced aversive sensation conditions the postprandial response to subsequent consumption of the same meal. Interestingly, aversive conditioning impaired the hedonic experience without significant impacts on homeostatic sensations or the physiological digestive response.

The target for conditioning was a comfort probe meal [17] that induced a pleasant and rewarding postprandial experience. The comfort probe meal was blindly paired with duodenal lipid infusion to induce a negative sensation of digestive well-being [27]. As expected [27,28], duodenal lipids induced a mild sensation of abdominal bloating, discomfort and nausea, as well as a reflex inhibition of gastric emptying with a prolonged residency of the meal in the stomach; gastric retention was associated with a sustained abdominal accommodation (elevation of the diaphragm) and sensation of satiety throughout the postprandial observation period.

Aversive conditioning (i.e., previous pairing of the comfort meal with lipid-induced aversive sensation) conditioned the subsequent postprandial response to the same meal, particularly affecting the reward experience. Various mechanisms may be involved in the impairment of the postprandial experience by conditioning.

In the first place, a satisfactory postprandial experience depends on a normal response of the digestive system, and conversely, digestive dysfunction deteriorates the postprandial experience [14], but conditioning did not affect the digestive function.

The conditioning paradigm used in the present experiments was analogous to that previously applied for conditioned taste aversion, pairing the rewarding meal with an aversive stimulus [29,30]. Remarkably, similar to conditioned taste aversion, postprandial conditioning was acquired after a single exposure [30], in contrast to the complex learning process with repeat pairing experiences required for other types of Pavlovian conditioning [6]. In previous studies, we showed that postprandial satisfaction is related to meal palatability [16], but a strong aversive taste was required to reduce postprandial well-being, to a much lesser extent than in the present study after conditioning.

Cognitive-emotive factors and expectations might be involved in conditioning the post-prandial experience. Indeed, a cognitive intervention (education) influenced the hedonic postprandial experience, without significant effects on homeostatic sensations [19], an effect similar to that produced by conditioning in the present study. Expectations are also important: mislabelled foods produce the effect expected by the (mis)information provided; for instance, a low-fat yoghurt mislabelled as high-fat induced similar symptoms to the real high-fat yoghurt in dyspeptic patients [31]. Anticipatory knowledge and attention have been shown to heighten visceral sensitivity and increase perception of intestinal stimuli; intestinal distention produced more intense perception when the stimuli were anticipated by a visual signal than when participants were distracted by a cognitive task [32].

5. Limitations

Our conditioning paradigm introduced a colour clue (coloured meal during and after conditioning versus non-coloured meal pre-conditioning), but we do not know whether conditioned postprandial dissatisfaction was selective to the colour or if it would also affect the non-coloured meal; indeed, other forms of conditioning express generalisation and affect related stimuli [33,34].

For this pilot study, a small sample size was included due to the complexity and invasiveness of the study; an interim sample size calculation justified no further inclusion for practical and ethical considerations, but once the concept is proven, a larger study with a less invasive methodology is indicated. Furthermore, only women were included and the effect of conditioning on men remains to be explored.

This pilot study, proving a new concept, opens a series of questions, particularly in relation to the specificity versus generalisation of the conditioned response, extinction interval and the relation between aversive stimulus/conditioned response [30,33,34], that remain to be addressed.

6. Conclusions and Inferences

Postprandial conditioning might have important implications and open relevant research avenues. Several conditions of great health impact, such as obesity, metabolic syndrome, diabetes or hypercholesterolemia, relate to consumption (or overconsumption) of specific foods, and in this context, aversive conditioning could be a tool to promote an avoidance behaviour.

The proof of aversive conditioning sustains the hypothesis of reward conditioning. If feasible, reinforcement of the postprandial reward and food valence could be applied to counteract natural neophobia (i.e., rejection of new or unknown foods) in children [30], and to promote ingestion in patients with anorexia and nutritional deficits, a common problem in oncological patients.

Patients with functional gut disorders, particularly with functional dyspepsia, complain of postprandial symptoms in the absence of a detectable cause and constitute about half of gastrointestinal consultations. Aversive food conditioning might be a mechanism of meal intolerance in these patients. Based on the present data, it could be speculated that an analogous technique could be applied to deconstruct aversive conditioning in these patients [33]; de-conditioning of food intolerances may have important applications as a mechanistic treatment in patients with food-related symptoms.

Author Contributions: A.N.: investigation, data curation, formal analysis, methodology, D.M.L.: conceptualisation (supporting), formal analysis (lead), investigation, methodology, visualisation, writing—draft preparation, F.A.: conceptualisation (lead), funding acquisition, methodology (lead), project administration, writing—review and editing. All authors have read and agreed to the published version of the manuscript.

Funding: The present study was supported in part by the Ministerio de Ciencia e Innovación (Agencia Estatal de Investigación, PID2021-122295OB-I00). Ciberehd is funded by the Instituto de Salud Carlos III. D.M.L received support from the Israeli Medical Association and from the Israel Gastroenterological Association.

Institutional Review Board Statement: The clinical study was conducted according to the Declaration of Helsinki. The study protocol had previously been approved by the Institutional Review Board of the University Hospital Vall d'Hebron (Comitè d'Ètica d'Investigació Clinica, Vall d'Hebron Institut de Recerca; protocol number PR(AG)338/2016M approved 28 October 2016, revised 11 December 2020) and all participants provided written informed consent. The study protocol was registered with ClinicalTrials.gov NCT04938934.

Informed Consent Statement: Informed consent was obtained from all subjects involved in the study.

Data Availability Statement: The data presented in this study will be shared upon reasonable request from the corresponding author.

Acknowledgments: The authors thank Gloria Santaliestra for secretarial assistance and Benjamin Koslowsky for English editing and proofreading.

Conflicts of Interest: The authors declare no conflict of interest.

References

1. Livovsky, D.M.; Pribic, T.; Azpiroz, F. Food, eating, and the gastrointestinal tract. *Nutrients* **2020**, *12*, 986. [CrossRef] [PubMed]
2. Livovsky, D.M.; Azpiroz, F. Gastrointestinal contributions to the postprandial experience. *Nutrients* **2021**, *13*, 893. [CrossRef] [PubMed]
3. Ceunen, E.; Zaman, J.; Weltens, N.; Sarafanova, E.; Arijs, V.; Vlaeyen, J.W.S.; Van Oudenhove, L.; Van Diest, I. Learned fear of gastrointestinal sensations in healthy adults. *Clin. Gastroenterol. Hepatol.* **2016**, *14*, 1552.e2–1558.e2. [CrossRef] [PubMed]
4. Icenhour, A.; Labrenz, F.; Ritter, C.; Theysohn, N.; Forsting, M.; Bingel, U.; Elsenbruch, S. Learning by experience? Visceral pain-related neural and behavioral responses in a classical conditioning paradigm. *Neurogastroenterol. Motil.* **2017**, *29*, e13026. [CrossRef]
5. Koenen, L.R.; Icenhour, A.; Forkmann, K.; Theysohn, N.; Forsting, M.; Bingel, U.; Elsenbruch, S. From anticipation to the experience of pain: The importance of visceral versus somatic pain modality in neural and behavioral responses to pain-predictive cues. *Psychosom. Med.* **2018**, *80*, 826–835. [CrossRef]
6. Meulders, A. Fear in the context of pain: Lessons learned from 100 years of fear conditioning research. *Behav. Res. Ther.* **2020**, *131*, 103635. [CrossRef]
7. Schier, L.A.; Hyde, K.M.; Spector, A.C. Conditioned taste aversion versus avoidance: A re-examination of the separate processes hypothesis. *PLoS ONE* **2019**, *14*, e0217458. [CrossRef]
8. Boeckxstaens, G.; Camilleri, M.; Sifrim, D.; Houghton, L.A.; Elsenbruch, S.; Lindberg, G. Fundamentals of neurogastroenterology: Physiology/motility—Sensation. *Gastroenterology* **2016**, *150*, 1292–1304. [CrossRef]
9. Enck, P.; Azpiroz, F.; Boeckxstaens, G.; Elsenbruch, S.; Feinle-Bisset, C.; Holtmann, G.; Lackner, J.M.; Ronkainen, J.; Schemann, M.; Stengel, A.; et al. Functional dyspepsia. *Nat. Rev. Dis. Prim.* **2017**, *3*, 17081. [CrossRef]
10. Masihy, M.; Monrroy, H.; Borghi, G.; Pribic, T.; Galan, C.; Nieto, A.; Accarino, A.; Azpiroz, F. Influence of eating schedule on the postprandial response: Gender differences. *Nutrients* **2019**, *11*, 401. [CrossRef]

11. Zigmond, A.S.; Snaith, R.P. The hospital anxiety and depression scale. *Acta Psychiatr. Scand.* **1983**, *67*, 361–370. [CrossRef] [PubMed]
12. Baños, R.M.; Cebolla, A.; Moragrega, I.; Van Strien, T.; Fernández-Aranda, F.; Agüera, Z.; de la Torre, R.; Casanueva, F.F.; Fernández-Real, J.M.; Fernández-García, J.C.; et al. Relationship between eating styles and temperament in an anorexia nervosa, healthy control, and morbid obesity female sample. *Appetite* **2014**, *76*, 76–83. [CrossRef] [PubMed]
13. Pribic, T.; Azpiroz, F. Biogastronomy: Factors that determine the biological response to meal ingestion. *Neurogastroenterol. Motil.* **2018**, *30*, e13309. [CrossRef] [PubMed]
14. Malagelada, C.; Accarino, A.; Molne, L.; Mendez, S.; Campos, E.; Gonzalez, A.; Malagelada, J.R.; Azpiroz, F. Digestive, cognitive and hedonic responses to a meal. *Neurogastroenterol. Motil.* **2015**, *27*, 389–396. [CrossRef]
15. Ciccantelli, B.; Pribic, T.; Malagelada, C.; Accarino, A.; Azpiroz, F. Relation between cognitive and hedonic responses to a meal. *Neurogastroenterol. Motil.* **2017**, *29*, e13011. [CrossRef]
16. Pribic, T.; Hernandez, L.; Nieto, A.; Malagelada, C.; Accarino, A.; Azpiroz, F. Effects of meal palatability on postprandial sensations. *Neurogastroenterol. Motil.* **2018**, *30*, e13248. [CrossRef]
17. Pribic, T.; Vilaseca, H.; Nieto, A.; Hernandez, L.; Monrroy, H.; Malagelada, C.; Accarino, A.; Roca, J.; Azpiroz, F. Meal composition influences postprandial sensations independently of valence and gustation. *Neurogastroenterol. Motil.* **2018**, *30*, e13337. [CrossRef]
18. Pribic, T.; Nieto, A.; Hernandez, L.; Malagelada, C.; Accarino, A.; Azpiroz, F. Appetite influences the responses to meal ingestion. *Neurogastroenterol. Motil. Off. J. Eur. Gastrointest. Motil. Soc.* **2017**, *29*, e13072. [CrossRef]
19. Pribic, T.; Vilaseca, H.; Nieto, A.; Hernandez, L.; Malagelada, C.; Accarino, A.; Roca, J.; Azpiroz, F. Education of the postprandial experience by a sensory-cognitive intervention. *Neurogastroenterol. Motil.* **2018**, *30*, e13197. [CrossRef]
20. Malagelada, C.; Barba, I.; Accarino, A.; Molne, L.; Mendez, S.; Campos, E.; Gonzalez, A.; Alonso-Cotoner, C.; Santos, J.; Malagelada, J.-R.; et al. Cognitive and hedonic responses to meal ingestion correlate with changes in circulating metabolites. *Neurogastroenterol. Motil.* **2016**, *28*, 1806–1814. [CrossRef]
21. Malagelada, C.; Pribic, T.; Ciccantelli, B.; Cañellas, N.; Gomez, J.; Amigo, N.; Accarino, A.; Correig, X.; Azpiroz, F. Metabolomic signature of the postprandial experience. *Neurogastroenterol. Motil.* **2018**, *30*, e13447. [CrossRef] [PubMed]
22. Pribic, T.; Kilpatrick, L.; Ciccantelli, B.; Malagelada, C.; Accarino, A.; Rovira, A.; Pareto, D.; Mayer, E.; Azpiroz, F. Brain networks associated with cognitive and hedonic responses to a meal. *Neurogastroenterol. Motil.* **2017**, *29*, e13031. [CrossRef] [PubMed]
23. Monrroy, H.; Pribic, T.; Galan, C.; Nieto, A.; Amigo, N.; Accarino, A.; Correig, X.; Azpiroz, F. Meal enjoyment and tolerance in women and men. *Nutrients* **2019**, *11*, 119. [CrossRef] [PubMed]
24. Barber, C.; Mego, M.; Sabater, C.; Vallejo, F.; Bendezu, R.A.; Masihy, M.; Guarner, F.; Espín, J.C.; Margolles, A.; Azpiroz, F. Differential effects of western and mediterranean-type diets on gut microbiota: A metagenomics and metabolomics approach. *Nutrients* **2021**, *13*, 2638. [CrossRef] [PubMed]
25. Van de Putte, P.; Perlas, A. Ultrasound assessment of gastric content and volume. *Br. J. Anaesth* **2014**, *113*, 12–22. [CrossRef]
26. North American Association for the Study of Obesity, National Heart, Lung, Blood Institute and NHLBI Obesity Education Initiative. *The Practical Guide: Identification, Evaluation, and Treatment of Overweight and Obesity in Adults*; National Institutes of Health, National Heart, Lung, and Blood Institute, NHLBI Obesity Education Initiative, North American Association for the Study of Obesity: Bethesda, MD, USA, 2000.
27. Feinle-Bisset, C.; Azpiroz, F. Dietary lipids and functional gastrointestinal disorders. *Am. J. Gastroenterol.* **2013**, *108*, 737–747. [CrossRef]
28. Caldarella, M.P.; Azpiroz, F.; Malagelada, J.-R. Selective effects of nutrients on gut sensitivity and reflexes. *Gut* **2007**, *56*, 37–42. [CrossRef]
29. Chambers, K.C. Conditioned taste aversions. *World J. Otorhinolaryngol. Head Neck Surg.* **2018**, *4*, 92–100. [CrossRef]
30. Lin, J.-Y.; Arthurs, J.; Reilly, S. Conditioned taste aversions: From poisons to pain to drugs of abuse. *Psychon. Bull Rev.* **2017**, *24*, 335–351. [CrossRef]
31. Feinle-Bisset, C.; Meier, B.; Fried, M.; Beglinger, C. Role of cognitive factors in symptom induction following high and low fat meals in patients with functional dyspepsia. *Gut* **2003**, *52*, 1414–1418. [CrossRef]
32. Accarino, A.M.; Azpiroz, F.; Malagelada, J.R. Attention and distraction: Effects on gut perception. *Gastroenterology* **1997**, *113*, 415–422. [CrossRef] [PubMed]
33. Bouton, M.E.; Maren, S.; McNally, G.P. Behavioral and neurobiological mechanisms of pavlovian and instrumental extinction learning. *Physiol. Rev.* **2021**, *101*, 611–681. [CrossRef] [PubMed]
34. Ramos, R.; Wu, C.-H.; Turrigiano, G.G. Strong aversive conditioning triggers a long-lasting generalized aversion. *Front. Cell Neurosci.* **2022**, *16*, 854315. [CrossRef] [PubMed]

Disclaimer/Publisher's Note: The statements, opinions and data contained in all publications are solely those of the individual author(s) and contributor(s) and not of MDPI and/or the editor(s). MDPI and/or the editor(s) disclaim responsibility for any injury to people or property resulting from any ideas, methods, instructions or products referred to in the content.

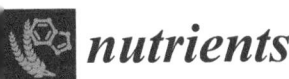

Article

Are Signals Regulating Energy Homeostasis Related to Neuropsychological and Clinical Features of Gambling Disorder? A Case–Control Study

Mikel Etxandi [1,2,†], Isabel Baenas [1,3,4,†], Bernat Mora-Maltas [1,4], Roser Granero [3,4,5], Fernando Fernández-Aranda [1,3,4,6], Sulay Tovar [3,7], Neus Solé-Morata [1,4], Ignacio Lucas [1,4], Sabela Casado [3,7], Mónica Gómez-Peña [1,4], Laura Moragas [1,4], Amparo del Pino-Gutiérrez [3,4,8], Ester Codina [1], Eduardo Valenciano-Mendoza [1], Marc N. Potenza [9,10,11,12,13], Carlos Diéguez [3,7] and Susana Jiménez-Murcia [1,3,4,6,*]

1. Department of Psychiatry, Bellvitge University Hospital-Bellvitge Institute for Biomedical Research (IDIBELL), 08907 Barcelona, Spain
2. Department of Psychiatry, Hospital Universitari Germans Trias i Pujol, IGTP Campus Can Ruti, 08916 Badalona, Spain
3. Ciber Fisiopatología Obesidad y Nutrición (CIBERObn), Instituto de Salud Carlos III, 28029 Madrid, Spain
4. Psychoneurobiology of Eating and Addictive Behaviors Group, Neurosciences Programme, Bellvitge Institute for Biomedical Research (IDIBELL), 08908 Barcelona, Spain
5. Department of Psychobiology and Methodology, Autonomous University of Barcelona, 08193 Barcelona, Spain
6. Department of Clinical Sciences, School of Medicine and Health Sciences, University of Barcelona, 08907 Barcelona, Spain
7. Department of Physiology, CIMUS, Instituto de Investigación Sanitaria, University of Santiago de Compostela, 15782 Santiago de Compostela, Spain
8. Department of Public Health, Mental Health and Perinatal Nursing, School of Nursing, University of Barcelona, 08907 Barcelona, Spain
9. Department of Psychiatry, Yale University School of Medicine, New Haven, CT 06510, USA
10. Child Study Center, Yale University School of Medicine, New Haven, CT 06510, USA
11. Connecticut Mental Health Center, New Haven, CT 06519, USA
12. Connecticut Council on Problem Gambling, Wethersfield, CT 06106, USA
13. Department of Neuroscience, Yale University, New Haven, CT 06520, USA
* Correspondence: sjimenez@bellvitgehospital.cat
† These authors contributed equally to this work.

Abstract: Gambling disorder (GD) is a modestly prevalent and severe condition for which neurobiology is not yet fully understood. Although alterations in signals involved in energy homeostasis have been studied in substance use disorders, they have yet to be examined in detail in GD. The aims of the present study were to compare different endocrine and neuropsychological factors between individuals with GD and healthy controls (HC) and to explore endocrine interactions with neuropsychological and clinical variables. A case–control design was performed in 297 individuals with GD and 41 individuals without (healthy controls; HCs), assessed through a semi-structured clinical interview and a psychometric battery. For the evaluation of endocrine and anthropometric variables, 38 HCs were added to the 41 HCs initially evaluated. Individuals with GD presented higher fasting plasma ghrelin ($p < 0.001$) and lower LEAP2 and adiponectin concentrations ($p < 0.001$) than HCs, after adjusting for body mass index (BMI). The GD group reported higher cognitive impairment regarding cognitive flexibility and decision-making strategies, a worse psychological state, higher impulsivity levels, and a more dysfunctional personality profile. Despite failing to find significant associations between endocrine factors and either neuropsychological or clinical aspects in the GD group, some impaired cognitive dimensions (i.e., WAIS Vocabulary test and WCST Perseverative errors) and lower LEAP2 concentrations statistically predicted GD presence. The findings from the present study suggest that distinctive neuropsychological and endocrine dysfunctions may operate in individuals with GD and predict GD presence. Further exploration of endophenotypic vulnerability pathways in GD appear warranted, especially with respect to etiological and therapeutic potentials.

Keywords: gambling disorder; addictive behavior; impulsive–compulsive behavior; gut hormones; adipocytokines; neuropsychology

1. Introduction

Gambling disorder (GD) has been classified as a behavioral addiction (BA) in the Diagnostic and Statistical Manual of Mental Disorders, Fifth Edition (DSM-5) [1], being characterized by recurrent maladaptive gambling behavior, leading to negative consequences in one or more areas of life functioning [2]. Diagnostic criteria include the need to gamble with increasing amounts of money (i.e., tolerance), the tendency to chase losses, irritability when attempting to stop the behavior (i.e., abstinence), the presence of unsuccessful efforts to control gambling behavior, a predominance of thoughts focused on the gambling behavior, the presence of lies or the loss of a significant relationship or job/educational opportunity because of gambling, and the propensity to gamble when feeling distressed or to rely on others to provide money to relieve desperate financial situations caused by gambling [1]. From an etiological perspective, neuroimaging, genetic, and biochemical studies have suggested shared vulnerability factors between addictive-related disorders, such as GD and substance use disorders (SUDs) [3,4]. For instance, dysfunctional neurobiological pathways involved in reward processing [5], which may underlie impulsive and compulsive tendencies, have been described [6].

Several endocrine factors have been implicated in brain responses to rewards and gratification [7,8] including gut hormones (e.g., ghrelin) and adipocytokines (e.g., leptin and adiponectin) [9,10], classically associated with food intake regulation and energy balance [11]. Despite its stimulating appetite role, ghrelin has been described as a hedonic neural reinforcer for natural (e.g., food) and non-natural rewards (e.g., drugs) by its interaction with dopamine signaling in the mesolimbic circuit and other neuroendocrine pathways (e.g., linked to stress, appetite, and metabolic processing) [12]. Ghrelin has been extensively studied in different addictive-related disorders, such as binge eating disorder (BED) and obesity [13,14], as well as in SUDs [15], especially involving alcohol [16,17].

Noticeably, ghrelin up-regulation has been described in SUDs, which positively correlates with craving, abstinence, and relapse [17–19]. Accordingly, exogenous ghrelin administration increases craving and drug consumption [9], contrary to ghrelin antagonists [20,21]. An antagonist of ghrelin named liver enriched antimicrobial peptide 2 (LEAP2) has been recently described [22,23]. It has been related to impulsivity and cognitive functioning [24] and may contribute to addictions due to its interplay with ghrelin. Furthermore, genetic alterations related to the ghrelin system, such as receptor polymorphisms, have been associated with reward-seeking behaviors and consumption [25], which together may have potential therapeutic implications [26,27]. In GD, a study by Sztainert et al. [28] suggests ghrelin as a potential predictor of gambling craving and persistence.

Adipocytokines have also been studied in relation to impulsivity [29] and addiction [30,31]. As in the case of regulation of food intake, opposite effects on craving and abstinence have been attributed to leptin compared with ghrelin [32]. Leptin concentrations have been inversely correlated with consumption severity [33], being proposed as a possible biomarker in SUDs involving alcohol and cocaine [10,34]. However, studies regarding alcohol consumption have shown inconsistent results [30], even describing higher leptin concentrations in individuals with alcohol use disorder than in HCs, positively associated with alcohol intake [30,34]. A single study exploring leptin concentrations in GD did not find significant differences compared with those in HCs [35]. Despite there are fewer studies related to adiponectin and addictions, decreased serum concentrations have been reported in obesity with and without eating disorders and in opioid use disorder [14,36]. Adiponectin has also been proposed as a biomarker of craving, like ghrelin, in alcohol use disorder [37]. Similar to other addictive-related disorders, these endocrine substrates represent potential candidates involved in the pathogenesis of BAs, such as GD [35]. However, this area remains underexplored in GD, and further research is needed.

Other neurobiological features linked to addictive-related disorders include impaired neuropsychological processes not only regarding executive functions, such as response inhibition, self-regulation, decision-making, cognitive flexibility, and planning but also working memory [38–42]. These cognitive functions have been described as core symptoms in BAs [39] and are especially related to impulse control [41]. More severe neuropsychological impairment has been described among older patients with GD and preferences for non-strategic gambling [41,43,44]. Neuropsychological impairment has statistically predicted poorer treatment outcome, with more frequent dropout and relapse [41,45].

Beyond neuropsychological factors, other psychological and clinical features have been implicated in the development of addictive disorders [46]. In GD, for example, certain personality traits such as high levels of novelty-seeking (related to impulsivity) and harm avoidance, especially in women [46,47], together with low self-directedness have been linked to both GD and SUDs [48,49]. Difficulties in emotion regulation and poorer psychological states have been linked to GD [50], particularly in women and older individuals with non-strategic gambling [43,44]. A more dysfunctional psychological profile has been associated with greater neuropsychological impairment [41,43,44]. However, studies have largely not explored relationships between different neurobiological features (i.e., endocrine, and neuropsychological factors) and psychological and clinical variables.

To the best of our knowledge, this is the first study that explores the roles of multiple specific signals implicated in addiction and energy homeostasis, meaning food intake and energy expenditure, and clinical and psychological measures among a clinical population with GD. We aimed to explore and compare plasma concentrations of specific metabolic hormones (i.e., leptin, ghrelin, adiponectin, and LEAP2) between patients with GD and HCs. As a second aim, we analyzed correlations between the mentioned endocrine factors and neuropsychological and clinical features. In line with previous literature in addictive disorders, we hypothesized the existence of significant differences in plasma hormonal concentrations between the GD and HC groups. We also hypothesized poorer cognitive functioning, worse psychopathological state, and a more dysfunctional personality profile among individuals with GD. These features were also hypothesized to be related to endocrine alterations, including being able to statistically predict GD presence.

2. Materials and Methods

2.1. Participants

The sample consisted of $n = 297$ treatment-seeking adult outpatients with GD (93.6% males) with a mean age of 39.58 years (SD = 14.16), voluntarily recruited at the Behavioral Addictions Unit-Psychiatry Department of Bellvitge University Hospital (Barcelona, Spain). As inclusion criteria, all the patients had a diagnosis of GD according to DSM-5 criteria [1]. The HC group was composed by 41 individuals without GD (90.2% males), with a mean age of 49.27 years (SD = 15.23) and was recruited via advertisement from the same catchment area. Regarding anthropometric and endocrine variables, 79 HCs were evaluated by adding to the initial sample 38 healthy adults from CIMUS, University of Santiago de Compostela (Santiago de Compostela, Spain). General exclusion criteria for all participants were the presence of an organic mental disorder, an intellectual disability, a neurodegenerative disorder (such as Parkinson's disease) or an active psychotic disorder. Recruitment of participants occurred from April 2018 to September 2021, and the evaluation of individuals with GD took place before starting treatment at the Behavioral Addictions Unit-Psychiatry Department of Bellvitge University Hospital (Barcelona, Spain).

Supplementary Materials Table S1 contains the complete description for the participants in the study.

2.2. Measures

2.2.1. Hormonal Assays

Endocrine variables were quantified from peripheral blood sample extraction by venous aspiration with ethylenediamine tetraacetic acid (EDTA; 25 mM final concentration), all samples were collected at 9 am, after at least 8 h of fasting. The blood was centrifuged at 1700 g in a refrigerated centrifuge (4 °C) for 20 min. Plasma was immediately separated from serum and stored at −80 °C until analysis. Parameter determinations were conducted using commercial kits according to the manufacturer's instructions and in a single analysis to reduce inter-assay variability. The quantitative measurement of LEAP-2 in plasma was performed using a commercial enzyme-linked immunosorbent assay (ELISA) kit (Human LEAP-2 [37–76] ELISA kit, Phoenix Pharmaceuticals, Inc., Burlingame, CA, USA), previously validated [51,52]. Intra-assay and inter-assay variation coefficients were <10% and <15%, respectively. The assay sensitivity limit was 0.15 ng/mL. Total ghrelin (pg/mL) was measured by ELISA kit (Invitrogen-Thermo Fisher Scientific, Madrid, Spain) for detection of human ghrelin, with a specificity of 100%. Intra-assay variation coefficient was <6% and inter-assay <8.5%. The assay sensitivity limit was 11.8 pg/mL [53]. Adiponectin (ng/mL) and leptin (ng/mL) plasma measurements were performed using a solid-phase sandwich ELISA kit (Invitrogen-Thermo Fisher Scientific, Madrid, Spain) with a specificity of 100%. Intra-assay and inter-assay variation coefficients were <4% and <5%, respectively, and assay sensitivity limit was 100 pg/mL for adiponectin and <3.5 pg/mL for leptin. The absorbance from each sample was measured in duplicate using a spectrophotometric microplate reader at a wavelength of 450 nm (Epoch 2 microplate reader, Biotek Instruments, Inc., Winooski, VT, USA).

2.2.2. Neuropsychological Variables

Iowa Gambling Task (IGT) [54]. A computerized task to evaluate decision-making, risk, reward, and punishment value. The participant must select 100 cards from four decks (i.e., A, B, C, and D), and after each card selection, an output is given either a gain or a loss of money. The participant is instructed that the aim of the task is to win as much money as possible. This test is scored by subtracting the number of cards selected from decks A and B from the number of cards selected from decks C and D. While decks A and B are not advantageous as the final loss is higher than the final gain, decks C and D are advantageous since the punishments are smaller. Higher scores point to better performance, while negative scores point to persistently choosing disadvantageous decks.

Wisconsin Card Sorting Test (WCST) [55] is a task for assessing cognitive flexibility and inhibitory control, composed of four stimulus cards and 128 response cards showing different shapes, colors, and numbers of figures in each one. The participant must match response cards with the stimulus cards in a way that it seems justifiable before receiving the feedback (i.e., correct, or incorrect). After ten sequential correct answers the categorization criteria changes. The number of complete categories, percentage of perseverative errors, and percentage of non-perseverative errors are recorded.

Stroop Color and Word Test (SCWT) [56] consists of three different lists, beginning with a word list containing the names of colors printed in black ink; then, a color list that comprises letter "X" printed in color; and, finally, a color-word list constituted of names of colors in a color ink that does not match the written name. Three final scores are obtained based on the number of items that the participant can read on naming on each list in 45 s. It assesses the ability to inhibit cognitive interference, which occurs when the processing of a stimulus feature affects the simultaneous processing of another attribute of the same stimulus.

Trail Making Test (TMT) [57] consists of 25 circles spread out over two sheets of paper (Parts A and B). The participant is told to connect these circles drawing a line between consecutive numbers (part A) and alternating numbers and letters following a sequential order (part B). The task assesses visual conceptual and visual-motor tracking, entailing motor speed, attention, and the capacity to alternate between cognitive categories (set-shifting). Each part is scored according to the spent time to complete the task.

Digits backward task of the Wechsler Memory Scale-Third Edition (WMS-III) [58] consists of two lists of digits presented verbally by the examiner. The participant is asked to repeat the digits in the same order (first list) and in reverse order (second list). It assesses verbal working memory due to internal manipulation of mnemonic representations of verbal information that is required in the absence of external cues.

Vocabulary subtest of the Wechsler Adult Intelligence Scale, 3rd ed. (WAIS-III) [59] requires defining words of increasing difficulty orally presented, to assess the vocabulary expression and to estimate intellectual capacity [60].

2.2.3. Clinical Variables

South Oaks Gambling Screen (SOGS) [61], Spanish validation [62], is a 20-item instrument for screening past-year gambling problems and related negative consequences. The total score is a measure of problem-gambling severity, with a score of five or more suggestive of "probable pathological gambling". Its internal consistency in the study sample was Cronbach's alpha (α) = 0.735.

Diagnostic Questionnaire for Pathological Gambling According to DSM criteria [63], Spanish validation [64], is a self-report questionnaire with 19 items coded in a binary fashion (yes-no), used for diagnosing GD according to the DSM-IV-TR and DSM-5 criteria [1]. Its internal consistency in the study sample was α = 0.796.

Symptom Checklist-90-Revised (SCL-90-R) [65], Spanish validation [66], is a 90-item self-report questionnaire measured on an ordinal 3-point scale, evaluating a broad range of psychological problems and psychopathology, based on nine primary symptomatic dimensions (Somatization, Obsession–Compulsion, Interpersonal Sensitivity, Depression, Anxiety, Hostility, Phobic Anxiety, Paranoid Ideation, and Psychoticism). It includes three global indices (global severity index, positive symptom distress index, and total positive symptom). The internal consistency in the study was α = 0.979.

Temperament and Character Inventory-Revised (TCI-R) [67], Spanish validation [68], is a questionnaire with 240-items scored on a 5-point Likert scale, measuring personality derived from three character dimensions (Self-Directedness, Cooperativeness, and Self-Transcendence) and four temperament dimensions (Harm Avoidance, Novelty Seeking, Reward Dependence, and Persistence). It is used only for research purposes in a public non-profit hospital, in its Spanish adaptation in which the original author participated [68]. The internal consistency in the study was between α = 0.702 (Novelty Seeking) and α = 0.876 (Persistence).

Impulsive Behavior Scale (UPPS-P) [69], Spanish validation [70], measures five facets of impulsive behavior through self-report on 59 items: negative urgency; positive urgency; lack of premeditation; lack of perseverance; and sensation-seeking. The internal consistency in the study was between α = 0.799 (lack of perseverance) and α = 0.928 (positive urgency).

2.2.4. Other Variables

Additional data (e.g., socio-demographic, socio-economic, anthropometric variables, and GD-related characteristics) were collected in a semi-structured face-to-face clinical interview as described elsewhere [71].

2.3. Procedure

All patients and HCs from the same catchment area were evaluated at the Behavioral Addictions Unit-Psychiatry Department of Bellvitge University Hospital (Barcelona, Spain), by an expert multidisciplinary team in the field of GD. In the first session, a comprehensive semi-structured clinical interview was conducted, in which all aspects related to gambling behavior were assessed. During the second session, the extraction of blood samples occurred. Samples were analyzed in CIMUS, University of Santiago de Compostela (Santiago de Compostela, Spain), where 38 out of 79 HCs were evaluated regarding endocrine and anthropometric measures. The neuropsychological assessment was performed in a third session.

2.4. Statistical Analysis

The statistical analysis was conducted with Stata17 for Windows [72]. Comparison between groups (GD versus HC) were made by Analysis of Covariance (ANCOVA), adjusting for sex, age, and body mass index (BMI) for endocrine variables, and adjusting for sex, age, and education level for neuropsychological variables. The effect size for the mean comparisons was obtained with the standardized Cohen's-d, considering moderate-mild effect values $0.50 < |d| < 0.80$ and high-large effect values $|d| > 0.80$ [73].

Associations between endocrine and neuropsychological and clinical variables were estimated with partial correlation coefficients, adjusting for sex, age, and BMI (associations with the neuropsychological tasks also included adjustment for the education level). Due to strong associations between the null-significance test for the correlation models given the sample sizes (low correlations achieve significance in large samples, and vice versa), in this study mild-moderate correlation was considered for values $|R| > 0.24$ and high-large correlation for values $|R| > 0.37$ [74].

A predictive model was obtained to select the variables with discriminative capacity to identify the presence of GD, through logistic regression. The criterion for the modeling was the diagnosis of GD (presence/absence), and potential predictors included sociodemographic measures, global psychopathological distress, impulsivity levels, personality features, and neuropsychological and endocrine measures. A stepwise selection method was used to automatically select significant contributors. Sex, age, and BMI were included as adjustment/covariables. The goodness-of-fit was measured with the Hosmer–Lemeshow test, the overall predictive capacity with the Cox-Snell's pseudo-R2, and the overall discriminative capacity with the area under the Receiver Operating Curve (ROC).

In this study, the increase in the Type-I error due to the performance of multiple significance tests was controlled with the familywise error Finner's procedure, which has shown greater efficiency than the classic Bonferroni adjustment method [75].

3. Results

3.1. Comparison of Endocrine Measures

Adjusting for sex, age, and BMI, the GD group reported higher ghrelin and lower LEAP2 and adiponectin values compared with HCs (Table 1 and first panel of Figure 1). No differences were found regarding leptin values.

3.2. Comparison of Neuropsychological and Clinical Measures

ANCOVAs comparing the mean values of the neuropsychological measures and clinical variables are displayed in Table 2 (see also second panel of Figure 1). Compared to HCs, the GD group displayed worse performance on the WCST, WAIS-vocabulary test, and performance-learning curve during IGT performance (Figure 2). The GD group also reported worse psychopathological states (higher mean scores on the SCL-90 R), higher impulsivity (except on the UPPS-P sensation-seeking scale) and more dysfunctional personality profiles (except on the TCI-R persistence scale).

Table 1. Comparison of clinical characteristics via ANCOVA.

	Control (N = 79)		GD (N = 297)			
	Mean	SD	Mean	SD	p	|d|
1 Ghrelin (pg/mL)	544.92	673.59	958.48	753.26	<0.001 *	0.58 †
1 LEAP2 (ng/mL)	8.41	3.99	5.28	2.88	<0.001 *	0.90 †
1 Leptin (ng/mL)	9.00	8.13	8.18	7.85	0.402	0.10
1 Adiponectin (ng/mL)	12784.98	14084.20	8381.47	4374.29	<0.001 *	0.42
2 BMI (kg/m^2)	24.99	2.36	26.57	5.04	0.005 *	0.40

Note. GD: gambling disorder. LEAP2: liver enriched antimicrobial peptide 2. BMI: body mass index. SD: standard deviation. |d|: Cohen's-d coefficient. * Bold: significant comparison. 1 Adjustment by sex, age, and BMI. 2 Adjustment by sex and age. † Bold: effect size into the range mild-moderate (|d| > 0.50 and <0.80) to high-large (|d| > 0.80).

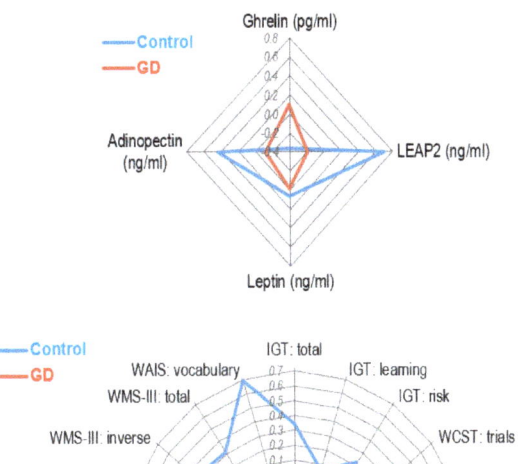

Figure 1. Radar-charts (z-standardized means are plotted). Note. GD: gambling disorder (n = 297). Control (n = 41). LEAP2: liver enriched antimicrobial peptide 2. IGT: Iowa Gambling Test. WCST: Wisconsin Card Sorting Test. TMT: Trail Making Test. WMS-III: Wechsler Memory Scale Third Edition. WAIS: Wechsler Adult Intelligence Scale. Due the different measurement scale for the variables in the graph, Z-standardized means are plotted to facilitate interpretation.

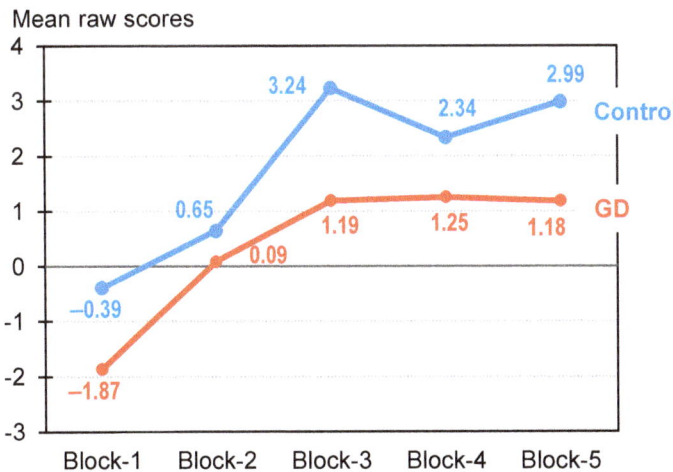

Figure 2. Performance-learning curve in the Iowa Gambling Test task. Note. GD: gambling disorder (n = 297). Control (n = 41).

Table 2. Comparison of the clinical characteristics via ANCOVA.

1 Neuropsychological Measures	Control (N = 41)		GD (N = 297)		p	|d|
	Mean	SD	Mean	SD		
IGT: block-1	−0.39	4.87	−1.87	5.16	0.115	0.30
IGT: block-2	0.65	5.87	0.09	5.52	0.583	0.10
IGT: block-3	3.24	9.50	1.19	6.97	0.126	0.25
IGT: block-4	2.34	9.85	1.25	7.46	0.446	0.12
IGT: block-5	2.99	8.33	1.18	8.56	0.249	0.21
IGT: total	8.88	28.10	2.10	21.94	0.104	0.27
IGT: learning	5.07	15.12	4.22	13.77	0.739	0.06
IGT: risk	5.33	15.78	2.44	13.64	0.257	0.20
WCST: trials	91.61	19.76	102.98	19.58	**0.001 ***	**0.58 †**
WCST: errors	20.04	16.28	33.14	21.77	**<0.001 ***	**0.68 †**
WCST: errors perseverative	9.13	6.27	15.09	10.06	**<0.001 ***	**0.71 †**
WCST: conceptual	65.77	8.66	60.60	16.25	0.063	0.40
WCST: categories completed	5.59	1.07	4.76	1.80	**0.006 ***	**0.56 †**
WCST: trials to complete 1-cat	17.64	6.52	26.79	28.09	0.053	0.45
TMT: A	28.81	8.10	31.77	10.51	0.088	0.32
TMT: B	70.67	22.07	78.41	36.38	0.202	0.26
TMT: Diff	41.74	18.48	47.75	32.35	0.271	0.23
Stroop: words	101.50	13.27	98.13	13.91	0.173	0.25
Stroop: colors	67.82	9.97	68.28	11.00	0.812	0.04
Stroop: words-colors	43.07	10.25	42.97	10.55	0.955	0.01
Stroop: estimated	40.48	5.20	40.11	5.53	0.700	0.07
Stroop: interference	2.59	7.71	2.86	7.75	0.838	0.04
WMS-III: direct	8.91	1.93	8.96	2.02	0.902	0.02
WMS-III: direct-span	5.99	1.12	6.01	1.16	0.947	0.01
WMS-III: inverse	6.55	1.89	6.18	1.99	0.304	0.19
WMS-III: inverse-span	4.80	0.98	4.64	1.15	0.427	0.15
WMS-III: total	15.46	3.36	15.14	3.62	0.617	0.09
WAIS: vocabulary	45.30	5.29	38.50	8.52	**<0.001 ***	**0.96 †**
2 Psychological measures	Mean	SD	Mean	SD	p	|d|
SCL-90R Somatization	0.43	0.35	0.99	0.78	**<0.001 ***	**0.92 †**
SCL-90R Obsessive/compul.	0.68	0.52	1.19	0.84	**<0.001 ***	**0.74 †**
SCL-90R Interp.sensitivity	0.40	0.38	0.99	0.80	**<0.001 ***	**0.95 †**
SCL-90R Depressive	0.51	0.59	1.54	0.93	**<0.001 ***	**1.32 †**
SCL-90R Anxiety	0.36	0.34	1.00	0.80	**<0.001 ***	**1.05 †**
SCL-90R Hostility	0.43	0.50	0.96	0.87	**<0.001 ***	**0.76 †**
SCL-90R Phobic anxiety	0.06	0.16	0.41	0.61	**<0.001 ***	**0.77 †**
SCL-90R Paranoid Ideation	0.46	0.47	0.95	0.79	**<0.001 ***	**0.75 †**
SCL-90R Psychotic	0.22	0.26	0.90	0.75	**<0.001 ***	**1.20 †**
SCL-90R GSI score	0.43	0.34	1.08	0.70	**<0.001 ***	**1.18 †**
SCL-90R PST score	26.37	16.45	47.53	20.77	**<0.001 ***	**1.13 †**
SCL-90R PSDI score	1.41	0.33	1.86	0.59	**<0.001 ***	**0.95 †**
UPPS-P Lack premeditation	20.98	4.02	24.32	5.51	**<0.001 ***	**0.69 †**
UPPS-P Lack perseverance	19.26	4.13	21.97	4.83	**0.001**	**0.60 †**
UPPS-P Sensation seeking	28.13	7.41	28.51	7.89	0.770	0.05
UPPS-P Positive urgency	20.70	5.85	31.92	9.22	**<0.001 ***	**1.45 †**
UPPS-P Negative urgency	23.02	5.55	32.25	6.44	**<0.001 ***	**1.54 †**
UPPS-P Total	112.13	18.36	138.83	22.37	**<0.001 ***	**1.30 †**
TCI-R Novelty seeking	99.34	10.63	110.82	13.13	**<0.001 ***	**0.96 †**
TCI-R Harm avoidance	88.04	17.86	98.79	16.83	**<0.001 ***	**0.62 †**
TCI-R Reward dependence	103.95	13.99	97.97	13.50	**0.009 ***	0.43
TCI-R Persistence	112.65	18.18	109.02	18.90	0.259	0.20
TCI-R Self-directedness	148.17	19.03	130.13	20.52	**<0.001 ***	**0.91 †**
TCI-R Cooperativeness	136.98	15.25	130.18	15.42	**0.010 ***	0.44
TCI-R Self-transcendence	66.73	15.93	61.38	13.83	**0.025 ***	0.36

Note. GD: gambling disorder. SD: standard deviation. IGT: Iowa Gambling Test. WCST: Wisconsin Card Sorting Test. TMT: Trail Making Test. WMS-III: Wechsler Memory Scale Third Edition. WAIS: Wechsler Adult Intelligence Scale. SCL-90R: Symptom Checklist-90-Revised. UPPS-P: Impulsive Behavior Scale. TCI-R: Temperament and Character Inventory-Revised. * Bold: significant comparison. 1 Adjustment by sex, age, and education. 2 Adjustment by sex and age. † Bold: effect size into the range mild-moderate (|d| > 0.50) to high-large (|d| > 0.80).

3.3. Associations between Endocrine Variables and Neuropsychological and Clinical Measures

Supplementary Materials Table S2 displays the partial correlation matrix between the endocrine profile with neuropsychological and clinical variables (psychopathology, impulsivity, and problem-gambling severity). No relevant associations were found within the GD subsample. Among HCs, lower ghrelin values were related to higher values on the IGT-block 5 and, on the WCST scales, number of trials and number of perseverative errors. Higher LEAP2 values were associated with worse psychological states and poorer performance on the TMT, Stroop task, and WMS digits-direct task. Higher leptin was also related to higher levels of phobic anxiety and worse performance on the IGT, WCST conceptual portion, and TMT. Finally, higher adiponectin values were correlated with lower scores on the UPPS-P lack of premeditation scale, and worse performance on the WMS direct and total scales.

3.4. Predictive Model for GD Presence

Table 3 shows the results of the logistic regression. The likelihood of being identified as GD was higher for individuals with lower education levels, lower social position indexes, greater psychopathological distress, higher impulsivity, lower self-transcendence, worse neuropsychological performance (specifically for WCST perseverative errors and on the Stroop color and WAIS vocabulary tasks), and lower LEAP2 levels.

Table 3. Predictive logistic regression model for identifying GD.

Dependent Variable: 1 = GD vs. 0 = HC	B	SE	p	OR	95% CI OR	
Covariates Sex (0 = women; 1 = men)	−0.781	1.498	0.602	0.458	0.024	8.623
Age (years-old)	−0.100	0.033	0.002	0.905	0.848	0.965
BMI (kg/m^2)	0.508	0.149	0.001	1.662	1.241	2.226
Education (low levels)	2.875	0.754	0.001	17.724	4.045	77.665
Socioeconomic status (low levels)	1.099	0.543	0.043	3.000	1.035	8.696
Psychopathology distress (SCL-90R GSI)	2.483	0.896	0.006	11.973	2.069	69.290
Impulsivity (UPPS-P total)	0.082	0.023	0.001	1.086	1.038	1.135
Personality: TCI-R self-transcendence	−0.071	0.031	0.023	0.932	0.877	0.990
WCST Perseverative errors	0.180	0.068	0.008	1.198	1.048	1.368
Stroop Color	0.093	0.047	0.046	1.098	1.002	1.203
WAIS Vocabulary	−0.175	0.064	0.007	0.840	0.740	0.953
LEAP2 (ng/mL)	−0.326	0.126	0.009	0.722	0.564	0.923
Fit statistics	H-L = 0.985; R2 = 0.427; AUC = 0.986 (95% CI: 0.973 to 0.998)					

Note. GD: gambling disorder (n = 297). HC: healthy control (n = 41). Stepwise logistic regression adjusted by sex, age, and BMI. SE: standard error. OR: odds ratio. H-L: Hosmer–Lemeshow test (p-value). R2: Cox-Snell R2. AUC: area under the ROC curve (95% confidence interval (CI)). List of statistical predictors: sociodemographics (marital status, studies levels, and socioeconomic position), psychopathology distress (SCL-90R GSI), impulsivity level (UPPS-total), personality features (TCI-R), psycho-neurological profile, and endocrine measures (ghrelin, leptin, LEAP2 and adinopectin).

4. Discussion

The present work studied gut hormones and adipocytokines, based on their association with reward and impulsive–compulsive processes, in people with GD compared with HCs. Likewise, neuropsychological, and clinical features were also evaluated, as well as its relationship with endocrine factors. Individuals with GD presented altered endocrine profiles compared to HCs, and regardless of BMI, were characterized by higher plasma ghrelin and lower LEAP2 and adiponectin concentrations, without significant differences in leptin levels. A worse neuropsychological performance, higher emotion dysregulation, greater psychopathological scores, higher impulsivity, and a more dysfunctional personality profile were also described in individuals with GD. Although significant correlations between endocrine factors and neuropsychological and clinical features were largely lacking, some neuropsychological domains and lower LEAP2 concentrations predicted GD presence. Implications are described below.

Increased plasma ghrelin concentrations in patients with GD seem consistent with results in SUDs, where ghrelin upregulation has been described [17,18], These findings suggest not only that this hormone could be involved in addictive processes [76] but also shared neurobiological substrates [3,4]. Despite not predicting GD presence, ghrelin upregulation could speculatively contribute to maintenance of gambling due to its reinforcing properties [28], as well as being a risk factor for relapse, related to intensify craving [28]. If such possibilities received empirical support, similar to in SUDs, they may have important therapeutic implications for GD [27].

Although this is the first study to explore LEAP2 in GD, lower concentrations among individuals with GD suggest a possible dysfunction in the ghrelin system also involving LEAP2. The findings raise the intriguing possibility as to whether altered ghrelin production may influence LEAP2 release, supporting LEAP2 antagonism [22] and favoring lower LEAP2 concentrations. Moreover, both ghrelin and LEAP2 concentrations are subject to BMI in both animals and humans but in opposite ways [52]. Thus, persistent differences in ghrelin and LEAP2 after adjustment by BMI between groups, together with the finding that lower LEAP2 concentrations statistically predicted the presence of GD, suggest that these potential disturbances may be intrinsically associated with GD. Going one step further, our results raise the question of whether LEAP2 could be a potential therapeutic target in GD and other addictive-related disorders because of the neutralization of ghrelin's possibly deleterious actions in craving, abstinence, and relapse. However, as LEAP2 has only been recently described and there is lack of extensive or consistent data in the literature, future research is needed [22].

The results regarding adiponectin agree with those reported in other addictive disorders [14,37]. Some protective functions have been linked to adiponectin, such as anti-inflammatory, anti-diabetic, and anti-atherogenic properties [77]. Thus, the results may in part explain a neurobiological basis for a worse metabolic state and a higher cardiometabolic risk associated with addiction, including individuals with GD, who had a significant higher BMI than HCs in our sample [77]. Speculatively, they may also in part explain incident cardiovascular conditions in relation to GD symptomatology in older adults [78]. Interestingly, our findings support the previous work by Geisel et al. [35], regarding leptin concentrations in GD. On the one hand, intrinsic compensatory mechanisms exist associated with endocrine dysfunctions in addiction, based on changes in receptors' activity and/or hormones' biosynthesis [79], which may be a possible rationale to explain the lack of differences between individuals with GD and HCs. Nevertheless, due to the heterogeneous methodology and mixed conclusions described in other addictive disorders, as well as limited work in GD, further studies are lacking to replicate these extend the current results.

Regarding neuropsychological performance, patients with GD had poorer cognitive flexibility and more perseverative errors than HCs, in line with previous findings [80]. Although we failed to find significant differences in the IGT trials, the GD group showed numerically less learning on the task, which may suggest a potential worse decision-making performance [41]. However, given the absence of statistically significant differences, the findings also resonate with prior reports showing similar patterns but no group differences in independent samples [81].

Patients with GD presented poorer estimated cognitive reserves compared to HCs. Lower scores on intellectual performance scales may be associated with a greater tendency to make risky decisions and may thus be a potential risk factor for the development of GD [82]. As a distinguishing finding, worse performance on the WAIS Vocabulary and WCST Perseverative errors predicted the presence of GD. Taken together, the results are in line with previous research suggesting that compulsive responding is in part mediated by impulsive decisions [39], since perseverative behavior has been "normalized" when feedback-response pause is increased in cognitive flexibility tasks [83]. One possibility is that low cognitive reserve may promote impulsivity, leading to an increase in perseverative behaviors in patients with GD. Even though significant correlations between endocrine and neuropsychological factors were largely absent, it may be worth further investigating possible common links based on relationships with reward-related neurocircuitry [84].

Patients with GD scored higher on general psychopathology and impulsivity measures [85], with more dysfunctional personality features (i.e., higher novelty-seeking and harm avoidance and lower reward dependence, self-directedness, cooperativeness, and self-transcendence) [85]. This profile has been linked to younger age of GD onset and problem-gambling severity [86,87]. Particularly, in our study, lower self-transcendence, and younger age, described as a possible risk factor of GD [2] also predicted the presence of GD. Self-transcendence seems to be a protective factor delaying the age of GD onset [86,88]. On the other hand, younger age has been positively linked to earlier GD onset, male sex, and higher novelty-seeking, and therefore, with problem-gambling severity [89]. Sociodemographic differences related to educational and socio-economic levels aligned with previous studies of our group [85]. From a social perspective, having a lower educational status and less social support have been previously implicated in GD [90].

Newly, relationships between endocrine and clinical variables were largely not observed. However, some previous studies revealed a relationship of appetite-related hormones with impulsivity domains and mood regulation [29,91]. Considering the complexity of addictive disorders and the limitations of cross-sectional studies, prospective studies with larger samples are warranted to understand better relationships over time.

Limitations and Strengths

Some limitations should be mentioned. As the cross-sectional nature of this study limits causal attributions, future longitudinal studies are needed to better understand the involvement of neuroendocrine alterations and their roles in GD. Moreover, endocrine measurements were analyzed from peripheral blood samples, which could limit the inference of their functioning at a neural level. The lower number of individuals in the HC group with respect to the GD group may also limit the interpretation of the results, studies with a larger sample size are necessary to confirm the findings. Moreover, the GD group was principally composed of treatment-seeking males referred to a specialized unit in Catalonia, Spain. As such, studies of other compositions from other jurisdictions are warranted to determine generalizability of the results. Nonetheless, the representation of women in the study is consistent with the prevalence estimates in clinical treatment-seeking samples in GD, and comparable to their frequency in the control group. On the other hand, other strengths of this work is an adequate sample size, the well-characterized clinical and neuropsychological profile of both groups, and the adjustment in models for potentially confounding factors.

5. Conclusions

The present study provides evidence about underlying neuropsychological and endocrine dysfunctions related to reward processing in GD. The results have identified specific endocrine, neuropsychological, and clinical factors statistically predicting the presence of GD. Despite the cross-sectional design, this study supports a multifactorial nature of GD. Additionally, it supports the existence of potential neurobiological targets, known for involvement in other addictive disorders, with possible therapeutic implications. Hence, future research in this area may contribute to the development of more specific psychological and biological treatment strategies in GD.

Supplementary Materials: The following supporting information can be downloaded at https://www.mdpi.com/article/10.3390/nu14235084/s1, Table S1: Characteristics of the sample; Table S2: Partial correlation matrix.

Author Contributions: M.E., I.B., B.M.-M. and S.J.-M. contributed to the development of the study concept and design. R.G. performed the statistical analysis. M.E., I.B., M.G.-P., L.M., A.d.P.-G., B.M.-M., E.V.-M. and S.J.-M. aided with data collection. I.B., A.d.P.-G., E.C., S.T., S.C. and C.D. carried out the procedures related to blood extraction and hormone analysis. M.E., I.B., B.M.-M., N.S.-M. and S.J.-M. aided in the interpretation of data and the writing of the manuscript. F.F.-A., M.N.P., C.D., S.J.-M. and I.L. revised the manuscript and provided substantial comments. F.F.-A. and S.J.-M. obtained funding. All authors have read and agreed to the published version of the manuscript.

Funding: CERCA Programme/Generalitat de Catalunya gave institutional support. This work was additionally supported by a grant from the Ministerio de Ciencia, Innovación y Universidades (grant RTI2018-101837-B-100), the Delegación del Gobierno para el Plan Nacional sobre Drogas (2019I47 and 2021I031), and Instituto de Salud Carlos III (ISCIII) (PI17/01167, PI20/00132) and co-funded by FEDER funds/European Regional Development Fund (ERDF), a way to build Europe. CIBERobn is an initiative of ISCIII. I.B. was partially supported by a Post-Residency Grant from the Research Committee of the University Hospital of Bellvitge (HUB; Barcelona, Spain) 2020–2021. This study has been also funded by Instituto de Salud Carlos III through the grant CM21/00172 (Co-funded by European Social Fund. ESF investing in your future). R.G. is supported by the Catalan Institution for Research and Advanced Studies (ICREA-Academia, 2021-Programme). M.N.P. was supported by the Connecticut Council on Problem Gambling. The funders had no role in the study design, data collection and analysis, decision to publish, or preparation of the manuscript.

Institutional Review Board Statement: The latest version of the Declaration of Helsinki was used to conduct the present study. The Clinical Research Ethics Committee of the Bellvitge University Hospital approved this study (ref. PR329/19 and PR338/17), as part of the scientific production within national and competitive research projects developed by our research group (RTI2018-101837-B-I00; 2017I067, 2019I47, and 2021I031).

Informed Consent Statement: Informed consent was obtained from all subjects involved in the study.

Data Availability Statement: Individuals may inquire with Jiménez-Murcia regarding the availability of the data as there are ongoing studies using the data. To avoid overlapping research efforts, Jiménez-Murcia will consider requests on a case-by-case basis.

Acknowledgments: We thank CERCA Programme/Generalitat de Catalunya for the institutional support. We also thank the Ministerio de Ciencia, Innovación y Universidades and the Delegación del Gobierno para el Plan Nacional sobre Drogas, Instituto de Salud Carlos III (ISCIII), CIBERobn (initiative of ISCIII), FEDER funds/European Regional Development Fund (ERDF), a way to build Europe, the European Social Fund-ESF investing in your future, and Bellvitge Biomedical Research Institute (IDIBELL).

Conflicts of Interest: Authors Mikel Etxandi, Isabel Baenas, Bernat Mora-Malta, Roser Granero, Sulay Tovar, Neus Solé-Morata, Ignacio Lucas, Mónica Gómez-Peña, Laura Moragas, Amparo del Pino-Gutiérrez, Ester Codina, Eduardo Valenciano-Mendoza, Sabela Casado, Carlos Diéguez, and Susana Jiménez-Murcia declare that they have no conflicts of interest. Marc N. Potenza has consulted for and advised Opiant Pharmaceuticals, Idorsia Pharmaceuticals, Baria-Tek, AXA, Game Day Data and the Addiction Policy Forum; has been involved in a patent application with Yale University and Novartis; has received research support from the Mohegan Sun Casino and Connecticut Council on Problem Gambling; has participated in surveys, mailings, or telephone consultations related to drug addiction, impulse control disorders, or other health topics; and has consulted for law offices and gambling entities on issues related to impulse control or addictive disorders. Fernando Fernández-Aranda received consultancy honoraria from Novo Nordisk and editorial honoraria as EIC from Wiley.

References

1. APA American Psychiatric Association. *Diagnostic and Statistical Manual of Mental Disorders*; American Psychiatric Publishing: Washington, DC, USA, 2013.
2. Potenza, M.N.; Balodis, I.M.; Derevensky, J.; Grant, J.E.; Petry, N.M.; Verdejo-Garcia, A.; Yip, S.W. Gambling disorder. *Nat. Rev. Dis. Prim.* **2019**, *5*, 51. [CrossRef] [PubMed]
3. Solé-Morata, N.; Baenas, I.; Etxandi, M.; Granero, R.; Forcales, S.V.; Gené, M.; Barrot, C.; Gómez-Peña, M.; Menchón, J.M.; Ramoz, N.; et al. The role of neurotrophin genes involved in the vulnerability to gambling disorder. *Sci. Rep.* **2022**, *12*, 1–11. [CrossRef]
4. Linnet, J. The anticipatory dopamine response in addiction: A common neurobiological underpinning of gambling disorder and substance use disorder? *Prog. Neuropsychopharmacol. Biol. Psychiatry* **2020**, *98*, 109802. [CrossRef] [PubMed]
5. Shevchouk, O.T.; Tufvesson-Alm, M.; Jerlhag, E. An Overview of Appetite-Regulatory Peptides in Addiction Processes; From Bench to Bed Side. *Front. Neurosci.* **2021**, *15*, 774050. [CrossRef] [PubMed]
6. Lüscher, C.; Robbins, T.W.; Everitt, B.J. The transition to compulsion in addiction. *Nat. Rev. Neurosci.* **2021**, *21*, 247–263. [CrossRef] [PubMed]
7. Geisel, O.; Panneck, P.; Hellweg, R.; Wiedemann, K.; Müller, K.A. Hypothalamic-pituitary-adrenal axis activity in patients with pathological gambling and internet use disorder. *Psychiatry Res.* **2015**, *226*, 97–102. [CrossRef]

8. Pettorruso, M.; Zoratto, F.; Miuli, A.; De Risio, L.; Santorelli, M.; Pierotti, A.; Martinotti, G.; Adriani, W.; di Giannantonio, M. Exploring dopaminergic transmission in gambling addiction: A systematic translational review. *Neurosci. Biobehav. Rev.* **2020**, *119*, 481–511. [CrossRef]
9. Farokhnia, M.; Grodin, E.N.; Lee, M.R.; Oot, E.N.; Balckburn, A.N.; Stangl, B.L.; Schwandt, M.L.; Farinelli, L.A.; Momenan, R.; Ramchandani, V.A.; et al. Exogenous ghrelin administration increases alcohol self-administration and modulates brain functional activity in heavy-drinking alcohol-dependent individuals. *Mol. Psychiatry* **2018**, *23*, 2029–2038. [CrossRef]
10. Martinotti, G.; Montemitro, C.; Baroni, G.; Andreoli, S.; Alimonti, F.; Di Nicola, M.; Tonioni, F.; Leggio, L.; di Giannantonio, M.; Janiri, L. Relationship between craving and plasma leptin concentrations in patients with cocaine addiction. *Psychoneuroendocrinology* **2017**, *85*, 35–41. [CrossRef]
11. Iovino, M.; Messana, T.; Lisco, G.; Mariano, F.; Giagulli, V.A.; Guastamacchia, E.; De Pergola, G.; Triggiani, V. Neuroendocrine modulation of food intake and eating behavior. *Endocr. Metab. Immune Disord. Drug Targets* **2022**, *22*. [CrossRef]
12. Revitsky, A.R.; Klein, L.C. Role of ghrelin in drug abuse and reward-relevant behaviors: A burgeoning field and gaps in the literature. *Curr. Drug Abuse Rev.* **2013**, *6*, 231–244. [CrossRef]
13. Micioni Di Bonaventura, E.; Botticelli, L.; Del Bello, F.; Giorgioni, G.; Piergentili, A.; Quaglia, W.; Cifani, C.; Micioni Di Bonaventura, M.V. Assessing the role of ghrelin and the enzyme ghrelin O-acyltransferase (GOAT) system in food reward, food motivation, and binge eating behavior. *Pharmacol. Res.* **2021**, *172*, 105847. [CrossRef] [PubMed]
14. Yu, Y.; Fernandez, I.D.; Meng, Y.; Zhao, W.; Groth, S.W. Gut hormones, adipokines, and pro- and anti-inflammatory cytokines/markers in loss of control eating: A scoping review. *Appetite* **2021**, *166*, 105442. [CrossRef] [PubMed]
15. Sustkova-Fiserova, M.; Charalambous, C.; Khryakova, A.; Certilina, A.; Lapka, M.; Šlamberová, R. The Role of Ghrelin/GHS-R1A Signaling in Nonalcohol Drug Addictions. *Int. J. Mol. Sci.* **2022**, *23*, 761. [CrossRef]
16. Koopmann, A.; Schuster, R.; Kiefer, F. The impact of the appetite-regulating, orexigenic peptide ghrelin on alcohol use disorders: A systematic review of preclinical and clinical data. *Biol Psychol.* **2018**, *131*, 13–40. [CrossRef]
17. Leggio, L.; Ferrulli, A.; Cardone, S.; Nesci, A.; Micelo, A.; Malandrino, N.; Capristo, E.; Canestrelli, B.; Monteleone, P.; Kenna, G.A.; et al. Ghrelin system in alcohol-dependent subjects: Role of plasma ghrelin levels in alcohol drinking and craving. *Addict. Biol.* **2012**, *17*, 452–464. [CrossRef] [PubMed]
18. Addolorato, G.; Capristo, E.; Leggio, L.; Ferulli, A.; Abenavoli, L.; Malandrino, N.; Farnetti, S.; Domenicali, M.; D'Angelo, C.; Vonghia, L.; et al. Relationship between ghrelin levels, alcohol craving, and nutritional status in current alcoholic patients. *Alcohol. Clin. Exp. Res.* **2006**, *30*, 1933–1937. [CrossRef]
19. Tessari, M.; Catalano, A.; Pellitteri, M.; Di Francesco, C.; Marini, F.; Gerrard, P.A.; Heidbreder, C.A.; Melotto, S. Correlation between serum ghrelin levels and cocaine-seeking behaviour triggered by cocaine-associated conditioned stimuli in rats. *Addict Biol.* **2007**, *12*, 22–29. [CrossRef] [PubMed]
20. Edvardsson, C.E.; Vestlund, J.; Jerlhag, E. A ghrelin receptor antagonist reduces the ability of ghrelin, alcohol, or amphetamine to induce a dopamine release in the ventral tegmental area and in nucleus accumbens shell in rats. *Eur. J. Pharmacol.* **2021**, *899*, 174039. [CrossRef]
21. Suchankova, P.; Steensland, P.; Fredriksson, I.; Engel, J.A.; Jerlhag, E. Ghrelin Receptor (GHS-R1A) Antagonism Suppresses Both Alcohol Consumption and the Alcohol Deprivation Effect in Rats following Long-Term Voluntary Alcohol Consumption. *PLoS ONE* **2013**, *8*, e71284. [CrossRef]
22. Ge, X.; Yang, H.; Bednarek, M.A.; Galon-Tilleman, H.; Chen, P.; Chen, M.; Lichtman, J.S.; Wang, L.; Dalmas, O.; Yin, Y.; et al. LEAP2 Is an Endogenous Antagonist of the Ghrelin Receptor. *Cell Metab.* **2018**, *27*, 461–469.e6. [CrossRef] [PubMed]
23. Lugilde, J.; Casado, S.; Beiroa, D.; Cuñarro, J.; García-Lavandeira, M.; Álvarez, C.V.; Nogueiras, R.; Tovar, S.; Diéguez, C. LEAP-2 Counteracts Ghrelin-Induced Food Intake in a NutrientGrowth Hormone and Age Independent Manner. *Cells* **2022**, *11*, 324. [CrossRef] [PubMed]
24. Voigt, K.; Giddens, E.; Stark, R.; Frisch, E.; Moskovsky, N.; Kakoschke, N.; Stout, J.C.; Bellgrove, M.A.; Andrews, Z.B.; Verdejo García, A. The hunger games: Homeostatic state-dependent fluctuations in disinhibition measured with a novel gamified test battery. *Nutrients* **2021**, *13*, 2001. [CrossRef] [PubMed]
25. Zallar, L.J.; Beurmann, S.; Tunstall, B.J.; Fraser, C.M.; Koob, G.F.; Vendruscolo, L.F.; Leggio, L. Ghrelin receptor deletion reduces binge-like alcohol drinking in rats. *J. Neuroendocrinol.* **2019**, *31*, e12663. [CrossRef] [PubMed]
26. Engel, J.A.; Jerlhag, E. Role of appetite-regulating peptides in the pathophysiology of addiction: Implications for pharmacotherapy. *CNS Drugs* **2014**, *28*, 875–886. [CrossRef] [PubMed]
27. Farokhnia, M.; Lee, M.R.; Farinelli, L.A.; Ramchandani, V.; Akhlaghi, F.; Leggio, L. Pharmacological manipulation of the ghrelin system and alcohol hangover symptoms in heavy drinking individuals: Is there a link? *Pharmacol. Biochem. Behav.* **2018**, *172*, 39–49. [CrossRef]
28. Sztainert, T.; Hay, R.; Wohl, M.J.A.; Abizaid, A. Hungry to gamble? Ghrelin as a predictor of persistent gambling in the face of loss. *Biol. Psychol.* **2018**, *139*, 115–123. [CrossRef]
29. Sutin, A.R.; Zonderman, A.B.; Uda, M.; Deiana, B.; Taub, D.D.; Longo, D.L.; Ferrucci, L.; Schlessinger, D.; Cucca, F.; Terracciano, A. Personality traits and leptin. *Psychosom. Med.* **2013**, *75*, 505–509. [CrossRef]
30. Bach, P.; Koopmann, A.; Kiefer, F. The Impact of Appetite-Regulating Neuropeptide Leptin on Alcohol Use, Alcohol Craving and Addictive Behavior: A Systematic Review of Preclinical and Clinical Data. *Alcohol Alcohol.* **2021**, *56*, 149–165. [CrossRef]

31. Peters, T.; Antel, J.; Föcker, M.; Esber, S.; Hinney, A.; Schéle, E.; Dickson, S.L.; Albayrak, O.; Hebebrand, J. The association of serum leptin levels with food addiction is moderated by weight status in adolescent psychiatric inpatients. *Eur. Eat Disord. Rev.* **2018**, *26*, 618–628. [CrossRef]
32. Bach, P.; Bumb, J.M.; Schuster, R.; Vollstädt-Klein, S.; Reinhard, I.; Rietschel, M.; Witt, S.H.; Wiedemann, K.; Kiefer, F.; Koopmann, A. Effects of leptin and ghrelin on neural cue-reactivity in alcohol addiction: Two streams merge to one river? *Psychoneuroendocrinology* **2019**, *100*, 1–9. [CrossRef] [PubMed]
33. Escobar, M.; Scherer, J.N.; Ornell, F.; Bristot, G.; Medino-Soares, C.; Pinto-Guimarães, L.S.; Von Diemen, L.; Pechansky, F. Leptin levels and its correlation with crack-cocaine use severity: A preliminary study. *Neurosci. Lett.* **2018**, *671*, 56–59. [CrossRef] [PubMed]
34. Mehta, S.; Baruah, A.; Das, S.; Avinash, P.; Chetia, D.; Gupta, D. Leptin levels in alcohol dependent patients and their relationship with withdrawal and craving. *Asian J. Psychiatr.* **2020**, *51*, 101967. [CrossRef] [PubMed]
35. Geisel, O.; Hellweg, R.; Wiedemann, K.; Müller, C.A. Plasma levels of leptin in patients with pathological gambling, internet gaming disorder and alcohol use disorder. *Psychiatry Res.* **2018**, *268*, 193–197. [CrossRef]
36. Shahouzehi, B.; Shokoohi, M.; Najafipour, H. The effect of opium addiction on serum adiponectin and leptin levels in male subjects: A case control study from Kerman Coronary Artery disease risk factors study (KERCADRS). *EXCLI J.* **2013**, *12*, 916.
37. Hillemacher, T.; Weinland, C.; Heberlein, A.; Gröschl, M.; Schanze, A.; Frieling, H.; Wilhelm, J.; Kornhuber, J.; Bleich, S. Increased levels of adiponectin and resistin in alcohol dependence–possible link to craving. *Drug Alcohol. Depend.* **2009**, *99*, 333–337. [CrossRef]
38. Lozano-Madrid, M.; Bryan, D.C.; Granero, R.; Sánchez, I.; Riesco, N.; Mallorquí-Bagué, N.; Jiménez-Murcia, S.; Treasure, J.; Fernández-Aranda, F. Impulsivity, emotional dysregulation, and executive function deficits could be associated with alcohol and drug abuse in eating disorders. *J. Clin. Med.* **2020**, *9*, 1936. [CrossRef]
39. van Timmeren, T.; Daams, J.G.; van Holst, R.J.; Goudriaan, A.E. Compulsivity-related neurocognitive performance deficits in gambling disorder: A systematic review and meta-analysis. *Neurosci. Biobehav. Rev.* **2018**, *84*, 204–217. [CrossRef]
40. Hinson, J.M.; Jameson, T.L.; Whitney, P. Impulsive decision making and working memory. *J. Exp. Psychology. Learn. Mem. Cogn.* **2003**, *29*, 298–306. [CrossRef]
41. Mallorquí-Bagué, N.; Tolosa-Sola, I.; Fernández-Aranda, F.; Granero, R.; Fagundo, A.B.; Lozano-Madrid, M.; Mestre-Bach, G.; Gómez-Peña, M.; Aymamí, N.; Borrás-González, I.; et al. Cognitive Deficits in Executive Functions and Decision-Making Impairments Cluster Gambling Disorder Sub-types. *J. Gambl. Stud.* **2018**, *34*, 209–223. [CrossRef]
42. Mestre-Bach, G.; Fernández-Aranda, F.; Jiménez-Murcia, S.; Potenza, M.N. Decision-Making in Gambling Disorder, Problematic Pornography Use, and Binge Eating Disorder: Similarities and Differences. *Curr. Behav. Neurosci. Rep.* **2020**, *7*, 97–108. [CrossRef] [PubMed]
43. Granero, R.; Penelo, E.; Stinchfield, R.; Fernández-Aranda, F.; Savvidou, L.G.; Fröberg, F.; Aymamí, N.; Gómez-Peña, M.; Pérez-Serrano, M.; del Pino-Gutiérrez, A.; et al. Is Pathological Gambling Moderated by Age? *J. Gambl. Stud.* **2014**, *30*, 475–492. [CrossRef] [PubMed]
44. Jiménez-Murcia, S.; Granero, R.; Fernández-Aranda, F.; Menchón, J.M. Comparison of gambling profiles based on strategic versus non-strategic preferences. *Curr. Opin. Behav. Sci.* **2020**, *31*, 13–20. [CrossRef]
45. Álvarez-Moya, E.M.; Ochoa, C.; Jiménez-Murcia, S.; Aymamí, M.N.; Gómez-Peña, M.; Fernández-Aranda, F.; Santamaría, J.; Moragas, L.; Bove, F.; Menchón, J.M. Effect of executive functioning, decision-making and self-reported impulsivity on the treatment outcome of pathologic gambling. *J. Psychiatry Neurosci.* **2011**, *36*, 165–175. [CrossRef]
46. Del Pino-Gutiérrez, A.; Jiménez-Murcia, S.; Fernández-Aranda, F.; Agüera, Z.; Granero, R.; Hakansson, A.; Fagundo, A.B.; Bolao, F.; Valdepérez, A.; Mestre-Bach, G.; et al. The relevance of personality traits in impulsivity-related disorders: From substance use disorders and gambling disorder to bulimia nervosa. *J. Behav. Addict.* **2017**, *6*, 396–405. [CrossRef]
47. Lara-Huallipe, M.L.; Granero, R.; Fernández-Aranda, F.; Gónez-Peña, M.; Moragas, L.; del Pino-Gutiérrez, A.; Valenciano-Mendoza, E.; Mora-Maltas, B.; Baenas, I.; Etxandi, M.; et al. Clustering Treatment Outcomes in Women with Gambling Disorder. *J. Gambl. Stud.* **2021**, *38*, 1469–1491. [CrossRef] [PubMed]
48. Dash, G.F.; Slutske, W.S.; Martin, N.G.; Statham, D.J.; Agrawal, A.; Lynskey, M.T. Big Five personality traits and alcohol, nicotine, cannabis, and gambling disorder comorbidity. *Psychol. Addict. Behav.* **2019**, *33*, 420. [CrossRef]
49. Zilberman, N.; Yadid, G.; Efrati, Y.; Neumark, Y.; Rassovsky, I. Personality profiles of substance and behavioral addictions. *Addict. Behav.* **2018**, *82*, 174–181. [CrossRef]
50. Vintró-Alcaraz, C.; Mestre-Bach, G.; Granero, R.; Vázquez-Cobela, R.; Seoane, M.L.; Diéguez, C.; Leis, R.; Tovar, S. Do emotion regulation and impulsivity differ according to gambling preferences in clinical samples of gamblers? *Addict. Behav.* **2022**, *126*, 107176. [CrossRef]
51. Barja-Fernández, S.; Lugilde, J.; Castelao, C.; Vázquez-Cobela, R.; Seoane, L.M.; Diéguez, C.; Leis, R.; Tovar, S. Circulating LEAP-2 is associated with puberty in girls. *Int. J. Obes.* **2021**, *45*, 502–514. [CrossRef]
52. Mani, B.K.; Puzziferri, N.; He, Z.; Rodríguez, J.; Osborne-Lawrence, S.; Metzger, N.P.; Chhina, N.; Gaylinn, B.; Thorner, M.O.; Thomas, E.L.; et al. LEAP2 changes with body mass and food intake in humans and mice. *J. Clin. Investig.* **2019**, *129*, 3909–3923. [CrossRef] [PubMed]

53. Pena-Bello, L.; Pertega-Diaz, S.; Outeiriño-Blanco, E.; García-Buela, J.; Tovar, S.; Sangiao-Alvarellos, S.; Diéguez, C.; Cordido, F. Effect of oral glucose administration on rebound growth hormone release in normal and obese women: The role of adiposity, insulin sensitivity and ghrelin. *PLoS ONE.* **2015**, *10*, e121087. [CrossRef] [PubMed]
54. Bechara, A.; Damasio, A.R.; Damasio, H.; Anderson, S.W. Insensitivity to future consequences following damage to human prefrontal cortex. *Cognition* **1994**, *50*, 7–15. [CrossRef]
55. Grant, D.A.; Berg, E. A behavioral analysis of degree of reinforcement and ease of shifting to new responses in a Weigl-type card-sorting problem. *J. Exp. Psychol.* **1948**, *38*, 404–411. [CrossRef] [PubMed]
56. Golden, C.J. *Stroop Color and Word Test: A Manual for Clinical and Experimental Uses*; Stoelting: Chicago, IL, USA, 1978.
57. Reitan, R.M. Validity of the Trail Making Test as an Indicator of Organic Brain Damage Perceptual and Motor Skills. *Percept. Mot. Ski.* **1958**, *8*, 271–276. [CrossRef]
58. Wechsler, D. *Wechsler Memory Scale*, 3rd ed.; The Psychological Corporation: San Antonio, TX, USA, 1997.
59. Wechsler, D. *KA WAIS-III: Wechsler Adult Intelligence Scale*, 3rd ed.; [Book in Spanish]; TEA Ediciones SA: Madrid, Spain, 1999.
60. De Oliveira, M.O.; Nitrini, R.; Yassuda, M.S.; Brucki, S.M.D. Vocabulary is an appropriate measure of premorbid intelligence in a sample with heterogeneous educational level in Brazil. *Behav. Neurol.* **2014**, *2014*, 875960. [CrossRef]
61. Lesieur, H.R.; Blume, S.B. The South Oaks Gambling Screen (SOGS): A new instrument for the identification of pathological gamblers. *Am. J. Psychiatry* **1987**, *144*, 1184–1188. [CrossRef]
62. Echeburúa, E.; Baez, C.; Fernández-Montalvo, J.; Páez, D. Cuestionario de Juego Patológico de South Oaks (SOGS): Validación española. *Análisis Modif Conduct.* **1994**, *20*, 769–791.
63. Stinchfield, R. Reliability, validity, and classification accuracy of a measure of DSM-IV diagnostic criteria for pathological gambling. *Am. J. Psychiatry* **2003**, *160*, 180–182. [CrossRef]
64. Jiménez-Murcia, S.; Stinchfield, R.; Álvarez-Moya, E.; Jaurrieta, N.; Bueno, B.; Granero, R.; Aymamí, M.N.; Gómez-Peña, M.; Martínez-Giménez, R.; Fernández-Aranda, F.; et al. Reliability, validity, and classification accuracy of a Spanish translation of a measure of DSM-IV diagnostic criteria for pathological gambling. *J. Gambl. Stud.* **2009**, *25*, 93–104. [CrossRef]
65. Derogatis, L.R. *SCL-90-R: Symptom Checklist-90-R. Administration, Scoring and Procedures Manuall—II for the Revised Version*; Clinical Psychometric Research: Towson, MD, USA, 1994.
66. Derogatis, L.R. *SCL-90-R. Cuestionario de 90 Síntomas-Manual*; TEA Editorial: Madrid, Spain, 2002.
67. Cloninger, C.R. *The Temperament and Character Inventory—Revised. Center for Psychobiology of Personality*; Washington University: Washington, DC, USA, 1999.
68. Gutiérrez-Zotes, J.A.; Bayón, C.; Montserrat, C.; Valero, J.; Labad, A.; Cloninger, C.R.; Fernández-Aranda, F. Temperament and Character Inventory Revised (TCI-R). Standardization and normative data in a general population sample. *Actas Esp Psiquiatr.* **2004**, *32*, 8–15. [PubMed]
69. Whiteside, S.P.; Lynam, D.R.; Miller, J.D.; Reynolds, S.K. Validation of the UPPS impulsive behaviour scale: A four-factor model of impulsivity. *Eur. J. Pers.* **2005**, *19*, 559–574. [CrossRef]
70. Verdejo-García, A.; Lozano, Ó.; Moya, M.; Alcázar, M.A.; Pérez-García, M. Psychometric properties of a Spanish version of the UPPS-P impulsive behavior scale: Reliability, validity and association with trait and cognitive impulsivity. *J. Pers. Assess.* **2010**, *92*, 70–77. [CrossRef] [PubMed]
71. Jiménez-Murcia, S.; Aymamí-Sanromà, M.; Gómez-Pena, M.; Álvarez-Moya, E.; Vallejo, J. *Protocols de Tractament Cognitivoconductual pel joc Patològic i D'altres Addiccions no Tòxiques [Protocols of Cognitive-Behaviour Therapy for Pathological Gambling and Other Behavioural Addictions]*; Hospital Universitari de Bellvitge, Departament de Salut, Generalitat de Catalunya: Barcelona, Spain, 2006.
72. Stata-Corp. *Stata Statistical Software: Release 17*; Stata Press Publication (StataCorp LLC): College Station, TX, USA, 2021.
73. Kelley, K.; Preacher, K.J. On effect size. *Psychol. Methods* **2012**, *17*, 137–152. [CrossRef]
74. Rosnow, R.L.; Rosenthal, R. Computing contrasts, effect sizes and counternulls on other people's published data: General procedures for research consumers. *Psychol. Methods* **1996**, *1*, 331–340. [CrossRef]
75. Finner, H.; Roters, M. On the false discovery rate and expecte type I errors. *J. Am. Stat. Assoc.* **2001**, *88*, 920–923. [CrossRef]
76. Vengeliene, V. The role of ghrelin in drug and natural reward. *Addict Biol.* **2013**, *18*, 897–900. [CrossRef]
77. Benchebra, L.; Alexandre, J.M.; Dubernet, J.; Fatséas, M.; Auriacombe, M. Gambling and Gaming disorders and physical health of players: A critical review of the literature. *Presse Med.* **2019**, *48*, 1551–1568. [CrossRef]
78. Pilver, C.E.; Potenza, M.N. Increased incidence of cardiovascular conditions among older adults with pathological gambling features in a prospective study. *J. Addict. Med.* **2013**, *7*, 387–393. [CrossRef]
79. Firouzabadi, N.; Haghnegahdar, M.; Khalvati, B.; Dehshahri, A.; Bahramali, E. Overexpression of adiponectin receptors in opium users with and without cancer. *Clin. Pharmacol. Adv. Appl.* **2020**, *12*, 59. [CrossRef]
80. Álvarez-Moya, E.M.; Jiménez-Murcia, S.; Aymamí, M.N.; Gómez-Peña, M.; Granero, R.; Santamaría, J.; Menchón, J.M.; Fernández-Aranda, F. Subtyping study of a pathological gamblers sample. *Can. J. Psychiatry* **2010**, *55*, 498–506. [CrossRef] [PubMed]
81. Balodis, I.M.; Linnet, J.; Arshad, F.; Worhunsky, P.D.; Stevens, M.C.; Pearlson, G.D.; Potenza, M.N. Relating neural processing of reward and loss prospect to risky decision-making in individuals with and without Gambling Disorder. *Int. Gambl. Stud.* **2018**, *18*, 269–285. [CrossRef] [PubMed]
82. Bexkens, A.; Jansen, B.R.J.; Van der Molen, M.W.; Huizenga, H.M. Cool Decision-Making in Adolescents with Behavior Disorder and/or Mild-to-Borderline Intellectual Disability. *J. Abnorm. Child Psychol.* **2016**, *44*, 357–367. [CrossRef] [PubMed]

83. Thompson, S.J.; Corr, P.J. A Feedback-Response Pause Normalises Response Perseveration Deficits in Pathological Gamblers. *Int. J. Ment. Health Addict.* **2013**, *11*, 601–610. [CrossRef]
84. Novelle, M.G.; Diéguez, C. Unravelling the role and mechanism of adipokine and gastrointestinal signals in animal models in the nonhomeostatic control of energy homeostasis: Implications for binge eating disorder. *Eur. Eat. Disord. Rev.* **2018**, *26*, 551–568. [CrossRef]
85. Jiménez-Murcia, S.; Granero, R.; Fernández-Aranda, F.; Arcelus, J.; Aymamí, M.N.; Gómez-Peña, M.; Tárrega, S.; Moragas, L.; del Pino-Gutiérrez, A.; Sauchelli, S.; et al. Predictors of outcome among pathological gamblers receiving cognitive behavioral group therapy. *Eur. Addict. Res.* **2015**, *21*, 169–178. [CrossRef]
86. Jiménez-Murcia, S.; Granero, R.; Tarrega, S.; Angulo, A.; Fernández-Aranda, F.; Arcelus, J.; Fagundo, A.B.; Aymamí, N.; Moragas, L.; Sauvaget, A.; et al. Mediational Role of Age of Onset in Gambling Disorder, a Path Modeling Analysis. *J. Gambl. Stud.* **2016**, *32*, 327–340. [CrossRef]
87. Castrén, S.; Basnet, S.; Salonen, A.H.; Pankakoski, M.; Ronkainen, J.E.; Alho, H.; Lahti, T. Factors associated with disordered gambling in Finland. *Subst. Abus. Treat. Prev. Policy* **2013**, *8*, 1–10. [CrossRef]
88. Martinotti, G.; Andreoli, S.; Giametta, E.; Poli, V.; Bria, P.; Janiri, L. The dimensional assessment of personality in pathologic and social gamblers: The role of novelty seeking and self-transcendence. *Compr. Psychiatry* **2006**, *37*, 350–356. [CrossRef]
89. Valero-Solís, S.; Granero, R.; Fernández-Aranda, F.; Steward, T.; Mestre-Bach, G.; Mallorquí-Bagué, N.; Martín-Romera, V.; Aymamí, N.; Gómez-Peña, M.; del Pino-Gutiérrez, A.; et al. The contribution of sex, personality traits, age of onset and disorder duration to behavioral addictions. *Front. Psychiatry* **2018**, *9*, 497. [CrossRef]
90. Dodig, D. Assessment challenges and determinants of adolescents' adverse psychosocial consequences of gambling. *Kriminol. Soc. Integr.* **2013**, *21*, 1–29.
91. Misiak, B.; Kowalski, K.; Stańczykiewicz, B.; Bartoli, F.; Carrà, G.; Samochowiec, J.; Frydecka, D. Frontiers in Neuroendocrinology Appetite-regulating hormones in bipolar disorder: A systematic review and meta-analysis. *Front. Neuroendocrinol.* **2022**, *67*, 101013. [CrossRef] [PubMed]

MDPI
St. Alban-Anlage 66
4052 Basel
Switzerland
www.mdpi.com

Nutrients Editorial Office
E-mail: nutrients@mdpi.com
www.mdpi.com/journal/nutrients

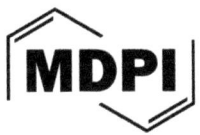

Disclaimer/Publisher's Note: The statements, opinions and data contained in all publications are solely those of the individual author(s) and contributor(s) and not of MDPI and/or the editor(s). MDPI and/or the editor(s) disclaim responsibility for any injury to people or property resulting from any ideas, methods, instructions or products referred to in the content.

www.ingramcontent.com/pod-product-compliance
Lightning Source LLC
LaVergne TN
LVHW070745100526
838202LV00013B/1304

9 7 8 3 7 2 5 8 0 5 7 5 4